S0-CEE-520

Cancers of the Head and Neck

Cancer Treatment and Research

WILLIAM L McGUIRE, *series editor*

Livingston RB (ed): Lung Cancer 1. 1981. ISBN 90-247-2394-9.
Bennett Humphrey G, Dehner LP, Grindey GB, Acton RT (eds): Pediatric Oncology 1. 1981. ISBN 90-247-2408-2.
DeCosse JJ, Sherlock P (eds): Gastrointestinal Cancer 1. 1981. ISBN 90-247-2461-9.
Bennett JM (ed): Lymphomas 1, including Hodgkin's Disease. 1981. ISBN 90-247-2479-1.
Bloomfield CD (ed): Adult Leukemias 1. 1982. ISBN 90-247-2478-3.
Paulson DF (ed): Genitourinary Cancer 1. 1982. ISBN 90-247-2480-5.
Muggia FM (ed): Cancer Chemotherapy 1. ISBN 90-247-2713-8.
Bennett Humphrey G, Grindey GB (eds): Pancreatic Tumors in Children. 1982. ISBN 90-247-2702-2.
Costanzi JJ (ed): Malignant Melanoma 1. 1983. ISBN 90-247-2706-5.
Griffiths CT, Fuller AF (eds): Gynecologic Oncology. 1983. ISBN 0-89838-555-5.
Greco AF (ed): Biology and Management of Lung Cancer. 1983. ISBN 0-89838-554-7.
Walker MD (ed): Oncology of the Nervous System. 1983. ISBN 0-89838-567-9.
Higby DJ (ed): Supportive Care in Cancer Therapy. 1983. ISBN 0-89838-569-5.
Herberman RB (ed): Basic and Clinical Tumor Immunology. 1983. ISBN 0-89838-579-2.
Baker LH (ed): Soft Tissue Sarcomas. 1983. ISBN 0-89838-584-9.
Bennett JM (ed): Controversies in the Management of Lymphomas. 1983. ISBN 0-89838-586-5.
Bennett Humphrey G, Grindey GB (eds): Adrenal and Endocrine Tumors in Children. 1983. ISBN 0-89838-590-3.
DeCosse JJ, Sherlock P (eds): Clinical Management of Gastrointestinal Cancer. 1984. ISBN 0-89838-601-2.
Catalona WJ, Ratliff TL (eds): Urologic Oncology. 1984. ISBN 0-89838-628-4.
Santen RJ, Manni A (eds): Diagnosis and Management of Endocrine-related Tumors. 1984. ISBN 0-89838-636-5.
Costanzi JJ (ed): Clinical Management of Malignant Melanoma. 1984. ISBN 0-89838-656-X.
Wolf GT (ed): Head and Neck Oncology. 1984. ISBN 0-89838-657-8.
Alberts DS, Surwit EA (eds): Ovarian Cancer. 1985. ISBN 0-89838-676-4.
Muggia FM (ed): Experimental and Clinical Progress in Cancer Chemotherapy. 1985. ISBN 0-89838-679-9.
Higby DJ (ed): The Cancer Patient and Supportive Care. 1985. ISBN 0-89838-690-X.
Bloomfield CD (ed): Chronic and Acute Leukemias in Adults. 1985. ISBN 0-89838-702-7.
Herberman RB (ed): Cancer Immunology: Innovative Approaches to Therapy. 1986. ISBN 0-89838-757-4.
Hansen HH (ed): Lung Cancer: Basic and Clinical Aspects. 1986. ISBN 0-89838-763-9.
Pinedo HM, Verweij J (eds): Clinical Management of Soft Tissue Sarcomas. 1986. ISBN 0-89838-808-2.
Higby DJ (ed): Issues in Supportive Care of Cancer Patients. 1986. ISBN 0-89838-816-3.
Surwit EA, Alberts DS (eds): Cervix Cancer. 1987. ISBN 0-89838-822-8.
Jacobs C (ed): Cancers of the Head and Neck. 1987. ISBN 0-89838-825-2.
MacDonald JS (ed): Gastrointestinal Oncology. 1987. ISBN 0-89838-829-5.
Ratliff TL, Catalona WJ (eds): Genitourinary Cancer. 1987. ISBN 0-89838-830-9.
Nathanson L (ed): Basic and Clinical Aspects of Malignant Melanoma. 1987. ISBN 0-89838-856-2.
Muggia FM (ed): Concepts, Clinical Developments, and Therapeutic Advances in Cancer Chemotherapy. 1987. ISBN 0-89838-879-5.

Cancers of the Head and Neck
Advances in Surgical Therapy, Radiation Therapy
and Chemotherapy

edited by

CHARLOTTE JACOBS, M.D.

Division of Oncology
Stanford University School of Medicine
Stanford, CA 94305-5306
U.S.A.

RC 280
H4
C 354
1987

1987 **MARTINUS NIJHOFF PUBLISHERS**
a member of the KLUWER ACADEMIC PUBLISHERS GROUP
BOSTON / DORDRECHT / LANCASTER

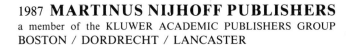

Distributors

for the United States and Canada: Kluwer Academic Publishers, P.O. Box 358,
Accord Station, Hingham, MA 02018-0358, USA
for the UK and Ireland: Kluwer Academic Publishers, MTP Press Limited,
Falcon House, Queen Square, Lancaster LA1 1RN, UK
for all other countries: Kluwer Academic Publishers Group, Distribution Center,
P.O. Box 322, 3300 AH Dordrecht, The Netherlands

Library of Congress Cataloging in Publication Data

Cancers of the head and neck.

  (Cancer treatment and research)
  Includes index.
  1. Head--Cancer--Treatment. 2. Neck--Cancer--
Treatment. I. Jacobs, Charlotte. II. Series.
[DNLM: 1. Head and Neck Neoplasms--therapy.
W1 CA693 / WE 707 C2153]
RC280.H4C354 1986   616.99'49106   86-17973

ISBN 0-89838-825-2 (this volume)
ISBN 90-247-2426-0 (series)

Copyright

© 1987 by Martinus Nijhoff Publishers, Boston.

All rights reserved. No part of this publication may be reproduced, stored in a
retrieval system, or transmitted in any form or by any means, mechanical,
photocopying, recording, or otherwise, without the prior written permission of
the publishers,
Martinus Nijhoff Publishers, P.O. Box 358, Accord Station, Hingham, MA
02018-0358, USA.

PRINTED IN THE NETHERLANDS

Table of contents

Cancer Treatment and Research

Foreword

Where do you begin to look for a recent, authoritative article on the diagnosis or management of a particular malignancy? The few general oncology textbooks are generally out of date. Single papers in specialized journals are informative but seldom comprehensive; these are more often preliminary reports on a very limited number of patients. Certain general journals frequently publish good indepth reviews of cancer topics, and published symposium lectures are often the best overviews available. Unfortunately, these reviews and supplements appear sporadically, and the reader can never be sure when a topic of special interest will be covered.

Cancer Treatment and Research is a series of authoritative volumes which aim to meet this need. It is an attempt to establish a critical mass of oncology literature covering virtually all oncology topics, revised frequently to keep the coverage up to date, easily available on a single library shelf or by a single personal subscription.

We have approached the problem in the following fashion. First, by dividing the oncology literature into specific subdivisions such as lung cancer, genitourinary cancer, pediatric oncology, etc. Second, by asking eminent authorities in each of these areas to edit a volume on the specific topic on an annual or biannual basis. Each topic and tumor type is covered in a volume appearing frequently and predictably, discussing current diagnosis, staging, markers, all forms of treatment modalities, basic biology, and more.

In *Cancer Treatment and Research*, we have an outstanding group of editors, each having made a major commitment to bring to this new series the very best literature in his of her field. Martinus Nijhoff Publishers has made an equally major commitment to the rapid publication of high quality books, and worldwide distribution.

Where can you go find quickly a recent authoritative article on any major oncology problem? We hope that *Cancer Treatment and Research* provides an answer.

WILLIAM L. MCGUIRE
Series Editor

Preface

Cancers of the head and neck are among the most morbid of cancers. Conventional surgery and/or radiation therapy have a high cure rate for patients with early stage disease. However, despite optimal treatment with surgery and radiotherapy, patients with nodal spread or extensive local disease have a low cure rate. Even if a cancer is cured, a patient is often left with long-term debilities from the treatment and/or cancer. The major causes for decreased survival in patients with advanced head and neck cancer include local recurrence, distant metastases, and second primaries. All of these need to be addressed if one is to improve upon the curability of advanced disease.

There are several new techniques, surgical and radiotherapeutic, designed to improve local control. Brachytherapy, or interstitial implantation, delivers a high dose of localized radiation with minimal normal tissue injury. This technique as discussed by Goffinet, may be even more efficacious when combined with hyperthermia. New, creative methods of radiation therapy delivery, such as the use of multiple fractions per day, as discussed by Parsons and Million, are also contributing to long-term local control. Laser therapy, discussed by Ossoff and Nemeroff, provides another tool for treatment of local disease.

In order to achieve an optimal treatment plan, the head an neck surgeon needs as much information as possible concerning the local extent of disease and prognostic factors which may influence outcome. Nuclear magnetic resonance, as discussed by Helsper, Bradley and Kortman, vastly improves the ability to evaluate the spread of disease. We must also seek to identify prognostic factors, such as extracapsular spread, as noted by Johnson and Myers, which change the prognosis and may alter our treatment plan.

In attempts to improve curability, chemotherapy has been added to combined modality programs. Although pilot studies have been encouraging, randomized trials have not yet confirmed a role for chemotherapy. However, some large trials, such as the Head and Neck Contracts Group, have suggested future directions for the use of the chemotherapy. The effectiveness of chemotherapy is in part dependent on the drug selection, dose, and timing of chemotherapy. Dr. Al-Sarraf addresses the issue of timing of chemotherapy as part of multimodality treatment in this volume.

Biologic modifiers and immunotherapy may in the future play a role in the control of this disease. Dr. Schuller addresses the role of the cervical lymphatic system in the immunologic reaction to cancer and the future of immunotherapy in the treatment of this disease. Biologic modifiers, such as interferon, are just beginning to be tested in head and neck cancer, and Connors and Jacobs describe their experience and that of others in the treatment of nasopharnx cancer.

For all head and neck oncologists, the goal of treatment is to eliminate the cancer, but with the least complex procedure and the best cosmetic and functional result. There are many innovative and creative new techniques geared to improve the quality of life for head and neck cancer patients. Dr. Cummings' chapter in this volume discusses the various procedures for mandibular reconstruction which afford optimal cosmesis while best maintaining the functions of mastication and articulation. The question of the necessity for a radical neck dissection continues to be debated, and Dr. Myers discusses those situations in which a modified neck dissection is appropriate. There are increased numbers of techniques for conservation laryngeal surgery, and Drs. Bailey and Stiernberg discuss the indications and results of these procedures. Innovative techniques in head and neck surgery increase patient options, but each case must be individualized.

Of course, it would be ideal to prevent head and neck cancer so that the above issues do not need to be addressed. Retinoids have been utilized to treat preneoplastic lesions, and Drs. Lotan, Stimson, Schantz and Hong discuss their potential role in chemoprevention.

The head and neck surgeon, radiotherapist and oncologist primarily treat squamous cell cancers, but increasingly are called upon the manage other cancers of the head and neck. The management of rhabdomyosarcoma has changed substantially in the last few yeras with improvement in the previously dismal prognosis. These advances are a result of the multimodality treatment of a large reserach group. New information concerning the etiology, evaluation, histologic subtypes and recommended treatment of rhabdomyosarcoma is presented in this volume by Drs. Wharam and Maurer. Likewise, the head and neck surgeon is often called upon to manage cutaneous melanomas, and there have been many advances in knowledge of the epidemiology, differential diagnosis, staging, and treatment as discussed by Drs. Fisher, Gillespie, Seigler, and Crocker. The head and neck surgeon may be first to evaluate a patient with a head and neck lymphoma, and it is imperative to understand the new staging systems and therapy for this disease.

Many of the innovative approaches in head and neck cancer will come from the laboratory or from pilot studies. However, randomized trials will be necessary to establish the superiority of any new approach over standard therapy. For combined modality programs, it is crucial to have a closely coordinated team of surgeons, radiation therapists, and oncologists. There are many biostatical pitfalls in the design and analysis of head and neck clinical trials, and Dr. Makuch and Johnson discuss methods to avoid these.

This current volume of head and neck oncology demonstrates marked progress in the treatment of head and neck cancer. There are several new, exciting approaches on the threshold of development. The current status of our management of this disease continues to serve as a stimulus for basic science and clinical research.

Charlotte Jacobs

List of contributors

AL-SARRAF, MUHYI, Department of Medicine, Wayne State University, Detroit, Michigan, USA

BAILEY, BYRON J., Department of ENT, University of Texas, Galveston, Texas, USA

BRADLEY, WILLIAM G., Huntington Medical Research Institutes and Department of Radiology, Huntington Memorial Hospital, Pasadena, California, USA

BYERS, ROBERT M., Head & Neck Surgery, University of Texas System Cancer Center, M.D. Anderson Hospital, Houston, Texas, USA

CONNORS JOSEPH M., Department of Medicine, Cancer Control Agency of British Columbia, University of British Columbia, Vancouver, BC, Canada

CROCKER, IAN R., Division of Radiation Oncology, Duke University Medical Center, Durham, North Carolina, USA

CUMMINGS, CHARLES W., Department of Otolaryngology, University of Washington Medical School, Seattle, Washington, USA

FISHER, SAMUEL R., Division of Otolaryngology, Duke University Medical Center, Durham, North Carolina, USA

GILLESPIE, CAMERON A., Division of Otolaryngology, Duke University Medical Center, Durham, North Carolina, USA

GOFFINET, DON R., Department of Radiation Therapy, Stanford University School of Medicine, Stanford, California, USA

HELSPER, JAMES T., Tumor Clinical Medical Group, Huntington Memorial Hospital, Pasadena, California, USA

HONG, WAUN KI, Head and Neck Oncology, University of Texas Systems Cancer Center, Houston, Texas, USA

JACOBS, CHARLOTTE, Department of Medicine/Oncology, Stanford University School of Medicine, Division of Oncology, Stanford, California, USA

JOHNSON, JONAS T., Department of Otolaryngology, University of Pittsburgh School of Medicine, Eye and Ear Hospital of Pittsburgh, Pittsburgh, Pennsylvania, USA

JOHNSON, MARY, G.H. Besselaar Associates, Inc., Princeton, New Yersey, USA

KORTMAN, KEITH E., Huntington Medical Research Institutes and Department of Radiology, Huntington Memorial Hospital, S. Pasadena, California, USA

LOTAN, REUBEN, Head and Nech Oncology, University of Texas Systems Cancer Center, Houston, Texas, USA

MAKUCH, Robert, Yale University School of Medicine, Department of Biostatistics, P.O. Box 3333, New Haven, CT 06510, USA

MAURER HAROLD M., Medical College of Virginia, Richmond, Virginia, USA

MILLION RODNEY R., Division of Radiation Therapy, Department of Radiology, University of Florida, Gainesville, Florida, USA

MYERS, EUGENE N., Department of Otolaryngology, University of Pittsburgh School of Medicine, Eye and Ear Hospital of Pittsburgh, Pittsburgh, Pennsylvania, USA

NEMEROFF, ROBERT F., Department of Otolaryngology, Head and Neck Surgery, Northwestern University Medical School, Chicago, Illinois, USA

OSSOFF, ROBERT H., Department of Otolaryngology, Vanderbilt University School of Medicine, Nashville, Tennesse, USA

PARSONS JAMES T., Radiation Therapy Department, University of Florida, Gainesville, Florida, USA

SCHANTZ, STIMSON P., Head and Neck Oncology, University of Texas Systems Cancer Center, Houston, Texas, USA

SCHULLER, DAVID E., Department of Otolaryngology, Comprehensive Cancer Center, Ohio State University, College of Medicine, Columbus, Ohio, USA

SEIGLER, HILLIARD F., Department of General and Thoracic Surgery, Duke University Medical Center, Durham, North Carolina, USA

STIERNBERG, CHARLES M., Department of ENT, University of Texas, Galveston, Texas, USA

WHARAM, Jr., MOODY D., Division of Radiation Therapy/Oncology. Johns Hopkins Hospital, Baltimore, Maryland, USA

WONG, WILSON S., Department of Radiology, Huntington Memorial Hospital, Pasadena, California, USA

1. Mandibular reconstruction in the surgical management of head and neck tumors

CHARLES W. CUMMINGS

Introduction

Tumor invasion of the mandible presents a virtual mandate for resection of the involved bone. These patients confront the head and neck surgeon with a taxing problem which requires careful assessment of the individual case and the selection of a reconstructive method from a host of options. Removal of the mandible increases the complexity of reconstruction, not only from the standpoint of cosmetic restitution but, in addition, and more importantly, restoration of the essential functions of mastication, alimentation, and articulation. The T-4 oral cavity lesions addressed here are entwined in a complex web of problems. Almost predictably, abuses of smoking and alcohol contribute to the medical and social disturbance. Frequently there is a poor social situation, such as a fragmented home, unemployment, or an absent support group. Suboptimal medical status is to be inspected, along with poor dental hygiene. Other major medical disorders frequently associated with oral cavity cancer include peripheral vascular disease, renal and hepatic disease, in addition to general inanition and malnutrition.

Another problem associated with management of tumors that involve the mandible is that surgery is only one of the components which comprise contemporary therapeutic management. Sequencing of the three major modalities (surgery, chemotherapy and radiation therapy) is being evaluated so as to establish the most beneficial order of delivery.

The goals of surgical management in the T-4 oral cavity tumor are straightforward. Primary, of course, is the elimination of tumor using the least complex surgical procedure, and, additionally, the fewest number of surgical procedures (if reconstruction is to be a staged event). Further, the surgeon is concerned with restoration of cosmesis, mandibular function, and dental competency.

The workup involved in T-4 carcinomas of the oral cavity is centered primarily about the imaging process. Initially, of course, a Panorex mandibular film and occlusal views are helpful if the tumor approximates the mandibular cortex and involves the periosteum. A Tc_{99} MDP bone scan may be used to document early

C. Jacobs (ed) Cancers of the head and neck.
© *1987, Martinus Nijhoff Publishers, Boston. ISBN 0–89838–825–2. Printed in the Netherlands.*

stage mandibular involvement as evidenced by an increase in uptake of the radioactive material but is subject to false positive interpretation. Computerized tomography plays an ever-increasing role in the staging process. In fact, some head and neck surgeons now prefer the CT scan to the exclusion of more routine radiological studies.

Every patient with oral cavity cancer should have the benefit of laryngoscopy, bronchoscopy, and esophagoscopy at the time of the initial clinical staging. The reason for this is the high association with synchronous second primary tumors which might alter significantly the surgical approach to the initial presenting tumor.

Surgical treatment: general concepts

There are some general concepts which apply to the surgical reconstruction of the involved mandible regardless of the specific procedure employed, and it is important to highlight these tenets prior to discussion of more specific methods of reconstruction.
1. Free bone grafts which are not vascularized or do not have an accompanying vascular pedicle take longer to establish continuity with the residual segments of the mandible. The process of reabsorption and deposition of new osteoid material is a dynamic one which occurs only in the presence of a viable periosteum and adequate vascular perfusion. Establishment of this environment takes several months.
2. It is also well established that intraoral contamination represents a true hazard to the successful outcome of free bone graft. In fact, contamination by saliva almost invariably results in failure of a devascularized graft. This is not the case with a vacularized bony segment. Grafts that bring with them an independent blood supply tend to heal more rapidly, as a fracture does.
3. It is also apparent, clinically, that the use of particulate marrow and cortical bone which is harvested from the iliac crest region enhances the establishment of new bone in devascularized bone grafts or alloplastic devices.
4. As with disruption of bone continuity by fracture, immobilization of the bone segments is essential to avoid ankylosis or pseudo-arthrosis and to establish good boney union.
The use of foreign materials as spanning devices, even those that elicit essentially no tissue reaction, fell into disrepute prior to the introduction of vascularized myocutaneous flaps because of the tremendously high incidence of intraoral breakdown and exposure of the alloplastic material. Gullane [1] has recently presented some encouraging results using metallic spanning devices in concert with reconstruction of the floor of the mouth with pectoralis myocutaneous flap. It is theorized that the bulk and vitality of the pectoralis muscle serves as a barrier between the intraoral cavity and the vitallium spanning device to allow the

establishment of proper healing. Most authors, however adhere to the principle of delayed reconstruction when using non-vascularized material or autografts to span surgically created mandibular defects. DeFries [2] and Lawson [3] demonstrate a much higher success rate in the patients with delayed repair as contrasted to those with immediate repair.

Other factors have had beneficial influence on mandibular reconstruction. One of the most significant is the introduction of effective antibiotics which I feel has decreased the incidence of postoperative wound infections and thus extrusion of the graft segment. Currently, the most effective perioperative antibiotic regime combines a fourth generation Cephalosporin and Flagyl. The avoidance of an irradiated recipient site is a theoretically important factor in the success of bone grafting. However, the use of vascularized bone flaps or myocutaneous flaps helps to counter the small vessel obliteration introduced by radiation therapy.

It has been stated [4] that hyperbaric oxygen contributes significantly to the survival of devitalized bone segments which have become exposed in the postoperative period. My experience with hyperbaric oxygen has not provided results that are sufficiently beneficial to warrant the expense of time and money associated with its use.

This discussion would not be complete without some brief mention of new materials that have been introduced as alloplastic grafts. Porous polyethylene [5] has been touted as advantageous because of its good formability, tissue tolerance and stability. Calcium phosphate [6] in the form of tricalcium phosphate is another material cited as advantageous because it can be carved with a scalpel and it allows for slow replacement by osteoid containing elements. It, as well, is nonreactive. The space age metallic compositions have assumed roles of significance in mandibular reconstruction. Vitallium is the most popular of these compounds. All of these new materials have potential for use if the early enthusiasm can be supported clinically.

Let us look now to the specific methods for mandibular reconstruction which are currently employed by today's head and neck reconstructive surgeons. The use of alloplastic spanning devices to bridge the defect created surgically between the two residual mandibular segments is one of the oldest methods of reconstitution. Originally a single stainless steel rod was inserted into the residual mandibular segments, and the mucosa was closed over it. The great problem with this early form of reconstruction was that the mucosa almost invariably was sewn so that the rod served as a focus for pressure, eventually resulting in breakdown and fistulization. As stated previously, the introduction of the myocutaneous flap has offered a vascularized buffer between the oral cavity and the spanning device. Now there are preformed and semi-malleable plates which can be formed to accomodate more exactly to the surgical defect. The design of these plates is similar to those which are used to stabilize mandibular fractures. Because of the multiple fenestrations there exists the opportunity to affix segments of cortical bone to the mandibular plates (Figure 1). In the absence of intraoral contami-

4

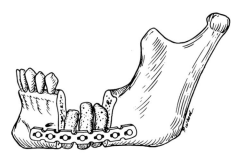

Figure 1. A fenestrated mandibular strut is positioned so as to span the surgically created gap in the mandible. As shown here, segments of cortical bone can held in place by screws affixed to the spanning device.

nation, this method must be considered to be a front-line procedure. It offers the advantages of internal stabilization of the mandibular segments, direct and quick mandibular stabilization, and additionally the opportunity to provide supplemental cortical bone to encourage the reformation of an osseous segment. Its disadvantages include the real potential for intraoral breakdown, exposure of a nonvascularized foreign body and creation of a need for removal of the alloplastic material.

Use of the alloplast-autograft in the form of preformed Vitallium or dacron mesh cribs has met with significant success and is uniquely appealing because the crib may be loaded with healthy cortical bone and particulate marrow which, in the presence of adequate extracellular fluid perfusion, will survive to lay down new bone and ultimately an intact osteoid bridge between the two mandibular segments (Figure 2). Giordano, Lawson, Schuller, Albert, *et al.* [7–10] have all reported relatively high levels of success. Delayed reconstruction is advocated by most authors because of the documented increase in success rate. The advantages of the alloplast autografts are that the tray allows for osteoid reestablishment while providing internal fixation and allowing for perfusion of the particulate marrow by extracellular nutrients. Another advantage is that radiation may be given with the crib in place. The polyurethane or dacron mesh contributes less to deflection of radiation energy than Vitallium, although both apparently can be used with a reasonable avoidance of complications. The disadvantages of the alloplast autograft in crib form are that this relatively bulky prosthesis and the additional employment of a thick myocutaneous flap may over-compensate for the defect created by the partial mandibulectomy. Occasionally infection, breakage, or discomfort will mandate removal of the crib as a delayed event. An appealing concept to me would be to employ the principles of alloplast-autograft mandibular replacement while utilizing a biodegradable material to formulate the crib. The potential for success with a slowly reabsorbable material would appear to be quite high.

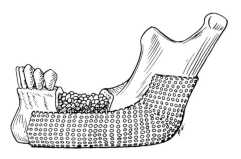

Figure 2. A preformed crib spans the surgically created defect and is filled with particulate and cancellous bone segments.

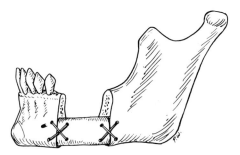

Figure 3. This drawing depicts a non-vascularized bony segment which is serving as an interface between the two remaining residual segments.

DeFries [2] has successfully used the homograft in the form of freeze dried bone. Modifications of this method for mandibular replacement have been proposed using an autograft (Figure 3), specifically the patient's own mandible which has been denuded of tumor and then totally devitalized either by sequential immersion in liquid nitrogen, as proposed by Cummings and Leipzig [11], or by intraoperative irradiation as proposed by Hamaker [12]. The advantages of this method are that one is utilizing a graft that is unique by its non-antigenicity and which conforms almost exactly to the defect at hand. An additional advantage is that there is less problem associated with the donor site. Particulate marrow can be harvested from the iliac bone with little disability compared to that caused by osteomyocutaneous flaps of free composite flaps where a large segment of the iliac crest, scapular spine, or rib are removed. One disadvantage of this method of reconstruction is almost uniform failure if intraoral contamination occurs. Although primary reconstruction has been used by Hamaker, his success rate hovers about 50%, which is unsatisfactory. Postoperative radiation must be delayed until one is assured that the grafted bone is well perfused and healthy. A further disadvantage is the observation that these autografts tend to undergo some delayed reabsorption, thus potentially diminishing the strenght of the grafted segment.

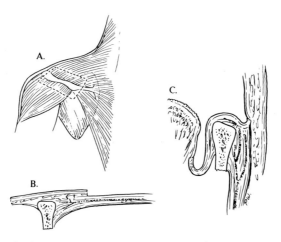

Figure 4. 'A' depicts the donor site of the trapezius scapular osteomyocutaneous flap. 'B' demonstrates the osteomyocutaneous segment prior to transport. 'C' depicts this composite graft placed in the intraoral recipient site.

Osteomyocutaneous flaps

With the general acceptance and greater use of myocutaneous flaps came the realization that in addition to muscle and overlying skin, cortical bone and its periosteum could be incorporated into a composite flap. Myocutaneous flaps are predominantly based on flat muscles which are supplied by named vessels that perforate the musculature and then proceed to supply the adjacent structures, be it periosteum or skin. There are two osteomyocutaneous flaps that are applicable to the head and neck region. The first is the pectoralis osteomyocutaneous flap which incorporates the lateral periosteum and underlying fifth rib, in addition to a large segment of pectoralis muscle [13]. The vascular supply for this composite flap is the pectoralis artery and its paired veins. The scope of this flap is such that the rib may be used to reconstitute the body or the mandibular arch, providing that the rib is shaped through fracture to accomodate for the curvature desired. A problem unique to the rib as a grafting material is that it is composed of thin bone which has marginal strength and is subject to some reabsorption, and thus it does not provide a strong foundation to support dentures. The morbidity of this specific flap includes the potential creation of a pneumothorax by penetration of the underlying pleura when harvesting the rib.

The second osteomyocutaneous flap involves the spine of the scapula (Figure 4). The vascular supply to this flap is predominantly from the occipital artery. The muscular pedicle is rather broad as it inserts into the posterior aspect of the neck and the occiput. With this flap, the scapular spine is separated from the body of the scapula so that the overlying skin, scapular spine, and trapezius muscle are moved as a composite flap. The arc provided by this flap allows for reconstruction of the lateral aspect of the mandible. Panje [14] has also recommended its use for reconstruction of the mandibular arch, although here, conformation to the surgical defect becomes a problem as does the length of the flap. The specific problems associated with the trapezius osteomyocutaneous flap include, an intraoperative position change as well as sacrifice of the spinal accessory nerve which severely impairs shoulder function. This problem also occurs with the pectoralis osteomyocutaneous flap, especially when a radical neck dissection (sacrifice of the spinal accessory nerve) is a component of the surgical procedure. In this setting, adduction and internal rotation of the arm compound the shoulder disability.

The advantages of the osteomyocutaneous flap are quite obvious. It is, of course, a single stage procedure, thus fulfilling the quest for the least number of hospitalizations. There is predictable vascularity, provided that the blood supply to the periosteum, and of course adherence of periosteum to cortical bone, is not disrupted. There is rapid healing with these grafts, so that at 4–6 weeks bone continuity is established. This is in stark contrast to the 3–4 months required by devascularized autografts or alloplast autografts. One can also transfer relatively large segments of bone and, in the case of the scapular spine, dense bone. An additional advantage is that the bony segments do not preclude postoperative radiation within the 6-week golden period. There are identifiable disadvantages to the osteomyocutaneous flap. There is no question that there is profound donor site morbidity which impairs function on a long-term basis. Compromise of shoulder function is recognized as an integral component of the end result of reconstruction when these flaps are utilized. Adaptation to the anatomical need is also a problem with these flaps. The scapular spine, being very dense bone, is very difficult to shape so as to conform to the curvature of the mandibular arch. Usually the general curvature of the arch is replaced by a rather straight-line bridging between the residual mandibular segments. An additional disadvantage is that these procedures become lengthy and, in the case of the scapular flap, require intraoperative position changes. Despite these disadvantages, the osteo-myocutaneous flaps do provide the surgeon with an opportunity to bring in already vascularized bone from a site removed from the focus of the surgical procedure.

Free flaps

The evolution of vascular microsurgery and a greater comprehension of small vessel vascular anatomy has given rise to the transfer of composite flaps as a bony muscular unit for insertion as a free graft at a distant site. Although several osseous sites have been identified and utilized to bridge the mandibular bony defect, only one – the iliac bone free gragt – has successfully survived clinical trials. Taylor [15] has provided beautiful documentation of the efficacy of the iliac composite graft, showing that with proper positioning, the composite graft

8

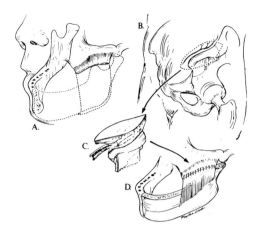

Figure 5. 'A' demonstrates the mandibular loss requiring reconstruction, 'B' the donor site involving the iliac crest, 'C' the free composite flap prior to transfer, and 'D' the free flap in place.

from a single iliac bone will reconstruct, with very acceptable confirmation, the entire half of the mandible (Figure 5). In addition, he has reconstructed an entire mandible using bilateral iliac bone composite grafts. Rosen and others have supported the concept of the free osteomyocutaneous graft in selected cases.

The advantages of the free flap are quite obvious [16, 17]. This method of reconstruction satisfied one requisite by being a single stage procedure. Secondarily, it allows for satisfactory fulfillment of the anatomical requisites. It, like the osteomyocutaneous flap, heals rapidly because of its intrinsic blood supply, and the patient may receive postoperative radiation within the previously established time frame. The disadvantages are, however, not insignificant. Foremost among them is the donor site morbidity. The patient experiences significant discomfort and compromise of function in the groin and lower abdominal regions, which requires weeks to resolve. Other donor sites, such as the foot, eliminate themselves from consideration because of the magnitude of the donor site disability. The most significant disadvantage to the free ostemyocutaneous flap is that it requires special expertise in microvascular anastomosis. It is physically impossible for every head and neck surgeon to develop and maintain the expertise necessary to achieve a high success rate with small vessel anastomosis. It therefore makes sense to have a small team of individuals at each regional head and neck facility who have and will maintain the expertise required to accomplish these procedures which are in very little demand clinically.

Summary

The technological explosion of both materials and procedures has resulted in major changes in mandibular reconstruction. Now, more than ever before, the variety of viable choices is broad. There is no standard method for reconstruction of the mandible, and infact, all of these various forms of reconstruction should be available to the head and neck surgeon. Certainly, however, the goals regarding reestablishment of function and cosmetic configuration are more achievable today than they were a decade ago. It is hoped that methods which assure proper sequencing of the other modes of therapy will continue to evolve, perhaps with the use of biodegradable materials in alloplast/autografts and the further ease of harvesting and establishment of microvascular anastomosis in free osteomyocutaneous flaps. Most assuredly, however, this type of reconstructive surgery, because of its inherent magnitude, will always carry significant levels of complication and of failure.

References

1. Holmes, H., Gullane, P., Personal communication: Mandibular reconstruction – new concepts.
2. DeFries, H.O. 1981. Reconstruction of the mandible: Use of combined homologous mandible and autologous bone. Otolaryngol. Head Neck Surg. 89: 694–697.
3. Lawson, W., Biller, H.F. 1982. Mandibular reconstruction: Bone graft techniques. Otolaryngol. Head Neck Surg. 90: 589–594.
4. Mainous, E.G. et al. 1973. Restoration of resected mandible by grafting with a combination of mandibular homograft and autogenous iliac marrow and postoperative treatment with hyperbaric oxygenation. Oral Surg. 35: 13–20.
5. Berghaus, A. 1905. Porous polyethylene in reconstructive head and neck surgery. Arch. Otolaryngol. 3: 154–160.
6. Ferraro, J.W. 1979. Experimental evaluation of ceramic calcium phosphate as a substitute for bone grafts. Plast. Reconstr. Surg. 63 (5): 634–640.
7. Giordano, A. et al. 1980. Particulate cancellous marrow crib graft reconstruction of mandibular defects. Laryngoscope 90: 2027–2036.
8. Lawson, W. et al. 1982. Experience with immediate and delayed mandibular reconstruction. Laryngoscope 92: 5–10.
9. Schuller, D. et al. 1982. Titanium tray mandibular reconstruction. Arch Otolaryngol. 108: 174–178.
10. Albert, T.W. 1986. Dacron mesh tray and cancellous bone in reconstruction of mandibular defects. Arch. Otolaryngol. Head Neck Surg. 112: 53–59.
11. Cummings, C.W., Leipzig, B. 1985. Mandibular reconstruction other than osteomyocutaneous homografts. In: Head and Neck Cancer, Vol. 1, B.C. Decker, Inc. and C.V. Mosby, St. Louis, Toronto, p. 501–505.
12. Hamaker, R.C. et al. 1983. Irradiated mandibular autografts. Cancer 52 (6): 1017–1022.
13. Ariyan, S., Finseth, F.J. 1978. The anterior chest approach for obtaining free osteocutaneous rib grafts. Plast. Reconstr. Surg. 62: 676–685.
14. Panje, W., Cutting C. 1900. Trapezius osteomyocutaneous island flap for reconstruction of the anterior floor of mouth and the mandible. Head Neck Surg. 3: 66–71.
15. Taylor, G.I. 1982. Reconstruction of the mandible with free composite iliac bone grafts. Ann Plast. Surg. 9 (5): 361–376.
16. Berggren, A., Weiland, A.J., Dorfman, H. 1982. Free vascularized bone grafts: factors affecting their survival and ability to heal to recipient bone defects. Plast. Reconstr. Surg. 69 (1): 19–29.
17. Panje, WR. 1981. Free compound groin flap reconstruction of anterior mandibular defect. Arch. Otolaryngol. 107: 17–22.

2. Extracapsular spread of squamous carcinoma in cervical metastasis

JONAS T. JOHNSON and EUGENE N. MYERS

Introduction

The unpredictable behavior of malignant disease has led many oncologists to search for factors which may be used to forecast prognosis. Histologic evidence of extracapsular spread (ECS) of metastatic disease in cervical lymph nodes has been recognized as a predictor of poor prognosis in patients with squamous cell carcinoma of the head and neck.

We do not currently understand the mechanism by which ECS develops in any particular patient. It may represent an observable feature of some as yet unrecognized aspect of tumor invasiveness, clonogenic capability or immunologic responsiveness. Current data only allows us to recognize ECS as an indication of the host-tumor relationship which predicts high risk for recurrent disease.

Staging

A tumor staging system is critical to the head and neck oncologist. Staging allows communication among investigators and comparison of treatment results among institutions and between historic periods. Additionally, staging has been developed and refined during the years to offer guidance in therapeutic decision making and patient counseling.

The staging of head and neck carcinoma has traditionally been based upon clinical findings alone. Statistical reporting and therapeutic decision making continue to be reflective of clinical staging. This, in part, reflects the fact that many patients are treated without benefit of pathologic staging. Also, most histologic and cytologic variables have not achieved wide acceptance as indicators of prognosis.

C. Jacobs (ed) Cancers of the head and neck.
© *1987, Martinus Nijhoff Publishers, Boston. ISBN 0–89838–825–2. Printed in the Netherlands.*

Differentiation

Tumor differentiation has been reported to be of prognostic importance by Bennett [1]. Cachin *et al.* [2] reviewed the clinical data (retrospectively) and histologic findings (prospectively) in a large group of patients with squamous carcinoma of the oropharynx. Thirty-nine percent of patients with well differentiated primary tumors did not develop cervical metastasis. In contrast, 80% of patients with poorly differentiated tumors had neck metastasis. Sessions [3] however, in a retrospective clinical-pathologic evaluation of 791 patients stated that differentiation was a reliable prognostic indicator only in patients with lesions of the inferior part of the hypopharynx. Johnson *et al.* [4] evaluated 177 neck dissections undertaken in 161 patients. All primary tumors were classified as either well differentiated, moderately well differentiated, or poorly differentiated. Differentiation did not correlate with the development of cervical metastasis or with survial. Noone *et al.* [5] retrospectively correlated the histologic findings in tumors of 62 patients. The survival data from patients with well differentiated tumors were compared to those with poorly differentiated tumors. The 5-year survival between the two groups (59% vs. 43%) was not deemed significant by statistical analysis (P > 0.10).

Similarly, the presence of sinus histocytosis, cellular inflammatory responses, lymphocytic infiltration, and germinal center hyperplasia are factors which are not reliable markers in predicting prognosis.

Multiple nodes

The demonstration of histologic evidence of involvement with tumor in multiple nodes has been believed to forebode a poor prognosis [6]. This issue is an integral part of the staging system. Is is interesting to note, however, that Sessions [3] observed that the number of nodes involved with malignancy did not correlate with survivorship in patients with carcinoma of the supraglottis or the glottis. Schuller *et al.* [7] substantianted this finding in a retrospective review of 242 patients. Neither the absolute number of involved cervical nodes nor the percentage of malignant nodes was found to correlate with ultimate survivorship. Johnson *et al.* [4] observed that the average number of nodes involved with malignancy was actually higher in the patients who survived with no evidence of disease when compared to a cohort group of patients who had died of recurrent disease.

Extracapsular spread

The presence of carcinoma in the cervical lymph node is said to reduce, for a given lesion, the number of patients who will survive disease-free by approximately 50%. The extension of cervical metastasis into the soft tissue of the neck has long been recognized as an indicator of poor prognosis. Bennett *et al.* [1] noted a 70% observed 5-year survival in patients with negative nodes as compared to a 26% 5-year survival in patients with positive nodes. A small number of these patients demonstrated extranodal spread of metastatic tumor. The survival in patients with ECS was 15%. Noone *et al.* [5] reported that 56% of patients with negative nodes survived disease-free for 5 years. In the group of patients with positive nodes, prognosis was improved if the metastasis was confined to the lymph node. Seventy percent of patients with tumor confined to the node survived 5 years. In contrast, when capsular involvement was noted the survival figure was 48%. Extracapsular spread of the tumor was associated with a 27% 5-year survival.

Shah *et al.* [8] commented that ECS of cervical metastasis and soft tissue involvement by tumor correlated with poor prognosis. Sessions [3] stated that the invasion of soft tissue by tumor decreased treatment success by a ratio of 5:1. Zoller *et al.* [9] reviewed a group of patients treated surgically. None of the survivors had had ECS in their lesions. Thirty-six percent of those who had died had lesions demonstrating ECS.

A prevailing concept in head and neck surgery has been the notion that ECS was a manifestation of large lymph nodes and that the TNM staging system addresses this issue. Fixation of cervical metastasis is felt to represent soft tissue invasion (ECS) and has been previously used as an integral part of the staging system. Currently, nodal size has been adopted as a more objective method by which to measure the aggressiveness of cervical metastasis. The presence of soft tissue invasion by cervical metastases has long been recognized as an indicator of poor prognosis. In turn, ECS has generally been assumed to correlate with nodal size and as such was a manifestation of late stage disease.

Cachin *et al.* [2] undertook a correlative study of lymph node size and histo-logic findings. It was noted that the presence of ECS was related to nodal size. Fourteen percent of nodes less than 1 cm demonstrated ECS. The incidence of ECS found in nodes 2 cm, 3 cm, 4 cm, and 5 cm was 26%, 49%, 71% and 76% respectively.

Snow *et al.* [10] substantiated these observations in a retrospective study in which 405 patients who had undergone 484 radical neck dissections were evaluat-ed. Specimens from 78 patients did not contain tumor. One hundred and seventy-six of the remaining patients (53.8%) had evidence of ECS. ECS was noted in 23% of nodes less than 1 cm in diameter. Forty-four percent of nodes 1–2 cm demonstrated ECS. Nodes 2 cm to 3 cm in diameter had ECS 53% of the time while 74% of nodes greater than 3 cm evidenced ECS.

Cachin *et al.* [2] compared the degree of lymph node involvement with survival three years after therapy. When 601 cases of carcinoma of the upper aerodigestive tract were considered 3-year survival was 65% in patients with no evidence of metastasis to the lymph nodes. In contrast, patients with carcinoma limited to the

14

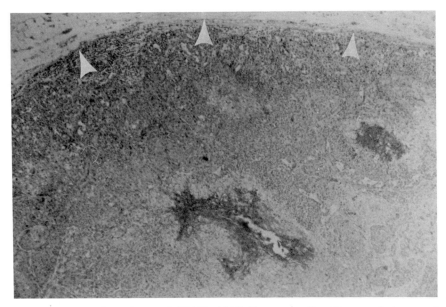

Figure 1. Low power photomicrograph (H & E × 187.5). Squamous cell carcinoma replacing a cervical lymph node. The capsule is intact (arrows). No ECS.

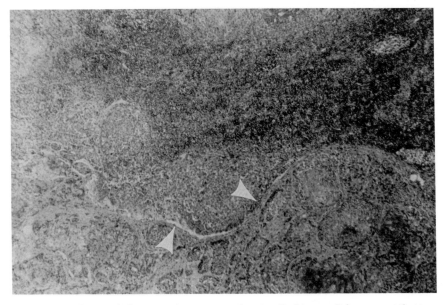

Figure 2. Photomicrograph demonstrating extracapsular spread of tumor. It is apparent that tumor has extended through the capsule of the node (arrowd indicate capsule).

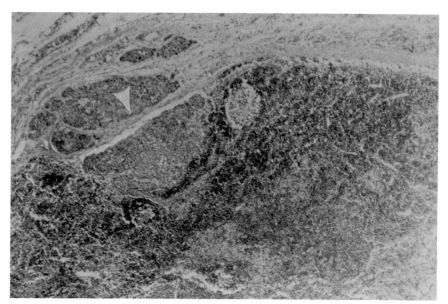

Figure 3. A small focus of tumor in this lymph node shows invasion of the capsule (arrow) with ECS (H & E × 300).

lymph nodes evidenced a 33% survivorship while patients with ECS experienced a 15% survivorship. These dramatic differences in survivorship based upon ECS were confirmed when smaller subsets of patients were examined with carcinoma of the tonsil and carcinoma of the tongue base individually.

In an initial report we retrospectively evaluated 161 patients treated with radical neck dissection [4]. Extracapsular spread was found in 65% of patients with cervical metastases who had been judged N_1 clinically. Seventy-five percent of patients with nodes greater than 3 cm in diameter had ECS. Patient survival following therapy was then correlated to histologic findings in the neck. Survivorship of patients who had no histologic disease in the neck was 70% which was comparable to survivorship of patients with histologic evidence of metastases in whom no evidence of ECS was noted (62% survival). In contrast, 37% of patients with cervical lymph node metastases demonstrating ECS survived with no evidence of disease. The differences in survivorship observed in the ECS group when compared to the former groups were statistically significant ($P < 0.05$).

These initial data were further examined to determine if ECS was a co-predictor reflective of some other determinant of survival. The average number of histologically proven malignant nodes per patient was examined. There was no difference in the number of nodes involved in the group of patients whose lesions showed ECS when compared to the group of patients whose lesion showed no ECS.

Patients with stage IV disease were, in fact, more likely to have histologic evidence of ECS in cervical metastasis than patients with stage III disease. When

16

the group of patients with stage IV disease was examined independently, however, it was demonstrated that a substantial decrease in survival was noted in patients with ECS (Table 1).

These preliminary observations led us to expand the scope of this initial study. We subsequently evaluated 349 more patients retrospectively [11]. ECS was noted in 59% of patients with cervical metastases. The scope of the larger study allowed more comprehensive review and comparison of survival data according to histologic findings in the neck. One hundred and twenty-six patients had stage III squamous cell carcinoma. Five patients were unavailable for further study because histologic slides were unavailable. Forty-nine patients (40.5%) had no evidence of cervical metastases. Of the remaining 72 patients with stage III disease 36 (50%) had ECS (Table 2).

In comparison 161 patients with stage IV disease were evaluated. In nine patients histologic findings could not be ascertained. Thirty-three percent of patients

Table 1. Survival status of patients stage IV disease

Characteristic	Number	NED[a]	DOD[b]	DOC[c]	Determinant survival (%)	Absolute survival (%)
No neck disease	19	10	9	0	52	52
Lesions showing no ECS	12	9	3	0	75	75
Lesions showed ECS	23	3	14	6	18	12

[a] NED = no evident disease.
[b] DOD = dead of disease.
[c] DOC = dead af other cause.

Table 2. Histological status of neck nodes in stage III patients

Site	Negative nodes[a]	No ECS[b]	+ ECS[c]	Unknown[d]
Tongue	2	1	3	–
Tonsil	11	8	10	2
Floor of mouth	4	1	2	–
Base of tongue	1	1	2	–
Epiglottis	15	11	11	–
Glottis	5	6	1	–
Hypopharynx	5	4	3	2
Miscellaneous	4	3	4	1
Unknown primary	2	1	0	–
Totals	49	36	36	5

[a] No histologic evidence of cervical metastasis.
[b] Cervical metastases limited to lymph node.
[c] Cervical metastasis has spread beyond lymph node capsule of soft tissue of neck.
[d] Histologic findings of extracapsular extent could not be ascertained.

had no histologic evidence of cervical metastases. Sixty-five percent of the 102 stage IV patients with cervical metastases evidenced ECS (Table 3).

Two-year disease free survival was then evaluated according to the histologic findings in the neck and stage of the primary tumor (Tables 4 and 5).

Survivorship in both stage III and stage IV disease was similar in patients with no evidence of cervical metastases when compared to patients with cervical metastases limited to the lymph nodes. When ECS was present, 2-year disease-free survivorship decreased by a factor of approximately one half. It should be noted that ultimate survivorship in these two groups of patients correlated better with ECS (or lack of ECS) than it did with the clinical stage of the disease.

Table 3. Histologic status of neck nodes in stage IV patients

Site	Negative nodes	No ECS	+ ECS	Unknown[a]
Tongue	7	3	6	1
Tonsil	6	1	11	2
Floor of mouth	4	4	6	2
Base of tongue	4	4	4	1
Epiglottis	11	12	12	2
Glottis	6	1	2	–
Hypopharynx	3	3	11	–
Miscellaneous	6	3	9	1
Unknown primary	3	0	1	–
Total	50	36	66	9

[a] Histologic findings of extracapsular extent could not be ascertained.

Table 4. Two-year disease-free survival according to histologic finding in Neck – stage III patients

	Patients	Died of disease	No evidence of disease	Died of second primary	Died other or lost to follow-up
Negative nodes	49	5 (13%)	34 (87%)	2	8
No ECS	36	8 (25%)	24 (75%)	1	3
+ ECS	36	20 (61%)	13 (39%)	1	2

Table 5. Two-year disease-free survival according to histologic finding in Neck – stage IV patients

	Patients	Died of disease	No evidence of disease	Died of second primary	Died other or lost to follow-up
Negative nodes	50	12 (29%)	30 (71%)	2	6
No ECS	36	10 (33%)	20 (67%)	1	4
+ ECS	66	34 (64%)	19 (36%)	2	11

18

Evaluation of treatment outcome in patients who had undergone a comprehensive treatment program involving surgery plus postoperative radiation therapy was undertaken. Patients with pathologic indication of surgical margins involved with tumor were excluded. Only patients with stage III or stage IV squamous cell carcinoma were included. A minimum dose of 50 gy of external beam radiation therapy delivered to the primary site and cervical lymphatics bilaterally had been undertaken within 6 weeks of surgery in every case. One hundred and five patients were identified who fulfilled these criteria. Two-year NED survival for patients with cervical metastasis limited to the lymph node was 73% (32 of 44 patients). In comparison, only 49% of patients with ECS (30 of 61 patients) remained free of disease. This difference in survivorship is statistically significant ($P < 0.03$) (Table 6). When further subdivided according to stage of disease, the impact of ECS upon treatment outcome in this group of patients who received combined therapy continue to demonstrate the negative effect of ECS upon ultimate outcome (Table 7).

Table 6. Surgery + post operative radiation survival according to cervical histology

	Patients	NED[a]	DOD[b]	
No ECS	44	32 (73%)	12	
				$P < 0.03$
ECS	61	30 (49%)	31	

[a] NED = no evident disease.
[b] DOD = dead of disease.

Table 7. Surgery + post operative radiation survival according to histology in the neck

	Patients	NED	DOD	
Stage III				
No ECS	20	16 (80%)	4	
				$P < 0.05$
ECS	25	12 (48%)	13	
Stage IV				
No ECS	24	16 (67%)	8	
				$P > 0.05$
ECS	36	18 (50%)	18	

Table 8. Surgery + post operative radiation survival according to stage

	Patients	NED	DOD	
Stage III	45	28 (62%)	17	
				$P < 0.05$
Stage IV	60	34 (57%)	26	

It is apparent that the prognostic value of the demonstration of ECS in cervical lymphatics is superior to the staging system currently employed (AJC) (Table 8).

Snyderman *et al.* [12] evaluated the impact of ECS in cervical lymph nodes in 96 patients with squamous cell carcinoma of the supraglottic larynx. Three-year NED survival was 71% in patients with no evidence of cervical metastasis. When metastases were confined to cervical lymphatics the 3 year NED rate was 79%. In contrast, the presence of ECS was associated with a 45% 3-year NED survivorship ($P < 0.05$).

Snyderman *et al.* [12] note that the clinical assessment of the extent of disease in cervical lymphatics correlates poorly with histologic findings. Forty one percent of patients clinically judged to have no evidence of cervical metastasis were found to have metastatic carcinoma histologically. Twenty percent of these patients with no palpable adenopathy were found to have ECS. In comparison of patients judged clinically to have a single cervical metastasis less than 3 cm (N_1), 17%, had no histologic evidence of disease. Seven percent of patients staged N_2 or N_3 had no evidence of metastases histologically. Fifty-three percent (32 of 60 patients) with histologic evidence of cervical metastases were found to have ECS.

Discussion

The interpretation of comparative therapeutic trials is predicated upon our belief that we can identify two truly comparable patient populations. In fact, we all readily acknowledge that patient populations are never truly 'equal'. Retrospective and non-randomized prospective trials assume that all factors which may influence the measured outcome can be adequately identified and evaluated. Perhaps the most important outcome of our experience with ECS is the recognition that previous unacknowledged factors may be operative and significantly influence outcome. ECS is an indicator of poor prognosis which is encountered in greater than one-half of patients with small (N_1) cervical adnopathy. These studies substantiate the glaring flaws in the clinical staging system as it currently exists. The continued investigation of the factors which influence the development of ECS are manditory.

All of the currently available data on the prognostic significance of ECS in cervical node metastases are based upon information gained through the retrospective evaluation of patient charts. It is clear that studies generated in this fashion may be methodologically flawed in many ways. Nevertheless, the histologic finding of ECS in cervical metastasis has served as a valuable tool in predicting treatment outcome. Current studies do not allow interpretation of the pathophysiology of this observation. ECS may reflect aggressiveness of the tumor or inadequacy of host response. ECS serves, nevertheless, as an indicator of poor prognosis.

The presence of ECS, or lack thereof, is an integral and necessary part of the

20

pathology report. Similarly, retrospective comparative studies should access the incidence of ECS in the treatment groups while prospective studies must stratify accordingly to maximize reliability.

References

1. Bennett, S.H., Futrell, J.W., Rogh, J.A., Hoye, R.C., Ketcham, A.S., 1971. Prognostic significance of histologic host response in cancer of the larynx or hypopharynx. Cancer 28: 1255–1265.
2. Cachin, Y., Sancho-Garnier, S., Micheau, C., Marandas, P. 1979. Nodal metastasis from carcinomas of the oropharynx. Otolaryngol. Clin. North Am. 12(1): 145–155.
3. Sessions, D.G., 1976. Surgical pathology of cancer of the larynx and hypopharynx. Laryngoscope 86: 814–839.
4. Johnson, J.T., Barnes, L., Myers, E.N., Schramm, V.L., Jr., Borochovitz, D., Sigler, B.A. 1981. The extracapsular spread of tumors in cervical node metastasis. Arch. Otolaryngol. 107: 725–729.
5. Noone, R.B., Bonner, H., Jr., Raymond, S., Brown, A.S., Graham, W.P., Lehr, H.B. 1974. Lymph node metastases in oral carcinoma. Plas. Reconstr. Surg. 53: 158–166.
6. Reed, G.F., Mueller, W., Snow, J.B. 1959. Radical neck dissection (a clinicopathological study of 200 cases). Laryngoscope 69: 702–743.
7. Schuller, D.E., McGuirt, W.F., McCabe, B.F., Young, D. 1980. The prognostic significance of metastatic cervical lymph nodes. Laryngoscope 90: 557–570.
8. Shah, J.P., Cendon, R.A., Farr, H.W., Strong, E.W. 1976. Carcinoma of the oral cavity – Factors affecting treatment failure at the primary site and neck. Am. J. Surg. 132: 504–507.
9. Zoller, M., Goodman, M.L., Cummings, C.W. 1970. Guidelines for prognosis in head and neck cancer with nodal metastasis. Laryngoscope 88: 135–140.
10. Snow, G.B., Annyas, A.A., Van Slooten, E.A., Bartelink, H., Hart, A.A.M. 1982. Prognostic factors of neck node metastasis. Clin. Otolaryngol. 7: 185–192.
11. Johnson, J.T., Myers, E.N., Bedetti, C.D., Barnes, E.L., Schramm, V.L., Jr., Thearle, P.B. 1985. Cervical lymph node metastases – Incidence and implications of extracapsular carcinoma. Arch. Otolaryngol. 111: 534–537.
12. Snyderman, N.L., Johnson, J.T., Schramm, V.L., Jr., Myers, E.N., Bedetti, C., Thearle, P. 1985. Extracapsular spread of carcinoma in cervical lymph nodes: Impact upon survival in patients with carcinoma of the supraglottic larynx. Cancer 56: 1587–1599.

3. The role of a modified neck dissection

ROBERT M. BYERS

Introduction

Since the 1960s, head and neck surgeons have gradually developed an understanding of how and when the lymph nodes in the cervical drainage areas for cancers of the oral cavity, oropharynx, larynx and hypopharynx, as well as for cancers of the skin can be removed while preserving functionally and cosmetically vital anatomic structures [1]. In addition, knowledge has been gained as to which regional nodal groups are at highest risk for containing metastatic cancer, depending upon the location of the primary cancer. Consequently, many regional lymphadenectomies have been suggested to fit the potential extent of the cervical metastasis. Although this approach has been applicable for squamous carcinoma, recently, modifications of the radical neck dissection have been reported for the treatment of melanoma and thyroid carcinomas [2, 3]. The use of immediate postoperative irradiation with the modified neck dissection is advised when certain adverse criteria have been identified which carry a high risk for local-regional recurrence if surgery is used as the only modality of treatment [4]. From a conceptual standpoint, the value of the various selective neck dissections is still evolving and hopefully will soon become standardized.

Definition

In order to gain widespread acceptance, a surgical procedure has to be an effective and reproducible technique for the majority of surgeons. The nonmenclature needs to be standardized so that each type of neck dissection is readily identifiable, and the results from different investigators can be compared.

Consequently, one of the most difficult problems in discussing the role of a modified neck dissection is actually defining what a modified neck dissection is. There have been many terms used to describe a modified neck dissection. Actually, many people feel that a modified neck dissection is merely something

C. Jacobs (ed) Cancers of the head and neck.
© 1987, Martinus Nijhoff Publishers, Boston. ISBN 0–89838–825–2. Printed in the Netherlands.

less radical than the classic neck dissection described by Crile and popularized by Hayes Martin. To define an operation merely by its conservatism or radicalism does not address the most vital issue, and that is its appropriateness. Perhaps the definition of a neck dissection should reflect a selectivity which is determined by the extent of the particular disease for which the operation is intended. Sometimes the scope of the modified dissection can be more extensive than the radical neck dissection. The proper selection is based on the site and stage of the primary, the predictability of the lymphatic drainage, the magnitude of the nodal drainage, and the surgeon's experience. The selected neck dissection will provide appropriate pathologic staging. It is important to understand that not every patient's neck needs to be dissected in the same manner. A modified neck dissection does not and should not portray a surgical procedure in which only the spinal accessory nerve, the sternocleidomastoid muscle and the internal jugular vein are routinely preserved. Many times it is equally valuable and feasible to preserve the external jugular vein, the greater auricular nerve, the cervical plexus, and many times even the ansa cervicalis. Discrimination can be exercised in preserving any of the anatomical structures in the neck which are not obviously involved with cancer, provided meticulous attention is paid to a clean and thorough removal of the lymphatic and connective tissue. This is of particular value and appropriate when bilateral dissections are indicated or if the neck is entered for exposure purposes in order to resect a primary cancer in the upper aerodigestive tract. Whenever the pathways of metastatic disease to cervical nodes are unclear, or perhaps altered by previous treatment or by large metastatic deposits, the effectiveness of a regional lymphadenectomy is questionable. The various modified neck dissections currently used at M.D. Anderson Hospital are: the functional, the supraomohyoid, the posterolateral, the anterior, the suprahyoid and the lower neck dissections. For purposes of clarity each of these types of dissections will be described in terms of the nodal groups which should be included and the more common primary cancers for which these operations would be most appropriate.

The functional neck dissection (Figure 1)

The functional neck dissection as described by Bocca *et al.* [1] implies that the patient is functionally better after this operation than if a radical neck dissection was performed. It is not an anatomically descriptive term. The nodal groups routinely removed are the same as with the radical neck dissection, however, the internal jugular vein, the sternocleidomastoid muscle and the 11th cranial nerve are preserved. This type of neck dissection would be inadequate for the following cancers: subglottic larynx or thyroid cancer with the paratracheal nodes at risk, the pyriform sinus or pharyngeal wall with retropharyngeal nodes involved, or a melanoma of the scalp with metastases to suboccipital nodes. Therefore, it is

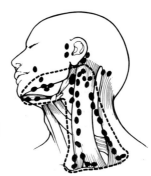

Functional: All sites.
Submental, submandibular, subdigastric,
mid and lower jugular, upper middle and
lower posterior cervical, paratracheal,
retropharyngeal, supraclavicular.

Figure 1. Nodes removed with functional neck dissection.

a selected type of dissection for cancers in the oral cavity, oropharynx and supraglottic and glottic larynx.

The supraomohyoid neck dissection (Figure 2)

This selected neck dissection is often confused with the suprahyoid dissection. The primary difference between the two operations involves the extent of the nodal groups removed, as you can see in comparing Figures 2 and 3. The supraomohyoid dissection, however, can incorporate the lower jugular nodes as well depending upon how far the omohyoid muscle is retracted inferiorly. The operation is designed for oral cavity or oropharynx primaries, particularly squamous carcinoma of the anterior floor of mouth when a bilateral dissection is indicated. The operation is not appropriate for lesions in the larynx and hypopharynx. Most of the time, the 11th cranial nerve is not disturbed except to visualize it in order to safely preserve it. The nodes in the upper portion of the posterior triangle are sometimes difficult to dissect when the spinal accessory nerve and the sternocleidomastoid muscle are not removed. If any question exists as to the necessity for adequate exposure in removing this group of nodes, the sternocleidomastoid muscle may be resected and the 11th nerve grafted.

The suprahyoid neck dissection (Figure 3)

This type of dissection is useful for masses in the submaxillary triangle with no histologic diagnosis. A frozen section of the mass will determine if a more extensive dissection is warranted, or if postoperative irradiation is preferable. The operation is definitive for benign tumors and low grade cancers of the submaxillary gland, if no submandibular nodes are involved. Since the operation does not include the subdigastric and midjugular nodes, it is not adequate as a staging procedure, nor appropriate therapy for cancers of the oral cavity or oropharynx.

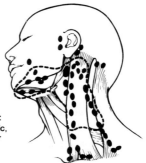

Supraomohyoid:
Lip, skin of face, oral cavity, oropharynx:
  submental, submandibular, subdigastric,
  midjugular, upper and middle posterior
  cervical.

Figure 2. Nodes removed with supraomohyoid neck dissection.

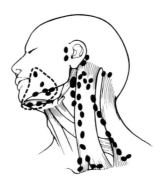

Suprahyoid:
Lip and skin of anterior face:
  Buccinator
  Submental
  Submandibular

Figure 3. Nodes removed with suprahyoid neck dissection.

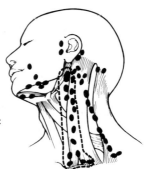

Anterior:
Larynx, hypopharynx, cervical esophagus:
  subdigastric, mid and lower jugular,
  paratracheal, retropharyngeal.

Figure 4. .Nodes removed with anterior neck dissection.

The anterior neck dissection (Figure 4)

Advanced cancers of the larynx and hypopharynx commonly metastasize to the upper, middle and lower jugular nodes bilaterally, but rarely involve nodes in the posterior triangle. Since most of these cancers are best treated with a combination

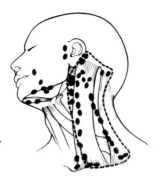

Posterior-Lateral:
Scalp, ear, posterior neck skin:
retroauricular, suboccipital, upper
middle and lower posterior
cervical.

Figure 5. Nodes removed with posterior-lateral neck dissection.

of surgery and radiation, the role of the anterior neck dissection is to remove any gross nodal disease. The spinal accessory nerve can usually be preserved, but the internal jugular vein and/or the sternocleidomastoid muscle on one or the other side of the neck may be invaded with cancerous nodes and necessitate its removal. The early lesions will probably not need combined treatment, and an anterior neck dissection will be adequate surgery for staging the N0 neck and resecting the unilateral or bilateral N1 neck. Of course, the paratracheal nodes would be included with lesions extending subglottically, and the retropharyngeal nodes would be included for hypopharyngeal cancers.

The posterior-lateral neck dissection (Figure 5)

The posterior-lateral neck dissection is a very specialized procedure designed to remove a group of nodes in the primary drainage area for skin cancers, particularly melanoma, of the posterior-lateral scalp, ear, and upper posterior neck. Cancers of the nasopharynx will metastasize to this area, but the nodes are not routinely treated with a surgical excision. These nodes are rarely involved as isolated metastases from other mucosal sites unless the anterior nodes are massively invaded as well. The removal of the retroauricular and suboccipital nodes illustrate the concept of a selected lymphadenectomy and certainly would not be included in the classic radical neck dissection.

The lower neck dissection (Figure 6)

When cancers of the thyroid metastasize regionally, the nodes of the lower posterior triangle, the lower and midjugular and the paratracheal areas are commonly involved. A selected neck dissection which will electively remove nodes at highest risk for metastases from well differentiated cancers of the thyroid, as well as squamous cancers of the cervical esophagus is useful from a staging

26

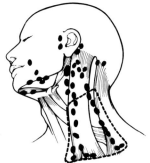

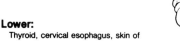

Lower:
Thyroid, cervical esophagus, skin of
lower neck:
   mid and lower jugular, middle and
   lower posterior cervical, supraclavicular,
   paratracheal.

Figure 6. Nodes removed with lower neck dissection.

standpoint. Very rarely do these cancers skip the first echelon of nodes and involve the upper jugular, subdigastric and submaxillary nodes.

Discussion

The effectiveness of a modified or selected neck dissection depends upon the expertise and experience of the head and neck surgeon. It is not surprising that it is more difficult to perform a modified neck dissection technically than a radical neck dissection. Adequate exposure is a must. The type of skin incision used varies with each neck dissection, depending upon the patient's anatomy and the extent of disease. A U-shaped incision is popular for ipsilateral suprahyoid, functional, supraomohyoid and anterior dissections. An apron-type incision is satisfactory for bilateral dissections. A hockey-stick incision works well for the posterior-lateral and lower neck dissections. Bifurcated or trifurcated type incisions should be avoided whenever possible.

The surgical specimen should be taken personally to the pathologist and each resected nodal group properly identified so that an accurate histologic assessment can be made of each node. The pathology report should reflect the total number of nodes removed, the number in each regional area, and the size and number of the nodes in each regional area which contained metastatic disease. The presence or absence of connective tissue disease should also be documented. The operative note must list the anatomic structures preserved and their relationship to the cancerous nodes.

The use of frozen section will occasionally help the surgeon in deciding intraoperatively on how extensive to perform the lymphadenectomy. If a unilateral supraomohyoid neck dissection is completed for an oral cavity primary, and a single suspiciously enlarged midjugular node is present, the lower jugular nodes need to be removed if the node is positive for metastatic disease. If it is negative, the operation is terminated. If there are multiple positive nodes in the specimen, the supraomohyoid neck dissection alone has staged the disease sufficiently to

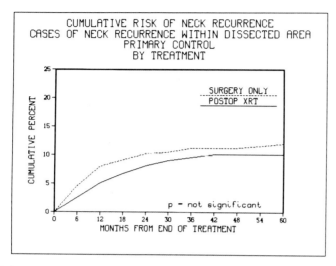

Figure 7. Neck recurrence with surgery versus surgery and XRT.

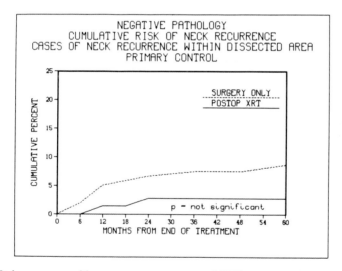

Figure 8. Neck recurrence with surgery versus surgery and XRT.

demonstrate the need for postoperative radiation, and no further dissection is indicated if all gross disease has been removed.

If, as a result of evaluation of the pathologic specimen, extracapsular nodal disease or multiple positive nodes are identified, the addition of postoperative radiation, ideally within 6 weeks following the surgical procedure, can decrease the incidence of regional recurrence (Figures 7–10). The radiation fields and dosage are tailored to the areas of highest risk for recurrence. When there are indications for postoperative irradiation from the dissection of one side of the neck or from findings as a result of resecting the primary, then the clinically N0

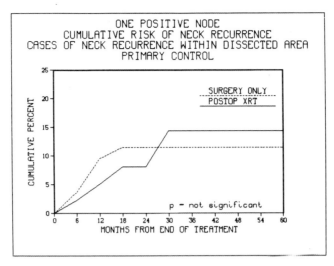

Figure 9. Neck recurrence with surgery versus surgery and XRT.

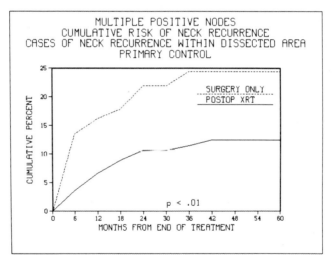

Figure 10. Neck recurrence with surgery versus surgery and XRT.

contralateral neck does not need to be dissected, but can be included in the postoperative radiation fields.

From a therapeutic standpoint, a modified or selected neck dissection if properly done is adequate treatment for the N0 and the N1 pathologically staged neck in the absence of extracapsular nodal extension [4]. Since the morbidity of a modified neck dissection alone is very minimal it can be useful for patients who are unreliable in their follow-up visits, or live at such distances that it would be difficult for them to return for regular routine follow-up. Therefore, instead of waiting for the nodal disease to evolve subsequent to the treatment of the primary, the neck can be electively dissected, pertinent pathologic information obtained which will maximize the patient's treatment, and thereby minimize the number of follow-up visits.

There are many instances in which to effectively resect the primary lesion, adequate exposure and safety is provided by entering the neck. In such a case it would be very detrimental to the patient, in the absence of any palpable disease, to perform a standard radical neck dissection. A modification of this, in which the surgeon selects the lymphadenectomy that is appropriate, will gain the needed exposure and certainly would be in the patient's best functional interest.

In summary, the modified neck dissection preserves function, provides pathologic staging and surgical exposure, and effectively eradicates metastatic disease in the neck either alone or in combination with radiation therapy.

References

1. Bocca, E., Pignataro, O. 1967. A conservation technique in radical neck dissection. Ann. Otol. Rhinol Laryngol. 76: 975–987.
2. Turkula, L., Woods, J. 1984. Limited or selective node dissection in malignant melanoma of the head and neck. Am. J. Surg. 148: 446–448.
3. Sako, K., Marchetta, F.C., Razack, M.S., Shedd, D.P. 1985. Modified radical neck disection for metastatic carcinoma of the thyroid. A reappraisal. Am. J. Surg. 150: 500–502.
4. Byers, R.M. 1985. Modified neck dissection: A study of 967 patients from 1970–1980. Am. J. Surg. 150: 414–421.

4. Extended partial laryngeal surgery

BYRON J. BAILEY and CHARLES M. STIERNBERG

Introduction

Partial laryngectomy is a procedure that was first performed over a century ago. H.B. Sands, in the United States, reported the first partial laryngectomy for the purpose of curing cancer. The patient was a young female, and she survived for 2 years and subsequently died of cancer of the kidney without any evidence of laryngeal recurrence [1]. In 1975, Bilroth, who is credited with performing the first total laryngectomy for cancer, reported a case in which a hemilaryngectomy was performed for cancer of the larynx [1]. It was not until the early part of this century, however, that surgeons began to refine and standardize the operative techniques for conservation surgery of the larynx. Popularization of several of these techniques and widespread acceptance by surgeons did not occur until the 1960s. At the present time, there are than a dozen varieties of partial laryngectomy techniques, and at least another dozen techniques that would be characterized as extended partial laryngectomy techniques. This chapter focuses on the latter type of laryngectomy.

The objectives of all of these procedures remain the same as they were when this evolution began in the last century. It is the goal of partial laryngectomy procedures to achieve the following:
1. adequate resection and cure of laryngeal cancer;
2. a satisfactory postoperative voice;
3. adequate respiratory function (avoidance of postoperative stenosis);
4. adequate postoperative deglution (avoidance of postoperative aspiration).
Extended partial laryngectomies are classified as extended vertical partial laryngectomy (EVPL) and extended supraglottic laryngectomy (ESGL) procedures. Just as the natural histories of glottic and supraglottic carcinomas are different, the indications and contraindications for these two types of laryngectomies are different. They will, therefore, be discussed separately.

C. Jacobs (ed) Cancers of the head and neck.
© *1987, Martinus Nijhoff Publishers, Boston. ISBN 0–89838–825–2. Printed in the Netherlands.*

Extended vertical partial laryngectomy

The contemporary practice of oncology requires the close cooperation of many diciplines. In a practical sense, at the present time, there are several options for the patient who presents with a lesion that is too extensive for standard vertical partial laryngectomy, but who might be cured with less than a total laryngectomy. The therapeutic options for such a patient with 'early advanced' laryngeal cancer include the following:
1. surgery alone, in the form of EVPL;
2. radiation therapy alone;
3. combined surgery and radiation therapy.
The particular problem areas that cause difficulty with the decision for optimum treatment have become known through the experience of many physicians dealing with laryngeal cancer. These problems have been reviewed recently by Guerrier [2] and may be summarized as follows:
1. squamous cell carcinoma at the anterior commissure of the larynx, where invasion of cartilage is not retarded by a perichondrial barrier;
2. subglottic extension;
3. carcinoma involving the laryngeal ventricle; this may present as a transglottic carcinoma;
4. laryngeal sarcoma;
5. cervical lymphadenopathy; a single node may not rule out the performance of a partial laryngectomy, but the presence of multiple nodes suggests the need for total laryngectomy and radical neck dissection;
6. metatstatic carcinoma; a single, small metastatic lesion (e.g., a small, solitary pulmonary upper lobe lesion) may be curable with partial laryngectomy plus lobectomy;
7. recurrence following radiation therapy for laryngeal carcinoma (radiation failure);
8. involvement of the paraglottic space of the larynx with cancer.
The relationship of these particular problems to the concept of extended vertical partial laryngectomy will be reviewed in the remainder of this chapter.

As reported by others, the key to success in regard to the use of extended vertical partial laryngectomy is the proper selection of patients for this technique. Attempts to 'stretch the rules' usually result in failure, and every effort should be made to avoid that particular misadventure.

Indications for extended vertical partial laryngectomy

The term extended vertical partial laryngectomy is used in this chapter as a broad designation for all procedures that involve more than a standard hemilaryngectomy or an other form of vertical partial laryngectomy that is confined to one-half of the larynx.

We have reported the indications we prefer previously [1]. The particular technique which we prefer for this group of lesions is usually an extended fronto-lateral vertical partial laryngectomy and laryngoplasty, and we use this technique, with modifications, in the following situations:

1. lesions that involve the anterior commissure;
2. tumor that invades the arytenoid cartilage;
3. selected, superficial, small transglottic lesions;
4. selected patients with recurrence after radiation therapy for large primary lesions;
5. large verrucous carcinomas;
6. bilateral vocal cord cancer (horseshoe lesions).

Others have added to this list, and we will continue with the understanding that indications 7 through 14 are gleaned from the literature, and that some of them are still in the process of documentation as far as their effectiveness in cancer control and their desirability relative to other treatment options.

7. Bulky transglottic lesions may be managed by a 'three-quarters extended vertical partial laryngectomy'. This technique is essentially a combination of vertical partial laryngectomy with supraglottic partial laryngectomy. This technique is indicated according to Biller and Lawson [3] under the following circumstances:
   a. when the tumor size is 2 cm or less in diameter,
   b. when there is no evidence of vocal cord fixation,
   c. in the absence of subglottic extension,
   d. in the absence of anterior commissure invasion,
   e. when there is no evidence of cartilage invasion on computerized tomography,
   f. when there has been no previous radiation therapy;
8. extended vertical partial laryngectomy has been recommended for certain patients with cord fixation (T3) glottic carcinoma. In a recent publication by Stell et al. [4] this topic was reviewed, with the observation that the original report of the work by Ogura and his colleagues [5] was quite successful, achieving an 85% 5-year survival. LeRoux-Robert in France achieved a 61% overall survival rate, and these two reports continue to generate interest in the further examination of this indication. At the present time, few surgeons in this country are utilizing extended vertical partial laryngectomy for patients with cord fixation. However, it is important to continue to clarify the situation, so that the controversy might be resolved;
9. glottic carcinoma with posterior subglottic extension is reported to be amenable to cure when a modified extended vertical partial laryngectomy is employed. The technique utilized involves resection of most of the cricoid cartilage on the ipsilateral side, and it is necessary to reconstruct the ary-

tenoid-cricoid defect in order to avoid postoperative aspiration problems. Biller and Som [6] have reported a technique that is useful for this purpose, and it will be described later in this chapter;

10. extended vertical partial laryngectomy may be employed in the management of radiation failure [7], in those patients with a small recurrence. Estimation of the size of a recurrent carcinoma after radiation therapy is often extremely difficult because of the postradiation tissue changes. However, when the lesions appear to be small, when there is no cord fixation, and when the other criteria for partial laryngectomy surgery are met, EVPL would appear to be a suitable management choice;

11. carcinoma invading the thyroid cartilage is associated with a poorer prognosis. When the invasion appears to be minimal, extended vertical partial laryngectomy may be attempted, but some authors [2] feel very strongly that wide resection with local laryngectomy is always indicated in the presence of cancer invasion of an ossified thyroid cartilage. Given the usual age group of patients with extensive laryngeal carcinoma, and the degree of ossification that is usually found in this age group, this latter recommendation would, if followed, rule out EVPL for any degree of thyroid cartilage invasion. This matter remains controversial and in need of further clarification;

12. chondrosarcoma is a less aggressive form of malignancy than invasive squamous cell carcinoma. For this reason, extended vertical partial laryngectomy has been reported by Cantrell *et al.* [8] to be an effective and more conservative form of treatment than total laryngectomy in certain instances;

13. piriform sinus cancer with laryngeal involvement is usually a condition requiring total laryngectomy and radical neck dissection. However, in certain selected cases [9] it appears that the technique of near-total laryngectomy (as popularized by Pearson and his colleagues at the Mayo Clinic) deserves careful consideration in the selection of the most appropriate treatment. Near-total laryngectomy is designed to provide the best possible voice and freedom from aspiration following cancer surgery, even though a tracheostomy is required for the adequate maintenance of respiratory function;

14. laryngotracheal invasion by thyroid carcinoma may present an opportunity for extended vertical partial laryngectomy. Thyroid malignancy may encroach upon the upper tracheal cartilaginous rings and the cricoid cartilage, and when this is the case, some of these structures must be sacrified in order to achieve a cure. Experimental work by Friedman *et al.* [10] has shown that 25% of the cricoid cartilage can be resected and reconstructed with preservation of satisfactory laryngeal function.

It is equally important to be familiar with the contraindications for extended vertical partial laryngectomy. The most common contraindications, with regard to the specific nature of the laryngeal cancer, are the following:

1. cancer invading the posterior commissure of the larynx;
2. cancer involving both arytenoid cartilages;

3. cancer invasion of ossified thyroid or cricoid cartilage;
4. fixation of the vocal cord;
5. bulky transglottic lesions (when there is high suspicion of paraglottic space involvement). The difficulty with bulky transglottic lesions is cancer recurrence after vertical partial laryngectomy. Analysis of the patients who have had recurrent tumor as reported by Biller [3] discloses four main areas of concern:
    a. persistent tumor at the superior margin,
    b. tumor invasion of the pre-epiglottic space,
    c. lateral extension to the paraglottic space,
    d. invasion at the posterior incision of the thyroid lamina.

This is a field of surgery that is in transition, and, just as is the case with radiation therapy and chemotherapy, the decision process is complex and evolving. Selection of treatment for each patient must be individualized and based upon careful attention to the best current information in regard to indications and contraindications of specific surgical procedures, as well as consideration of the changing role of combination therapy with adjuvant chemotherapu and adjuvant radiation therapy.

Technique of extended vertical partial laryngectomy

Vertical partial laryngectomy and laryngoplasty is a concept that deals with the conflict between excising as much tissue as possible in order to preserve function. When carcinoma involves the anterior commissure of the larynx, or when it is invading both true vocal cords (horseshoe lesion), a number of specific technical points must be considered. The absence of an internal perichondrium in the region of the anterior commissure tendon predisposes this area to local cancer invasion. When cartilage invasion has occurred, there are also technical problems with regard to its curability utilizing radiation therapy. This situation is clearly documented and repeatedly expressed in patient series analyses drawn from the experience of the last two decades. Because of the decreased protection against local tumor invasion in this region, a number of surgical technique modifications have been devised for resection of the cartilage region of the anterior commissure.

The technique that we employ begins with a curved, collar incision placed one finger breadth below the cricoid cartilage and curving superiorly for about three centimeters in order to create a flap that can be elevated deep to the platysma muscle and up to the level of the hyoid cartilage. The soft tissue is then incised in the midline down to the perichondrium on the surface of the thyroid cartilage. The external thyroid perichondrium is carefully elevated laterally and is sutured to the overlying sternohyoid, sternothyroid, muscle. The plane between the perichondrium and the overlying muscles is not dissected but is purposely left undisturbed in order to maximize the integrity of nutrient vessels. Two paramedian incisions are made through the thyroid cartilage as shown in Figure 1A.

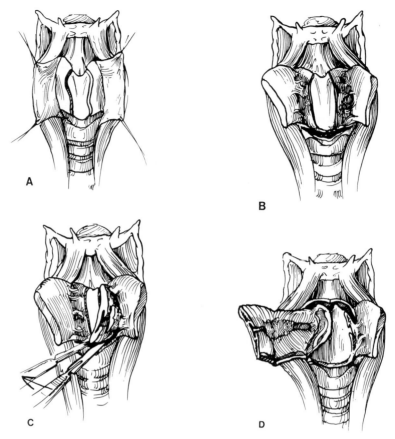

Figure 1. (A) Creation of a central cartilage segment in patients with anterior commissure carcinoma. (B) Elevation of the internal thyroid pericondirum on both sides. (C) Laryngeal entry away from the tumor as first step in resection. (D) Primary resected with adequate margins as exposure is gained.

The inner perichondrium is then exposed through these incisions and an elevation between the cartilage and perichondrium is carried back to the level of the superior and inferior cornua on each side (Figure 1B).

The airway is entered from inferiorly by means of an incision through the cricothyroid ligament. This incision is extended initially on the side of lesser tumor involvement, and as visualization of the tumor is gained from below, the surgeon is guided with regard to the subsequent superior dissection which procedes under direct visualisation. The exposure is increased by working on the side of lesser tumor involvement in order to avoid any risks of cutting across the tumor at this point. Further entry into the larynx is gained by continuing the dissection toward the side of greater tumor involvement as shown in Figure 1C. As this superior line of incision is increased and as the surgeon comes across the midportion of the false cord, the larynx can be opened in a manner comparable to the opening of a book. Direct inspection of the superior, posterior, and inferior margins of

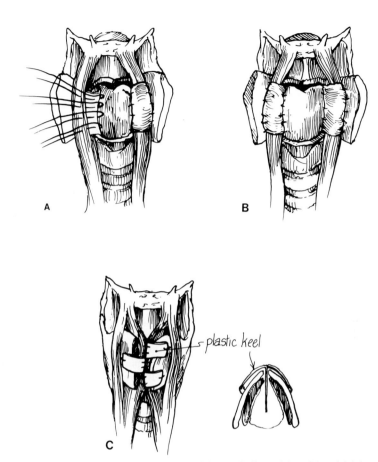

Figure 2. (A) Reconstruction using bilateral, bipedicle muscle flaps with perichondrial tissue preserved for surfacing the lumen. (B) Perichondrium sutured to mucosa bilaterally. (C) Silicone (Silastic) keel is placed in the anterior commissure to prevent anterior web formation.

the resection is accomplished (Figure 1D), and the tumor is excised, Tissue biopsy specimens approximately 2 mm in width are then obtained from each margin and are sent for frozen section analysis. When confirmation of adequate tumor resection has been received, the reconstructive phase is begun.

The reconstruction of the larynx is accomplished using bilateral, bipedicle muscle-perichondrium flaps on each side. These muscle flaps consist of the majority of the sternohyoid, sternothyroid, and thyrohyoid muscles along with the external thyroid perichondrium which will form the new lining of the laryngeal lumen.

The bipedicle muscle flaps are created by incising vertically from a point approximately 1 cm above the superior margin of the thyroid cartilage to a point one centimerter below the inferior margin of the thyroid cartilage. The major point of this reconstructive technique is the preservation of the thyroid alae and the reconstitution of the surgical defect by the bipedicle muscle flaps (Figure 2A).

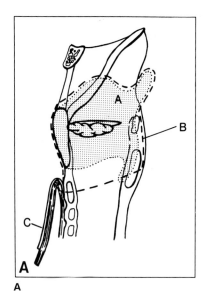

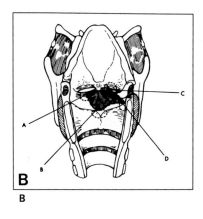

Figure 3. Maximum limits of resection, anatomical. (A) A indicates thyroid cartilage; B, maximum limits of cartilage resection (up to 1 cm beyond midline and upper one-half of ipsilateral cricoid hemisphere); and C, perichondrium adherent to inner aspect of strap muscles. (B) A indicates extension beyond one-third of opposite cord; B, greater than 10 mm anterior subglottic extension (risk of T4 through cricoid membrane); C, extension beyond midventricle (risk of T4 in lateral ventricle into thyroid ala); D, greater than 5 mm posterior subglottic extension (risk of T4 into cricoid cartilage).

The external perichondrium is sutured to the laryngeal mucosa at the posterior resection line (Figure 2B). The muscle flaps and cartilage are then brought together at the midline anteriorly, using a silastic keel to prevent anterior commissure web formation (Figure 2C). The closure anteriorly can be fairly loose, and the bulk of the two muscle flaps is positioned posteriorly, in order to avoid a posterior glottic defect.

The alternative form of hemilaryngectomy is a procedure which sacrifices the supporting thyroid cartilage. Standard hemilaryngectomy and an extended vertical frontolateral laryngectomy (for disease involving the anterior commissure or both vocal cords) involve removal of the hemithyroid cartilage with the possibility of extending the cartilage cut beyond the midline as appears to be necessary for more extensive lesions. This technique has been reported in a recent publication by Mohr, Quenelle, and Shumrick [11].

They feel that the procedure is indicated for selected T1, T2, and T3 glottic lesions and for any patient who refuses radiation therapy or experiences irradiation treatment failure. Specific indications for this procedure include the following:
1. T2 glottic lesions, including those which have impaired cord mobility and those patients who fail radiation. The anatomic limits are (a) involvement of one-third of the opposite cord, (b) extension to the mid ventricle, (c) up to 5 mm of posterior subglottic extension, (d) up to 10 mm of subglottic extension

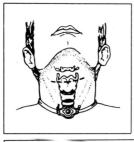

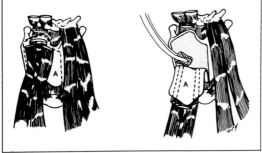
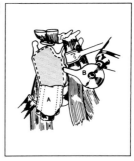

Figure 4. Beginning and initial skeletonization. A indicates perichondrium; B, saw cut.

anteriorly, and (e) the entire hemithyroid cartilage to 1 cm beyond the midline and up to as much as one-half of the ipsilateral cricoid hemisphere;

2. patients with T3 glottic lesions whose anatomic limits are as described above and who are felt to have cord fixation by bulk or muscle invasion;

3. T1 glottic lesions, particularly irradiation failures, irradiation refusals, and patients diagnosed before the age of 40 years.

The contraindications to the technique as reported by these authors include the following:

1. poor pulmonary reserve (Fev 1 less than 60%);

2. the inability to learn a new swallowing technique;

3. anatomic limitations such as greater than one-third of the contralateral cord being involved, greater than 10 mm of anterior subglottic extension, extension beyond the midportion of the ventricle, more than 5 mm of posterior subglottic extension, or when resection of greater than one-half of the upper cricoid hemisphere would be required. These limits are shown graphically in Figure 3.

The surgical technique is shown in Figures 4 through 8. The horizontal skin incision is made just below the level of the notch of the thyroid cartilage and extending from mid-sternocleidomastoid muscle on the side of the lesion to the anterior border of the sternocleidomastoid muscle on the contra-lateral side. A subplatysmal plane is employed to raise the upper flap to a point beyond the superior margin of the hyoid bone, and the lower flap is developed down to the inferior margin of the cricoid cartilage. These strap muscles are transected

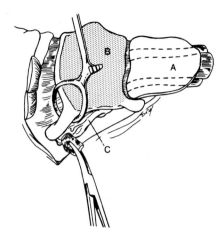

Figure 5. Piriform sinus mucosa reflected. A indicates perichondrium remains adherent to undersurface of strap muscles even though detached from inferior border of thyroid cartilage; B, denuded thyroid cartilage; C, piriform sinus mucosa being reflected from inner aspect of thyroid cartilage.

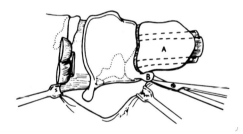

Figure 6. Cricothyroid joint being released. A indicates perichondrium; B, scissors transecting the joint.

halfway between the thyroid cartilage and hyoid bone, and a perichondrial incision is made along the margins of the hemithyroid. The perichondrium over the hemicartilage is reflected downward with the strap muscles remaining attached to it (Figure 4). The cartilage cuts are then made in accordance with the individual requirements for adequate resection, and the larynx is then skeletonized as with a total laryngectomy (Figure 5).

The cricothyroid joint is disarticulated (Figure 6), and an anterior, lateral pharyngotomy is performed on the side of the lesion (Figure 7). Under direct vision, the lesion is encircled as is consistent with obtaining adequate margins (Figure 8), and the specimen is delivered.

The margins are then biopsied and the tissue is sent for frozen section analysis to assess the adequacy of the operative procedure (Figure 9).

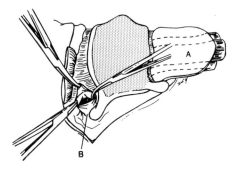

Figure 7. Entry through anterolateral pharyngotomy. A indicates perichondrium; B, anterolateral pharyngotomy site.

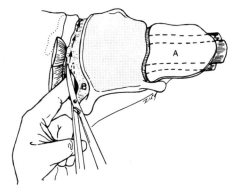

Figure 8. Entry into larynx viewed from inside. A indicates perichondrium; B, continuation of pharyngotomy.

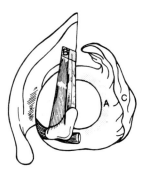

Figure 9. Frozen section biopsy specimens taken from stippled areas A (subglottic mucosa) and B (opposite cord). Incision is carried along subglottic margin.

42

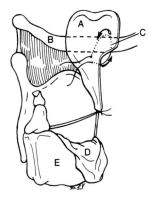

Figure 10. Beginning of reconstruction. A indicates epiglottis; B, hyoid; C, circumhyoidal suture; D, piriform sinus mucosa; and E, cricoid.

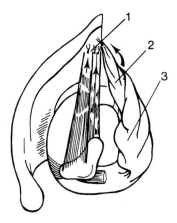

Figure 11. Recreating anterior commissure. 1 indicates true cord; 2 indicates attached neocord slightly above recreated anterior commissure; 3 indicates hypopharyngeal mucosa.

When it has been determined that adequate margins have been achieved, the reconstruction is begun. The epiglottis is stabilized by means of a circumhyoidal suture (Figure 10). A functional anterior commissure is recreated by suturing the retracted vocal cord remnant from the side of lesser involvement to the ipsilateral thyroid cartilage. The piriform sinus mucosa is elevated on the side of the tumor resection and then is pulled forward and sutured into place just above the reconstituted glottis as shown in Figure 11.

The perichondrium that remains attached to the inner aspect of the strap muscles is then used for the final surfacing and closure as shown in Figure 12.

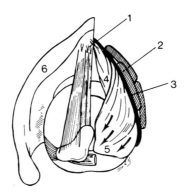

Figure 12. Near-completed reconstruction. 1 indicates reattached remaining cord; 2, strap muscles; 3, perichondrium; 4, hypopharyngeal mucosa – piriform sinus creating neocord; 5, remaining hypopharyngeal mucosa – can be used to close laryngopharyngotomy by itself or in combination with perichondrium; and 6, opposite thyroid cartilage.

Biller and Lawson [12] have reported a technique which is suitable for patients who present with glottic carcinoma even more extensive than we have just discussed. The procedure is recommended for those individuals with invasive carcinoma involving the anterior commissure and both vocal cords, and it may be employed when there is diminished vocal cord mobility bilaterally or even with fixation of one cord and diminished motion of the other. There should be subglottic involvement of less than one centimeter anteriorly and laterally and no subglottic involvement posteriorly. Tumor should involve no more than the arytenoid vocal processes and the anterior surface of the arytenoid cartilage (including the vocal process) must be free of tumor. There must not be vocal cord fixation on the side of the preserved arytenoid. The procedure is not recommended after radiation failure, but it may be employed when there is cartilage invasion anteriorly or anterolaterally.

The technique described might be termed a 'radical partial laryngectomy' in view of the fact that some patients will have only one arytenoid cartilage and the posterior commissure preserved. The surgeon then performs a staged reconstruction, which consists of rotating the remaining posterior border of thyroid cartilages 90° forward in order to obtain tissue that will provide anterior-posterior dimension length and support. A temporary of laryngostome is constructed using skin flaps turned in from the neck. This laryngostome is closed later.

Although decanulation was possible, the patients who underwent the most extensive resection had suboptimal respiratory function and were prone to respiratory infections. The procedure would seem to be justifiable and worthy of further investigation and development in view of the fact that these patients are confronted with no surgical alternative other than total laryngectomy.

Biller and Som [6] recommend another form of extended verical partial laryngectomy for glottic carcinoma when there is posterior subglottic extension. The

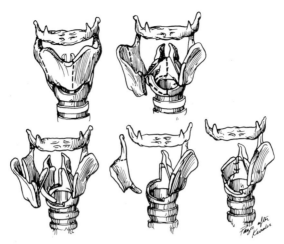

Figure 13. After resection of most of the ipsilateral cricoid cartilage, the defect is reconstructed using a pedicled myochondral flap (inferior constrictor muscle and thyroid cartilage).

concern with lesions of this type is that invasive squamous cell carcinoma which extends below the level of the vocal cord for more than 5 mm is very likely to invade the adjacent cricoid cartilage. For this reason, the condition has long been considered a contraindication for partial laryngectomy.

Resection of the upper portion of the posterior aspect of the cricoid cartilage is possible and is certainly essential if one is to achieve adequate tumor resection. When this has been attempted previously, there have been serious problems with persistent postoperative aspiration.

In the resection and reconstruction which these authors propose, the technique begins with a standard hemilaryngectomy, which is then combined with a resection of the upper portion of the cricoid cartilage as shown in Figure 13. The posterior one-third of the thyroid cartilage is separated from the superior and inferior cornua and is rotated into the cricoid defect that has been created. The thyroid cartilage graft is nourished by its inferior constrictor muscle pedicle, and serves to replace the cricoarytenoid complex so as to provide airway support and prevent postoperative aspiration.

Biller and Lawson [3] have reported their experience with the management of bulky transglottic lesions by means of a three-quarters extended vertical partial laryngectomy. They feel that this procedure is indicated when the following criteria are met:

1. a tumor 2 cm in diameter or less;
2. no evidence of vocal cord fixation;
3. absence of subglottic extension;
4. no involvement of the anterior commissure;
5. no evidence of cartilage invasion on CT scan;
6. no prior radiotherapy.

After adequate excision of these tumors, the posterior one-fourth of the ipsilateral thyroid ala is rotated and turned into position so that it bridges the gap from the cricoarytenoid area to the anterior commissure, thereby serving as a cushion for the opposite cord to meet. Their experience with five patients who were managed successfully is quite promising, and it is hoped that a conservative surgical procedure will prove to be adequate for this tumor which exhibits considerable biological agressiveness in many patients.

Extended vertical partial laryngectomy may be combined with a partial pharyngectomy and planned postoperative radiation therapy as described by Sessions [13]. He describes a patient in whom a horizontal subtotal supraglottic laryngectomy was combined with a vertical hemilaryngectomy and partial pharyngectomy. The patient underwent reconstruction utilizing a free sternocleidomastoid muscle graft and subsequently received 60 Gy of planned postoperative radiation therapy to the laryngopharynx in both sides of the neck.

His later course was complicated by atrophy of the reconstructed area, leading to aspiration pneumonia. The patient was subsequently reconstructed using a secondary cartilage implant to reconstitute the integrity of the glottis. The patient has done well since, with no evidence of recurrence. Further experience with this technique is required before its role in the standard management if this problem (T3NOMO laryngopharyngeal cancer) is firmly established, but the concept is quite intriguing.

More recently, near-total laryngectomy (as described by Pearson) has attracted widespread interest. This technique is not discussed in detail here, because it is felt to represent a different genre of surgical procedures. Respiratory function is sacrificed intentionally, in order to attempt to preserve better phonation and achieve a lower incidence of aspiration.

Surgical reconstruction after extended vertical partial laryngectomy

The term 'laryngoplasty' was coined by Pressman in 1954 [1]. It was a landmark concept in the field of laryngology, and it awakened laryngeal oncologic surgeons to the need to consider all appropriate steps that might be of value in restoring or preserving laryngeal function to a maximum degree. The bipedicle muscle flap that is utilizqed with the cartilage sparing vertical partial laryngectomy is one of several reconstructive techniques that have emerged during the past two decades.

Calcaterra [14] has noted that 'reconstruction of the larynx for vertical partial laryngectomy is of paramount importance in eventual voice and deglutition rehabilitation. Many different methods of laryngeal reconstruction have been tried, attesting to the challenge of minimizing hoarseness and aspiration after this type of surgery'. He reports on the use of a superiorly based sternohyoid myofascial flap to reconstruct the glottic defect after vertical partial laryngectomy. He has utilized this technique in 31 patients with good results over a 6-year

46

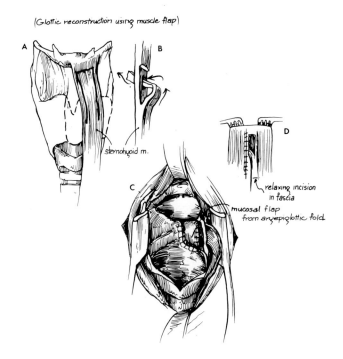

Figure 14. Inferiorly based sternohyoid muscle flap placed into the surgical defect and sutured to the cricoid cartilage posteriorly.

period and has noted that swallowing was resumed in all patients without significant aspiration. Decanulation was delayed in eight of the 31 patients, but they were eventually extubated.

Earlier, Sessions [15] and Hirano [16] reported their experience with the use of sternohyoid muscle flap to reconstitute the more extensive defect that follows extended vertical partial laryngectomy. Hirano employed a superiorly based flap, while Sessions prefers the inferiorly based flap as shown in Figure 14. These techniques are well within the capability of reconstructive surgeons, and they warrant consideration as a standard reconstructive step in patients who undergo hemilaryngectomy with sacrifice of the overlying thyroid cartilage.

Glottic reconstruction designed to enhance phonation and prevent aspiration has been proposed in a variety of other forms. These include the following:

1. the use of perichondrium and investing cervical fascia as proposed by Stegnja-jic [17];
2. utilization of the epiglottis to reconstruct large anterior glottic defects as proposed by Tucker *et al*. [18] and as illustrated in Figure 15;
3. utilization of composite nasal septal cartilage grafts as reported initially by Duncavage and Toohill, later by Laurian and Zohar, and recently summarized by Butcher and Dunham [19] and as illustrated in Figure 16.

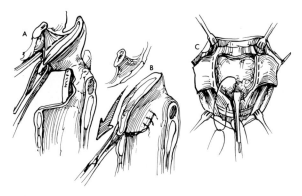

Figure 15. Laryngoplasty accomplished by mobilizing the epiglottis and displacing it inferiorly to reconstruct a large anterior glottic defect.

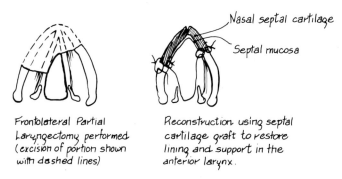

Frontolateral Partial
Laryngectomy performed
(excision of portion shown
with dashed lines)

Nasal septal cartilage

Septal mucosa

Reconstruction using septal
cartilage graft to restore
lining and support in the
anterior larynx.

Figure 16. Nasal mucoseptal graft to reconstruct the anterior one-half of the larynx following resection of anterior glottic stenosis.

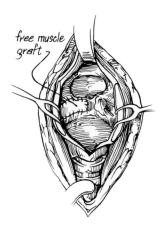

free muscle
graft

Figure 17. Free graft of the thyrohyoid muscle is sewn into the surgical defect after vertical partial laryngectomy.

48

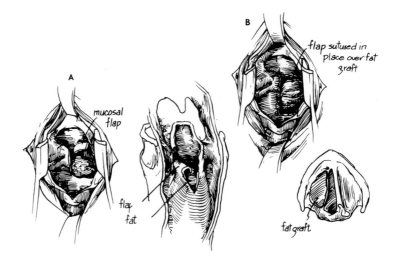

Figure 18. Free fat graft augmenting the glottic region after vertical partial laryngectomy.

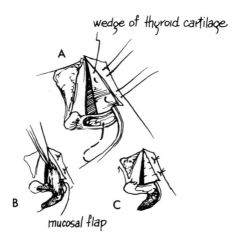

Figure 19. Creating a pseudocord by folding the superior portion of the thyroid cartilage medially to fill the defect after an extended supraglottic partial laryngectomy.

4. the use of free muscle graft as described by Quinn [1] and illustrated in Figure 17;
5. the use of a free fat graft as recommended by Dedo [1] and shown in Figure 18;
6. the cartilage fold-over operation as originally reported by Ogura and Dedo [1] and as illustrated in Figure 19.

When the anterior commissure technique of the vertical partial laryngectomy is used, there is sometimes a problem with postoperative web formation at the anterior commissure. A variation of the traditional McNaught keel is described

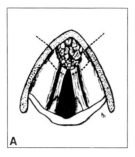 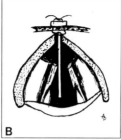

Figure 20. (A) Anterior commissure tumor with extent of resection outlined. (B) Silastic sheeting interposed between vocal cords and fixed with stitches through thyrohyoid and cricothyroid membranes, through skin and tied over buttons.

by Blitzer *et al.* [20] and shown in Figure 20. This adjunctive step is helpful in terms of prevention of the web, and it is easily removed by direct laryngoscopy during the early postoperative period.

The recurring theme that is noted throughout many of these reconstructive techniques, is that elaborate reconstruction steps are necessary in the event that there has been extensive local tissue removal, particularly when the arytenoid cartilage is excised. The concept of 'arytenoid unity' as described by Guerrier [2] must be understood by laryngeal surgeons. The integrity of arytenoid unity (proper form and function of the pharyngoepiglottic fold, the arytenoid, and the corresponding cord) must be reestablished. When the arytenoid unit is destroyed by surgery, aspiration is inevitable, and as Guerrier [2] points out, 'during deglutition, the base of the tongue and the arytenoid are everything, the epiglottis is nothing'. Careful attention to detail in regard to this one concept is probably the most important element of laryngeal reconstruction.

Results of surgical treatment

We have utilized vertical partial laryngectomy and extended vertical partial laryngectomy in the surgical management of 110 patients with glottic carcinoma during the past 23 years. The first 5 years of this experience involved patients at the University of California at Los Angeles and Harbor General Hospital (Torrance, California), and the past 18 years involved patients at the University of Texas Medical Branch in Galveston. Of this larger group of 110 patients, extended vertical partial laryngectomy was performed in 84 patients. Failure of radiation therapy for glottic carcinoma was the indication for surgery in 14 of these 84 patients. There was tumor invasion involving the anterior commissure and both cords in 71 patients, and superficial transglottic lesions were present in 13 patients. Most of the patients have been followed in excess of 10 years, and all of the subsequent data will pertain to the patients who have been followed for more than 3 years.

The overall cancer death rate is 7.2% (eight of 110 patients). The cause of death in this group was lung cancer in four patients, residual laryngeal cancer in three patients, and carcinoma of the liver in one patient. Seven of the 110 patients (6.3%) died of other causes. In this group there were five patients who died of cardiovascular disease and two patients who succumbed to respiratory disease. Death from cardiovascular disease is a predominant cause and probably reflects the pathology of the cardiovascular system that is often associated with the same etiological factor involved in the development of the glottic carcinoma – namely heavy smoking.

Vertical partial laryngectomy and extended vertical partial laryngectomy have been very effective in achieving local control. Laryngeal recurrence was observed in 11 of the 110 patients (10%). Of this group of 11 patients, four ultimately died of carcinoma (three larynx, one lung), two patients were succesfully salvaged by a second partial laryngectomy, and five patients were salvaged by total laryngectomy. Two patients developed cervical lymph node metastasis in association with their local laryngeal recurrence.

Postoperative morbidity consisted of transient aspiration (2 to 4 months in duration) in six patients. There were four patients who developed laryngeal stenosis, two patients with severe hoarseness (very breathy voice voice following vertical partial laryngectomy), and one patient early in the series who developed a serious local infection and who is also included among the patients with stenosis.

The present status of this patient group is that 90 patients are alive and well, with adequate voices and no evidence of disease. Five patients are alive without evidence of disease, with total laryngectomy being required for salvage. Most of the patients is this series have been followed for more than 10 years.

The experience with conservation laryngeal surgery for a 10-year period at the University of Michigan has been summarized in a recent article by Maceri *et al.* [21]. While this review does not analyze the patients with extended partial laryngectomy as a separate group, it does provide a helpful overview of the relationship of conservation laryngeal surgery to the total treatment picture. Between 1972 and 1982, 342 patients with glottic carcinoma were seen. Of this group, 82 were excluded because of poor follow-up or because their primary treatment was received elsewhere. This left a study group of 260 patients. Of this group, 110 patients presented with supraglottic carcinoma, and 33 of the 110 were managed by supraglottic partial laryngectomy. There were 150 of the 260 patients who presented with glottic carcinoma, and 21 vertical hemilaryngectomies were performed in this group. This provided total group of 54 patients who had undergone partial laryngectomy. Analysis of this group led to the following conclusions:

1. over 66% of the patients undergoing partial laryngectomy were ultimately decanulated;

2. completion laryngectomy was required in 21% of the patients in this group;
3. permanent tracheotomy was required for 30% of the patients undergoing supraglottic laryngectomy and 10% of the patients undergoing vertical hemilaryngectomy;
4. the ultimate vocal quality is independent of the type of conservation surgery utilized;
5. local control was not compromised by conservation surgery. The disease-free survival was equivalent for the partial laryngectomy group and a radiation therapy comparison group of similar patients;
6. persistant laryngeal edema requiring tracheotomy was associated with recurrent or with residual invasive carcinoma 60% of the time.

Extended vertical partial laryngectomy has been utilized in the management of T3 glottic carcinoma as reported in two major series. The first of these reports the experience of Ogura and his colleagues in St. Louis [5]. In this patient series, there were 18 patients who underwent hemilaryngectomy for T3 glottic carcinoma. This group experienced an 85% 5-year survival which probably represents the maximum curability for this lesion by any modality. It almost certainly reflects a very careful process of patient selection and excellent surgical technique.

In Europe, LeRoux-Robert [22] has been the primary proponent of extended vertical partial laryngectomy. He has been able to achieve an overall survival rate of 61% in the treatment of 127 patients with T3 (fixed cord) glottic carcinoma utilizing hemilaryngectomy. While this result is less dramatic than that reported by Lesinski, Bauer, and Ogura, the patient group is much larger, and the result is still better than that reported for total laryngectomy plus radiation therapy in many other series.

Mohr *et al.* [11] have utilized extended vertical partial laryngectomy in the treatment of 27 patients with T2 glottic carcinoma and five patients with T3 glottic carcinoma. In the patient group with T2 lesions, the 3 year adjusted survival rate was 100%; the 5 year rate was 94.1%; and the 10 year rate was 84.7%. The average survival in years was 5.48. The group of five patients with T3 lesions was followed for an average survival time of 8.4 years. One patient died of prostatic carcinoma, and the remaining four patients are alive and well without evidence of disease.

Biller and Lawson [3] utilized extended vertical partial laryngectomy for bulky transglottic carcinoma in a group of five patients whom were followed for 1 ½ to 2 ½ years. In this patient group, they achieved the following results:
1. four of five patients were able to swallow without aspiration;
2. all five patients were decannulated (two at 3 weeks, two at 5 months, and one at 9 months);
3. no recurrence of carcinoma had been observed at 1.5 to 2.5 years postoperatively.

Biller and Lawson [12] reported their experience with a group of five patients who underwent bilateral vertical hemilaryngectomy for extensive bilateral, invasive glottic carcinoma. These patients had a two-stage procedure consisting of wide local excision of the tumor and reconstruction as described previously in this chapter. The outcome in this group was quite favorable with regard to achieving a good airway, good glottic closure, and good vocal quality. One patient died of a pulmonary embolus, but the other four patients remained alive and well and free of disease for periods of 3, 6 (2 patients) and 7 years.

Tucker et al. [18] studied ten patients who underwent extended vertical partial laryngectomies for bilateral invasive glottic carcinomas. Many of these patients were left with only one arytenoid and the posterior commissure following the cancer resection. Utilization of the epiglottis to reconstitute the glottic complex resulted in the following outcome:

1. nine of the ten patients were decannulated within 17 days;
2. all patients were able to be fed orally at periods ranging from 1 to 18 days;
3. all but one patient was discharged within 23 days postoperatively (one patient developed aspiration pneumonia with delayed decannulation and was discharged from the hospital at 9 weeks);
4. no recurrence was observed in this patient group at follow-up ranging up to 23 months.

Biller and Som [6] described their experience in the surgical management of five patients with posterior subglottic extension. These patients would formerly have been considered to be inoperable in terms of extended vertical partial laryngectomy because of the need to resect the cricoid cartilage. The reconstruction employed in this report has been described previously in this chapter. The outcome results in these five patients are as follows:

1. deglutition was adequate at 14 days in all five patients, and there were no problems with long term aspiration;
2. four of the five patients were decannulated at 2 weeks, (3 patients) and 20 weeks (1 patient);
3. one patient developed recurrent carcinoma, but the remaining four patients were free of tumor at 2 years (1 patient), 4 years (2 patients), and 5 years (1 patient).

Extended supraglottic laryngectomy

The supraglottic laryngectomy procedure is a conservation laryngeal procedure that is now widely used with a high success rate in well selected patients. However, if cancer has spread beyond the limits of resection for this operation, a wide field total laryngectomy or an extended supraglottic laryngectomy is necessary for cure. Different techniques of the extended supraglottic laryngectomy are used when cancer involves areas such as an arytenoid, a piriform sinus, or the base of tongue. Knowledge of the regional anatomy will facilitate understanding these surgical procedures, and it is briefly reviewed here.

Anatomically, the border between the glottic and supraglottic regions of the larynx is the superior arcuate line where squamous epithelium meets respiratory epithelium. Clinically, an imaginary horizontal plane passing through the laryngeal ventricles divides these regions. The superior surfaces of the true cords form the floors of the ventricles and are in the glottic region. The undersurfaces of the false cords form the roofs of the ventricles and are in the supraglottic region. The supraglottic region of the larynx is subdivided into sites. These include false vocal cords, aryepiglottic folds, infrahyoid epiglottis, and arytenoids.

Another area of the supraglottis, the preepiglottic space, is a particularly important avenue for cancer spread. It is bordered anteriorly by the thyrohyoid membrane and upper portion of the thyroid cartilage, posteriorly by the epiglottis and quadrangular membrane, and superiorly by hyoepiglottic ligament. The space is filled predominately with adipose tissue and lymphatics and communicates posterolaterally with the paraglottic spaces. This area must be completely resected when excising supraglottic carcinomas, because natural dehiscences in the epiglottic cartilage at the petiole allow invasion in a high percentage of cases [23–25].

Indications and contraindications

The standard supraglottic laryngectomy is indicated for patients with supraglottic carcinomas confined to the supraglottic region of the larynx. A medical contraindication is pulmonary disease that causes the patient's forced expiratory volume in 1 s to be less than 60% of predicted value. Pulmonary function tests are essential for any patient who is a candidate for this operation or its extended version. Other contraindications include tumor involvement of the anterior or posterior commissure, both arytenoids, thyroid cartilage, floor or laryngeal ventricles, or glottis. True vocal cord fixation or impaired mobility is also a contraindication. When cancer spreads to the base of tongue, piriform sinus, or one arytenoid, an extended supraglottic laryngectomy can sometimes be performed. However, pririform sinus involvement cannot extend inferiorly to the apex because this is at the level of the glottis. Base of tongue involvement should not extend beyond a line 1 cm posterior to the circumvallate papillae. If it does, special techniques are necessary to suspend the larynx as described by Hillel and Goode [26] or to reconstruct the base of tongue defect.

Surgical techniques

An appreciation of the basic concepts of the standard supraglottic laryngectomy is necessary to understand the extended versions of this procedure (Figure 21). The standard supraglottic laryngectomy is begun by elevating the external perichondrium away from the superior half of both thyroid alae. Following this, a

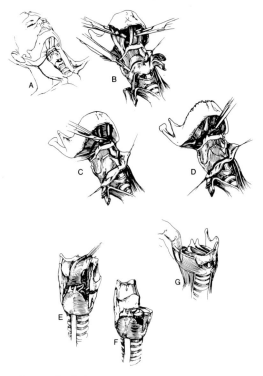

Figure 21. Technique of supraglottic laryngectomy.

horizontal cut is made through the thyroid cartilage at a level midway between the thyroid notch and inferior border of the thyroid cartilage in the midline. The pharynx is entered either through the vallecula above the hyoid bone or through one of the piriform sinuses, depending upon where the primary tumor is located. The principles are to enter the pharynx through a 'safe' area away from the primary tumor and to visualize it well initially. The opening into the vallecula is widened, and incisions are carried down both lateral pharyngeal walls to the base of the piriform sinuses. The epiglottis is then grasped with a tenaculum, and the larynx is pulled upward so that the primary tumor and supraglottic structures can be seen through the pharyngotomy. The incision is extended down each aryepi-glottic fold just anterior to the arytenoids. With one blade of the scissors placed in the laryngeal ventricle and the other in the piriform sinus of the same side, this incision is continued through the ventricle and the overlying cartilage incision toward the anterior commissure. This is done on both sides, and the specimen is removed. Before closure of the defect, frozen section biopsies are taken from several areas to insure that margins close to the tumor are negative for malignancy. These areas usually include the piriform sinuses, the laryngeal ventricles, and the area just above the anterior commissure. When a frozen section diagnosis is

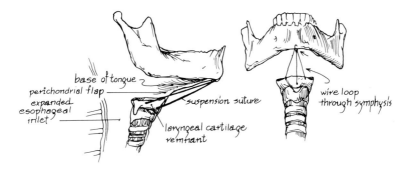

Figure 22. Suturing the laryngeal remnant to the mandible so that the postoperative glottic position will be placed as far superiorly and anteriorly as possible.

positive for malignancy, further excisions are performed until a negative report is obtained.

After tumor resection, meticulous reconstruction enhances a smooth postoperative course. The incisions down through the aryepiglottic folds leave denuded soft tissue and sometimes leave exposed arytenoid cartilage. Mucosal coverage of these areas is necessary to avoid fibrosis and possible supraglottic stenosis. Two or three chromic catgut sutures are used to reapproximate the mucosal edges. Care should be taken to avoid closing these areas too tightly, because this will tether the vocal cords. Closure of the pharyngotomy is accomplished by suturing the previously dissected perichondrium to the base of tongue and closing the lateral pharyngeal wall defects. Sutures that approximate the perichondrium to the base of tongue should pass through the tongue musculature approximately one centimeter away from the cut mucosal edge of the base of the tongue. This allows the base of tongue to act as a shelf over the glottis and keeps food from funneling directly into the glottis.

Extended supraglottic laryngectomy

When a supraglottic carcinoma extends into the base of tongue, the standard supraglottic laryngectomy can be extended to include this area. However, if greater than half of the base of tongue requires resection, special techniques are necessary for reconstruction. Regional myocutaneous flaps can be rotated into the defect, but these are adynamic and often too bulky, resulting in dysphagia with or without aspiration. An anterior tongue setback flap can also be performed to replace the resected portion of the tongue base. This may be more physiologic than a myocutaneous flap, but has been described for use after carcinoma resection of the base of the tongue without laryngectomy rather than for supraglottic carcinoma that invades the base of the tongue [27]. Another option is suspension of the larynx from the mandible. The objective of the procedure is

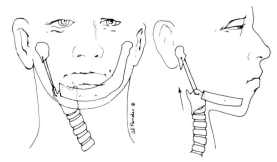

Figure 23. Frontal and lateral views showing the location of the laterally suspended larynx and the final placement of the suspension sutures (From Hillel, A.D., Goode, R.L. [26].).

to bring the glottis up to a more superior and anterior position, allowing food to pass lateral and posterior to it (Figure 22). Permanent suspension wires or sutures are passed through drill holes in the remaining thyroid alae. The larynx is suspended from the anterior mental area of the mandible [28], or if resection has largely been one side of the base of tongue and pharynx [26], the larynx is suspended from the ipsilateral mandibular condyle (Figure 23).

Supraglottic carcinomas that cross the laryngeal ventricles to involve at least one true vocal cord are by definition transglottic lesions. If the vocal cord is fixed, a total laryngectomy should be done. However, without fixation several techniques have been described for resecting the involved glottis with the supraglottic structures and maintaining glottic competence. Biller and Lawson [3] describe a technique for transglottic carcinomas in which the specimen includes epiglottis, false vocal cords, one true cord, an arytenoid, the adjacent cartilage, the subglottis to the lower border of the thyroid cartilage, and the paraglottic space to the medial aspect of the piriform sinus. The glottis is reconstructed by mobilizing the remaining posterior part of the thyroid lamina on the ipsilateral side, wiring it to the anterior commissure anteriorly and the midcricoid posteriorly, and covering this with piriform sinus mucosa.

Occasionally, supraglottic carcinoma involves the anterior face of one arytenoid but does not extend to the glottic region. Provided clear margins can be ontained, the involved arytenoid can be removed with the supraglottic specimen. In this case, the vocal process is left attached to the true vocal cord, and glottic competence is restored by suturing the vocal process posteriorly to the cricoid cartilage in the midline.

When a supraglottic carcinoma spreads outside the larynx to a piriform fossa, partial pharyngectomy can sometimes be performed in conjunction with supraglottic laryngectomy. However, this puts the patient at increased risk for dysphagia and aspiration. Involvement should be limited to the base of the piriform sinus. Since the apex is at the level of the glottis, extension here would require removal of the ipsilateral vocal cord. Near-total laryngectomy has recently been described for fixed cord glottic carcinomas [29]. This operation may also be used for

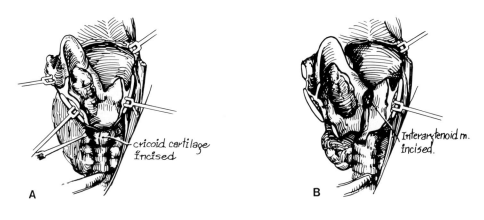

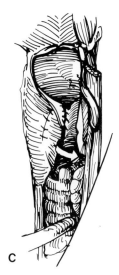

Figure 24. (A) The tumor is visible, obliterating the right vocal cord, ventricle, and false cord. The laryngeal incision continues down through the cricoid and swings around through the right upper trachea, deep to the thyroid gland. (B) The interarytenoid muscle is cut in the midline. (C) The myomucosal laryngeal remnant is tubed on itself. Note the flap from the pharynx, which is necessary to augment the tube when laryngeal mucosa in insufficient.

infrahyoid supraglottic carcinomas that involve the glottis or for transglottic lesions that extend to the piriform sinus (Figure 24A, B, C).

Whether by standard supraglottic laryngectomy or an extended version, cancer of the supraglottic latynx is curable with conservation laryngeal surgery. In a review of 260 cases of supraglottic cancer treated between 1971 and 1980, DeSanto concluded that surgery alone for this disease compared favorably to combined surgery and radiotherapy or radical radiation and surgical salvage. He found only a 2% local recurrence rate among the 98 patients treated by supraglottic laryngectomy [30].

Conclusion

The history of extended vertical partial laryngectomy is rich in terms of innovation and creativity. The examples we have described in this chapter are but a few of the many contributions that have been made to this field and which have served to improve the quality of surgical care and increase the options available to patients with laryngeal cancer. The field has reached a point in its evolution where it deserves support in terms of research funding for randomized prospective studies designed to assess the relative merits of the many different surgical procedures. This type of information would be of great value in clarifying the correlation between surgical techniques and functional outcome.

The ability to control advanced laryngeal cancer by means of conservation surgical techniques has been clearly established over the past two decades. The future of conservation laryngeal surgery appears bright, but we inevitably return to three fundamental conclusions when we assess the progress in this field:

1. surgeons who choose to perform conservation laryngeal surgery must follow all of the rules in regard to patient selection. This involves a very careful analysis of the patient's general health, laryngeal neoplasm, and psychological make-up;
2. the surgeon must individualize the treatment for each patient. Minor variations in tumor site may create major differences in the treatment outcome. Further, while some patients will accept readily the challenges of learning new strategies for speech and swallowing, others will not;
3. the surgeon must understand completely that case selection is the key to success in conservation surgery of the larynx. One must avoid the temptation to fit patients into a mold that you 'wish' were right for them.

Careful attention to the details of this type of surgery will bring great rewards to patients and physicians in terms of successful management of glottic carcinoma.

References

1 Bailey, B.J. 1985. Glottic carcinoma. In: Surgery of the larynx (B.J. Bailey, H.F. Biller, eds.).15 W.B. Saunders Company, Philadelphia.
2. Guerrier, Y. 1979. Difficult indications for partial laryngectomy. O.R.L. 41: 262–272.
3. Biller, H.F., Lawson, W. 1984. Partial laryngectomy for transglottic cancers. Ann. Otol. Rhinol. Laryngol. 93: 297–300.
4. Stell, P.M., Dalby, J.E., Singh, S.D., Ramadan, M.F., Bainton, R. 1982. The management of glottic T3 carcinoma. Clin. Otolaryngol. 7: 175–180.
5. Lesinski, S.G., Bauer, W.C., Ogura, J.H. 1976. Hemilaryngectomy for T3 (fixed cord) epidermoid carcinoma of larynx. Laryngoscope 86: 1563.
6. Biller, H.F., Som, M.L. 1977. Vertical partial laryngectomy for glottic carcinoma with posterior subglottic extension. Ann. Otol. Rhinol. Laryngol. 86: 715–718.

7. Burns, H., Bryce, D.P., Van Nostrand, A.W.P. 1979. Conservation surgery in laryngeal cancer and its role following failed radiotherapy. Arch. Otolaryngeol. 105: 234–239.

8. Cantrell, R.W., Reibel, J.F., Jahrsdoerfer, R.A., Johns, M.E.. 1980. Conservative surgical treatment of chondrosarcoma of the larynx. Ann. Otol. Rhinol. Laryngol. 89: 567–571.

9. Dumich, P.S., Pearson, B.W., Weiland, L.H.. 1984. Suitability of near-total laryngopharyngectomy in piriform carcinoma. Arch. Otolaryngol. 110: 664–669.

10. Friedman, M., Shelton, V.K., Skolnik, E.M., Berlinger, F.G., Arab, M. 1982. Laryngotracheal invasion by thyroid carcinoma. Ann. Otol. Rhinol. Laryngol. 91: 363–369.

11. Mohr, R.M., Quenelle, D.J., Shumrich, D.A. 1983. Verticofrontolateral laryngectomy (hemilaryngectomy). Arch. Otolaryngol. 109: 384–395.

12. Biller, H.F., Lawson, W., 1981. Bilateral vertical partial laryngectomy for bilateral vocal cord carcinoma. Ann. Otol. Rhinol. Laryngol. 90: 489–491.

13. Sessions, D.G. 1980. Extended partial laryngectomy. Ann. Otol. Rhinol. Laryngol. 89: 556–557.

14. Calcaterra, T.C. 1983. Sternohyoid myofascial flap reconstruction of the larynx for vertical partial laryngectomy. Laryngoscope 93: 422–424.

15. Bailey, B.J. 1985. Glottic reconstruction. In: Surgery of the larynx (B.J. Bailey, H.F. Biller, eds.). W.B. Saunders Company, Philadelphia.

16. Hirano, M. 1976. Technique for glottic reconstruction following vertical partial laryngectomy: a preliminary report. Ann. Otol. Rhinol. Laryngol. 85: 25–31.

17. Stegnjajic, A.,Wenig, B.L., Guberina, L., Abramson, A.L. 1985. Glottic reconstruction with thyroid perichondrium and investing cervical fascia. Arch. Otolaryngol. 111: 462–475.

18. Tucker, H.M., Wood, B.G., Levine, H., Katz, R. 1979. Glottic reconstruction after near total laryngectomy. Laryngoscope 89: 609–618.

19. Butcher, R.B., Dunham, M. 1984. Composite nasal septal cartilage graft for reconstruction after extended frontolateral hemilaryngectomy. Laryngoscope 94: 959–962.

20. Blitzer, A., Pang, M., Som, M, Cho, H.1980. Modification of the anterior commissure technique of partial laryngectomy. Arch. Otolaryngol. 106: 503–504.

21. Maceri, D.R., Lampe, H.B., Makielski, K.H., Passamani, P.P., Krause, C.J. 1985. Conservation laryngeal surgery: a critical analysis. Arch. Otolaryngol. 111: 361–365.

22. LeRoux, R.J. 1975. Panel discussion on glottic tumours. IV. A statistical study of 620 laryngeal carcinomas of the glottic region personally operated upon more than 5 years ago. Laryngoscope 85: 1440.

23. Kirchner, J.A. 1969. One hundred laryngeal cancers studied by serial sections. Ann. Otol. Rhinol. Laryngol. 78: 497–505.

24. Olofsson, J. 1976. Growth and spread of laryngeal carcinoma. In: Workshops from the Centennial Conference on Laryngeal Cancer (P.W. Alberti, D.P. Bryce, eds.). Appleton-Century-Crofts, New York.

25. Olofsson, J., Van Nostrand, A.W.P. 1973. Growth and spread of laryngeal and hypopharyngeal carcinoma with reflections on the effect of preoperative irradiation: 139 Cases studied by whole organ serial sectioning. Acta Otolaryngol. (Suppl.), 308.

26. Hillel, A.D., Goode, R.L. 1983. Lateral laryngeal suspension. Laryngoscope 93: 26–31.

27. Schechter, G.L., Sly, D.E., Roper II, A.L., Jackson, R.T., Bumatay, J. 1980. Set-back tongue flap for carcinoma of the tongue base. Arch. Otolaryngol. 106: 668–671.

28. Calcaterra, T. 1976. Laryngeal suspension after supraglottic laryngectomy. Arch. Otolaryngol. 102: 716.

29. Pearson, B.W. 1985. The theory and technique of near-total laryngectomy. In: Surgery of the larynx (B.J. Bailey, H.F. Biller, eds.). W.B. Saunders Company, Philadelphia.

30. DeSanto, L.W. 1985. Cancer of the supraglottic larynx: A review of 260 patients. Otolaryngol. Head Neck Surg. 93 (6): 705–711.

5. Laser surgery for head and neck cancer

ROBERT H. OSSOFF and ROBERT F. NEMEROFF

Introduction

Laser is an acronym that means light amplification by the stimulated emission of radiation. A laser is an electro-optical device that is usually a gas or crystal. The atoms of this lasing medium typically exist in nature at several different energy levels across the electromagnetic spectrum. When these atoms are stimulated by an extrinsic energy source, they will emit electromagnetic radiation oar photons in a narrow, intense beam. The light emitted from a laser, then, is organized light in direct contrast to the random pattern light that is emitted from the common light bulb. The key to this organization is stimulated emission.

The first laser, a pulsed ruby laser, was discovered by Maiman in 1960 [1]; this laser had a wavelength of 0.69 µm and emitted light in short pulses lasting only 1 ms or less. Soon after Maiman's discovery, the output power of the ruby laser was increased, and the neodymium (Nd)-in-glass laser was developed [2].

Preliminary work with these two lasers stimulated interest in the field of medical research regarding the possible application of laser energy to treat and cure cancer. Investigators began to use both of these lasers on various tumor lines implanted in experimental animals, and it was quickly determined that the entire tumor had to be destroyed if a cure was to be achieved. This was relatively difficult with the low powered ruby and Nd-in-glass lasers because of the low absorption of these wavelengths in nonpigmented biologic tissue. To facilitate tumor destruction, therefore, researchers began to use higher and higher power densities of these two pulsed lasers. Mechanical tissue disruption occured at these higher power densities, causing viable cancer cells to be propelled into the laboratory environment as well as elsewhere in the animal [3]. Needless to say, these findings had a significantly negative effect on the use of lasers in cancer research. However, the concept of differential absorption of laser light by biologic tissue was learned from these early experiments, and this concept stimulated research and development of other lasers.

Interest in the carbon dioxide laser was stimulated by Yahr and Strully when

C. Jacobs (ed) Cancers of the head and neck.
© *1987, Martinus Nijhoff Publishers, Boston. ISBN 0–89838–825–2. Printed in the Netherlands.*

they discovered that they could make a fine incision in skin and also perform a partial liver resection with minimal blood loss utilizing this laser [4]. Encouraged by these findings, researchers in the laboratories of the American Optical Corporation developed a carbon dioxide laser system for surgical research [5]. Between 1967 and 1972, numerous concurrent investigations were undertaken in the various surgical specialities utilizing this laser.

Interest in using this laser for laryngeal surgery began in 1967 when Jako discovered that he could produce discrete lesions in a cadaver larynx with the focused beam of a carbon dioxide laser. Development of an endoscopic attachment and micromanipulator by Bredemeier [6] allowed this laser to be utilized with the operating microscope for laryngeal surgery. Jako [7] utilized this micromanipulator attachment with the microscope to study vocal cord surgery with the laser in the canine model. He demonstrated that the depth and extent of tissue removal could be precisely controlled with the carbon dioxide laser and that tissue excision was bloodless and healing was uneventful. Jako concluded his research in 1970 suggesting that 'vocal cord surgery with the carbon dioxide laser was ready for clinical trials'.

In 1971, Strong and Jako began using the carbon dioxide laser in laryngeal surgery; they presented their first fourteen cases treated with this laser at the 1972 annual meeting of the American Broncho-Esophagological Association [8]. Two years later, Strong reported on 15 patients with tracheobronchial disease treated 70 times with the bronchoscopic attachment to the carbon dioxide laser [9]. At the Centennial Conference on Laryngeal Cancer held in Toronto, Canada in May 1974, Strong reported for the first time on the use of the carbon dioxide laser in the treatment of patients with selected early cancers of the glottic larynx [10].

This pioneering report helped to establish the carbon dioxide laser as a therapeutic instrument in the curative treatment of early squamous cell cancers of the head and neck. Other lasers have now found a place in the surgical armamentarium for treating patients with malignant neoplasms of the upper aerodigestive tract, either therapeutically or palliatively. This article will describe the currently accepted role of the carbon dioxide laser in the therapeutic management of squamous cell carcinoma of the upper aerodigestive tract. Additionally, the role of the Neodymium: Yttrium Aluminum Garnet (Nd: YAG) laser in the palliation of patients with tracheobronchial airway obstruction and the argon pumped tunable dye laser used for photodynamic therapy (PDT) in the management of patients with early, superficial squamous cell carcinoma of the upper aerodigestive tract will be briefly discussed.

Carbon dioxide laser

Carbon dioxide lasers produce light with a wavelength of 10.6 µm in the invisible range of the electromagnetic spectrum. A second, built-in, coaxial helium neon laser is necessary to indicate with its red color the site where the invisible CO_2 laser beam will impact the target tissue. This laser, then, acts as an aiming beam for the invisible carbon dioxide laser beam. The radiant energy produced by the carbon dioxide laser is strongly absorbed by pure, homogeneous water and by all biological soft tissues. The extinction length of this wavelength is 0.03 mm in water and in soft tissue; reflection and scattering are negligible. Because absorption of the radiant energy produced by the CO_2 laser is independent of tissue color, and because the thermal effects produced by this wavelength on adjacent nontarget tissues are minimal, the carbon dioxide laser has become extremely versatile for use in otolaryngology-head and neck surgery.

With current technology, light from this laser cannot be transmitted through existing flexible fiberoptic endoscopes, although research and development of a suitable flexible fiber for transmission of this wavelength is being carried out on an international level. Presently, the radiant energy of this laser is transmitted from the optical resonating chamber to the target tissue via a series of mirrors through an articulating arm to the target tissue. This laser can be used free-hand for macroscopic surgery, attached to the operating microscope for microscopic surgery, and adapted to an endoscopic coupler for bronchoscopic surgery [11]; in this application, rigid, nonfiberoptic bronchoscopes must be used [12].

Larynx

Endoscopic management of squamous cell carcinoma of the glottic larynx is not a new concept. Lynch [13] reported on 39 patients with early glottic cancers managed by transoral excision in 1920. New and Dorton [14] in 1941 reported a 90% cure rate in ten patients managed with transoral excision and diathermy. Lillie and DeSanto [15] reported on 98 patients with early glottic carcinoma who were treated with transoral excision in 1973; all were cures, although five of these patients required further treatment.

The transoral excision of squamous cell carcinoma of the larynx utilizing the carbon dioxide laser is, therefore, an obvious extension of the application of this surgical instrument. The advantages of precision, hemostasis and decreased post-operative edema allow the laryngologist to perform exquisitely accurate and relatively bloodless endoscopic surgery of the larynx.

Three distinct roles exist for the use of the carbon dioxide laser in the management of patients with early squamous cell carcinomas of the glottis. First, with the laser it is possible to excise bulky tumors located on the anterior commissure or vocal fold; this aids in obtaining an accurate assessment of the size and depth of invasion of the tumor for purposes of staging and treatment. Additionally, previously biopsied tumors of the vocal cord may represent a diagnostic problem with respect to their extent. Here the laser may be used to excise the area surrounding the biopsy site. Inexact staging following direct laryngoscopy is fairly common.

T_1 glottic carcinoma represents a family of early cancers confined to one or both vocal cords. The extent of disease can be variable but requires vocal cord mobility as determined by indirect or direct examination. This implies that the tumor is confined to the surface epithelium and has not deeply invaded the vocalis muscle. However, deep invasion of the vocalis muscle has been found after excisional biopsy with the carbon dioxide laser in patients who were staged T_1 by indirect exam [16]. Therefore, excisional biopsy with the laser allows the surgeon to differentiate those early glottic lesions which are superficial from those which have deeply invaded the vocalis muscle.

Airway reestablishment is the second role of the carbon dioxide laser in the management of patients with squamous cell carcinoma of the larynx. Here, the laser can be used to reduce the amount of tumor obstructing the airway, thereby avoiding the need for a preoperative tracheotomy [17].

Endoscopic laser excision of early laryngeal squamous cell carcinoma confined to the true vocal cords may be curative. This represents the third role of the carbon dioxide laser in the management of patients with carcinoma of the larynx. Reports by Blakeslee [18] and Koufman [19] support the previous nonlaser series of Lillie and De Santo, New and Dorton, and Lynch, and a recent paper by Ossoff *et al.* [20] demonstrates the efficacy (96% 3-year absolute survival rate) of endoscopic excisional biopsy of early glottic carcinoma with this laser.

Our current treatment plan for the management of patients with early cancers confined to the true vocal cords includes an excisional biopsy with the carbon dioxide laser. Supravital staining with toluidine blue is performed as a diagnostic aid prior to biopsy. The surgical specimen is labeled and oriented prior to being sent for frozen section examination. Any questionable margins are controlled by frozen section to the limits of endoscopic cordectomy [21]. If the tumor is found to be histologically a T_3 or T_4, the patient is later treated by traditional surgical techniques (partial or total laryngectomy) or by external beam radiation therapy.

Treatment of selected, early glottic carcinomas can be approached with optimism because of several factors. First, true vocal cord cancers cause early symptoms and are relatively easy to diagnose. Second, they are the most common of laryngeal carcinomas, making up about 70% in one series [22]. Third, at the level of the glottic larynx, early midcordal cancers are limited to the confines of the laryngeal framework, and the lymphatic system is not readily invaded. Fewer than 1% of patients with T_1 glottic carcinomas present with cervical metastasis [23]. Fourth, therapeutic expertise in the management of these early glottic cancers is highly developed, and about 90% of patients with this disease will recuperate regardless of the treatment modality used. Therefore, considerations other than cure rate should be thought of when planning the initial treatment of these patients with T_1 glottic carcinomas. Factors worthy of consideration include the quality of posttreatment voice, the cost of treatment, the time lost by the patient during treatment, and the anticipated posttreatment morbidity, if any.

Advantages associated with the endoscopic management of patients with early laryngeal cancer include accuracy associated with the use of the operating microscope, minimal morbidity associated with the characteristic tissue interaction of the carbon dioxide laser and the laryngeal soft tissues, and cost-effectiveness. Because the diagnosis and therapeutic management of these early laryngeal cancers can be performed on an ambulatory (outpatient) basis at the same time when the carbon dioxide laser is utilized, this advantage will most probably cause more head and neck surgeons to treat these early glottic cancers endoscopically with the laser.

Two questions must be answered, however. First, which treatment option (endoscopic laser excision or external beam radiation therapy) yields better posttreatment voice quality, both short- and long-term? Second, which treatment option is associated with less posttreatment morbidity? The author has recently been funded by the National Cancer Institute to conduct a randomized, prospective study over the next five years to attempt to answer these questions. Hopefully, at that time the answers to these two questions will have emerged and the controversies surrounding the use of the carbon dioxide laser for the management of patients with selected, early glottic carcinomas will be put to rest.

Oral cavity

The indications for transoral resection of squamous cell carcinoma of the oral cavity are limited to superficial lesions up to 4 cm in diameter (T_2) anterior to the faucial arch. Sites that can be safely resected include the floor of the mouth, tongue, buccal mucosa, gingiva, gingivobuccal sulcus and the soft palate. Periosteum may be stripped off of mandible or hard palate, but bone should not be resected transorally.

Only those lesions that are superficial should be attempted by transoral resection with the laser. Resection of deep or moderately deep lesions is contraindicated using this technique. Additional contraindications include lesions of the retromolar trigone, lesions with cervical metastases, patients with trismus (indicates deep invasion), patients with mandibular or maxillary involvement, recurrences after radiation therapy, and patients where exposure is poor because of lesion location or general inaccessibility.

Transoral management of superficial cancers of the oral cavity involves excision of the lesion and frozen section control. Supravital staining with toluidine blue is performed in a manner similar to that for glottic lesions. Specimens should be sent to pathology labeled and oriented on a specimen mount. Although transoral resection of oral cavity squamous cell carcinomas can be performed free-hand with the laser hand-piece, use of the operating microscope provides excellent illumination and magnification and more control of the actual excision.

Strong [24] reported 57 cases of primary squamous cell carcinoma of the oral cavity excised transorally with the carbon dioxide laser in 1979. There were no significant postoperative complications described in this series. Twenty-one of these patients were followed for 30 months with two dead of local disease, two dead of cervical metastasis, and one dead of a myocardial infarction.

The advantages of the transoral excision of squamous cell carcinoma of the oral cavity with the carbon dioxide laser inclue precise dissection with microscopic control, frozen section control of margins, decreased blood loss, minimal postoperative pain, decreased morbidity, and reduced hospitalization time. Because of this latter advantage, this technique will probably be utilized more frequently in the future for properly selected lesions.

Nd:YAG laser

Nd:YAG lasers produce light with a wavelength of 1.060 μm in the invisible range of the electromagnetic spectrum. The radiant energy of the ND:YAG laser is weakly absorbed by pure water in which the extinction length is 60 mm. Therefore, its radiant energy can be transmitted through clear liquids facilitating its use in the eye or other water filled cavities such as the urinary bladder. The absorption of light from this laser is slightly color dependent with increased absorption in darkly pigmented tissues and carbonaceous debris. In biological tissue, strong scattering, both forward and backward, determines the effective extinction length which is usually 2 to 4 mm. Back scattering can account for up to 40% of the total amount of scattering. The zone of damage produced by the incident beam of a Nd:YAG laser produces a homogeneous zone of thermal coagulation and necrosis which may extend up to 4 mm deep and lateral from the surface, making precise control impossible.

This laser is an excellent surgical instrument with which to perform tissue coagulation; vaporization and incision can also be performed with this wavelength. When utilized for these two functions, however, precision is lacking, and tissue damage is unpredictable.

The radiant energy from the Nd:YAG laser can be transmitted through flexible fiberoptic delivery systems allowing its use with flexible endoscopes. When utilized in the management of patients with obstructing neoplasms of the tracheobronchial tree, it is considered safer to employ a rigid, ventilating bronchoscope, rather than a flexible fiberoptic bronchoscope [25]. With this approach, the laser fiber is passed down the lumen of the rigid bronchoscope with a rod lens telescope and suction catheter [26]. Control of hemorrhage has been reported to be more secure with the Nd:YAG laser because of its deeper penetration and scattering effect in soft tissue [27]. Because hemorrhage is the most dangerous complication

associated with laser bronchoscopy, the ability to control it is extremely important. Therefore, we now favor the Nd:YAG laser to treat vascular lesions such
as obstructing carcinoma of the tracheobronchial tree.

Otolaryngologists may begin to use this laser in conjunction with the carbon
dioxide laser when performing bronchoscopic laser surgery. Here, the effective
coagulating properties of the Nd:YAG laser have been shown in our laboratory
research to augment the predictable vaporizing properties of the carbon dioxide
laser. Less soft tissue manipulation and shorter operative times may result from
such a combined wavelength approach to bronchoscopic laser surgery.

Argon tunable dye laser system

The argon tunable dye laser system works on the principle of the argon laser
making a high intensity beam which is focused on dye that is continuously
circulating in a second laser optically coupled to the argon laser. The argon laser
beam energizes the dye, causing it to emit laser energy. By varying the type of
dye and using a tuning system, different desired wavelengths can be obtained. The
laser energy from this dye laser can then be transmitted through flexible fiberop-
tics and delivered through endoscopic systems or inserted directly into tumors.
The major clinical use of this laser at the present time is in conjunction with
selective photodynamic therapy of malignant tumors following the intravenous
injection of the photosensitizer, hematoporphyrin derivative [28].

After the intravenous injection, the hematoporphyrin derivative disseminates
to all the cells of the body, rapidly moving out of normal tissue, but remaining
longer in neoplastic tissue. After a few days, there is a differential in concentration
between the tumor cells and the normal cells. When the tumor is exposed to red
light (630 μm), the dye absorbs the light; the absorption of this red light causes
a photochemical reaction to occur. Toxic oxygen radicals such as singlet oxygen
are produced within the exposed cells causing selective tissue destruction and
cellular death. Since there is less photosensitizer in the normal tissues, a much
less severe or no reaction occurs. The main technical problem is getting enough
light to the target area. The argon tunable dye laser system has helped to solve
this problem [29].

From the results obtained by many investigators in this country, it is obvious
that the premise of treating selected neoplasms with hematoporphyrin derivative
followed by activation with red light is valid [30–32]. The overall potential and
exact place of maximum value of this form of treatment remains to be established.
Areas that appear to be very promising include carcinoma of the urinary bladder [33], endobronchial lesions of the lung [34], selected carcinomas of the upper
aerodigestive tract [35], skin cancers [36], and metastatic dermal breast cancers [37]. The potential for this compound to serve as a tumor marker in sites
where multicentric tumors are common, such as the mucosal surfaces lining the

upper aerodigestive tract, has been recently discussed [38]. The Department of Otolaryngology at Vanderbilt University Medical Center and the Department of Otolaryngology-Head and Neck Surgery at Northwestern University Medical School are two of ten centers in the United States currently involved in a randomized clinical trial studying the efficacy of dihematoporphyrin ether (Photofrin^{TM} II) in the management of patients with selected, superficial mucosal carcinomas of the upper aerodigestive tract. The control arm in this investigation calls for excision of the carcinoma with the carbon dioxide laser.

Conclusions

The carbon dioxide laser has established itself as a therapeutic instrument in the management of selected squamous cell carcinomas of the head and neck. Cure rates with this instrument parallel those obtained with traditional surgical instruments or external beam radiation therapy for selected lesions of the glottic larynx and oral cavity. There is a definite learning curve associated with the use of the carbon dioxide laser; therefore, surgeons not familiar with its use should attend a hands-on training course prior to beginning the most simple procedures on human subjects. Because of the cost-effectiveness associated with the transoral excision of laryngeal and oral cavity cancers with the carbon dioxide laser, it is expected that the management of appropriate lesions with this laser will increase over the next few years. Laser excision of obstructing neoplasms of the tracheobronchial tree has a place in the palliative management of patients with lung cancer. The role of photodynamic therapy in the management of patients with selected, superficial mucosal carcinomas is currently being assessed.

References

1. Maiman, T.H. 1960. Stimulated optical radiation in ruby. Nature 187: 493–494.
2. Snitzer, E. 1961. Optical maser action of $Nd^{3}+$ in Ba crown glass. Phys. Rev. Lett. 7: 444.
3. Ketcham, A.S., Hoye, R.C., Riggle, G.C. 1964. A surgeon's appraisal of the laser. Surg. Clin. North Am. 47: 1249–1263.
4. Yahr, W.Z., Strully, K.J. 1966. Blood vessel anastomosis and other biomedical applications. J. Assoc. Adv. Med. Instr. 1: 28–31.
5. Polanyi, T.G., Bredemeier, H.C., Davis, T.W., Jr. 1970. CO_2 laser for surgical research. Med. Biol. Eng. Comput. 8: 548–558.
6. Bredemeier, H.C. 1973. Stereo Laser Endoscope. US Patent.
7. Jako, G.J. 1972. Laser surgery of the vocal cords: An experimental study with carbon dioxide lasers on dogs. Laryngoscope 82: 2204–2216.
8. Strong, M.S., Jako, G.J. 1972. Laser surgery in the larynx, early clinical experience with continuous CO_2 laser. Ann. Otol. Rhinol. Laryngol. 81: 791–798.
9. Strong, M.S., Vaughan, C.W., Polanyi, T.G. et al. 1974. Bronchoscopic CO_2 laser surgery. Ann. Otol. Rhinol. Laryngol. 83: 769–776.

10. Strong, M.S. 1974. Laser management of premalignant lesions of the larynx. Can. J. Otolaryngol. 3(4): 560–563.
11. Ossoff, R.H., Karlan, M.S. 1982. Universal endoscopic coupler for carbon dioxide laser surgery. Ann. Otol. Rhinol. Laryngol. 91: 608–609.
12. Ossoff, R.H., Karlan, M.S. 1983. A set of bronchoscopes for carbon dioxide laser surgery. Otolaryngol. Head Neck Surg. 91: 336–337.
13. Lynch, R.C. 1920. Intrinsic carcinoma of the larynx with a second report of the cases operated on by suspension and dissection. Trans. Am. Laryngol. Assoc. 43: 119–126.
14. New, G.U., Dorton, H.E. 1941. Suspension laryngoscopy and the treatment of malignant disease of the hypopharynx and larynx. Mayo Clin. Proc. 16: 411–416.
15. Lillie, J., DeSanto, L. 1973. Transoral surgery of early cordal carcinoma. Trans. Am. Acad. Ophthalmol. Otolaryngol. 77: 92–96.
16. Vaughan, C.W., Strong, M.S., Jako, G.J. 1978. Laryngeal carcinoma: Transoral treatment utilizing the CO_2 laser. Am. J. Surg. 136: 490–493.
17. Davis, R.K., Shapshay, S.M., Vaughan, C.W. et al. 1981. Pretreatment airway management in obstructing carcinoma of the larynx. Otolaryngol. Head Neck Surg. 89: 209–214.
18. Blakeslee, D., Vaughan, C.W., Shapshay, S.M. 1984. Excisional biopsy in the selective management of T_1 glottic cancer: A three-year follow-up study. Laryngoscope 94: 488–494.
19. Koufman, J.A. The endoscopic management of early cord carcinoma with the carbon dioxide surgical laser: Clinical experience and a proposed subclassification. Otolarynfol. Head Neck Surg. (in press).
20. Ossoff, R.H., Sisson, G.A., Shapshay, S.M. 1985. Endoscopic management of selected early laryngeal malignancies. Ann. Otol. Rhinol. Laryngol. 94: 560–564.
21. Davis, R.K., Jako, G.J., Hyams, V.J. et al. 1982. The anatomic limits of CO_2 laser cordectomy. Laryngoscope 92: 980–984.
22. DeSanto, L.W., Devine, K.D., Lillie, J.C. 1977. Cancers of the larynx: glottic cancer. Surg. Clin. North Am. 57: 611–620.
23. DeSanto, L.W., Pearson, B.W. 1981. Initial treatment of laryngeal cancer: principles of selection. Minn. Med. 64: 691–698.
24. Strong, M.S., Vaughan, C.W., Healy, G.B. et al. 1979. Transoral management of localized carcinoma of the oral cavity using the CO_2 laser. Laryngoscope 89: 897–905.
25. Dumon, J.F., Shapshay, S., Bourcereau, J., Cavaliere, S., Meric, B., Garbi, N., Beamis, J. 1984. Principles for safety in application of Neodymium-YAG laser in bronchology. Chest 86: 163–168.
26. Dumon, J.F., Reboud, E., Garbe, L., Aucomte, F., Meric, B. 1982. Treatment of tracheobronchial lesions by laser photoresection. Chest 81: 278–284.
27. Shapshay, S.M., Simpson, G.T. 1983. Lasers in bronchology. Otolaryngh. Clin. North Am. 16: 879–886.
28. Dougherty, T.J., Grindley, G.B., Fiel, R., Weishaupt, K.R., Boyle, D.G. 1975. Photoradiation therapy II. Cure of animal tumors with hematoporphyrin and light. J.N.C.I. 55: 115–121.
29. Hayata, Y., Kato, H., Konaka, C., Ono, J., Takizawa, N. 1982. Hematoporphyrin derivative and laser photoradiation in the treatment of lung canver. Chest 81: 269–277.
30. Dougherty, T.J., Kaufman, J.E., Goldfarb, A., Weishaupt, K.R., Boyle, D., Mittleman, A. 1978. Photoradiation therapy for the treatment of malignant tumors. Cancer Res. 38: 2628–2635.
31. Cortese, D.A., Kinsey, J.H. 1982. Hematoporphyrin-derivative phototherapy for local treatment of cancer of the tracheobronchial tree. Ann. Otol. Rhinol. Laryngol. 91: 652–655.
32. Wile, A.G., Coffey, J., Nahabedian, M.Y., Baghdassarian, R., Mason, G.R., Berns, M.W. 1984. Laser photoradiation therapy of cancer: an update of the experience at the University of California, Irvine. Lasers Surg. Med. 4: 5–12.
33. Tsuchiya, A., Obara, N., Miwa, M., Ohi, T., Kato, H., Hayata, Y. 1983. Hematoporphyrin derivative and laser photoradiation in the diagnosis and treatment of bladder cancer. J. Urol. 130: 79–82.

70

34. Hayata, Y., Kato, H., Konaka, C., Amemiya, R., Ono, J., Ogawa, I., Kinoshita, K., Sakai, H., Takahashi, H. 1984. Photoradiation therapy with hematoporphyrin derivative in early and stage 1 lung cancer. Chest 86: 169–177.
35. Wile, A.G., Novotny, J., Mason, G.R. 1984. Photoradiation therapy of head and neck cancer. Am. J. Clin. Oncol. 6: 39–43.
36. McCaughan, J.S., Guy, J.T., Hawley, P., Hicks, W., Inglis, W., Laufman, L., May, E., Nims, T.A., Sherman, R. 1983. Hematoporphyrin-derivative and photoradiation therapy of malignant tumors. Lasers Surg. Med. 3: 199–209.
37. Dougherty, T.J., Lawrence, G., Kaufman, J.H., Boyle, D., Weishaupt, K.R., Goldfarb, A. 1979. Photoradiation in the treatment of recurrent breast carcinoma. J.N.C.I. 62:231–237.
38. Ossoff, R.H., Pelzer, H.J., Atiyah, R.A., Berktold, R.E., Sisson, G.A. 1984. Potential applications of photoradiation therapy in head and neck surgery. Arch. Otolaryngol. 110: 728–730.

6. Radiation therapy with multiple fractions per day in the treatment of head and neck cancer

JAMES T. PARSONS and RODNEY R. MILLION

Introduction

In the United States, radiation therapy for mucosal lesions of the head and neck is most often delivered with a continuous course of irradiation consisting of five 180–200 rad fractions per week administered Monday through Friday. Deviations from this schedule have usually been done for one of three reasons.

Convenience

From a practical standpoint, both patient and physician would like for treatment to be completed in as short a time as is consistent with good results. Most clinical investigations of altered fractionation have involved delivery of a reduced number of high-dose fractions, administered once, twice, or thrice weekly, or occasionally even single-dose therapy. Such treatment, which has come to be known as 'hypofractionation' [1], is less expensive, results in less interruption of normal daily activities, and reduces the workload in a busy radiation therapy department compared to conventional treatment.

Various methods have been tried through the years to mathematically equate these abbreviated treatment schedules with conventional fractionation schemes. The best known of these methods is the nominal standard dose (NSD) formula of Ellis [2]. Other investigators have sought to devise new fractionation schemes that produce acute reactions equivalent to those produced by conventional schemes, on the assumption that the late effects and tumor control achieved by the two dose schedules would also be equivalent.

In the vast majority of instances, whether the new schedules were devised mathematically or by matching acute reactions, the late complications produced by dose schedules employing fewer, larger-dose fractions have been much more severe than had been predicted and tumor control has generally been poor [3–15].

Despite its description by Coutard in 1934 [16], the notion that there is a

C. Jacobs (ed) Cancers of the head and neck.
© *1987, Martinus Nijhoff Publishers, Boston. ISBN 0–89838–825–2. Printed in the Netherlands.*

dissociation between acute and late effects received little attention in the literature until the last decade. *It is now known that with X-rays, as one reduces the size of the dose per fraction, one achieves a differential sparing of the tissues responsible for late effects relative to those responsible for acute effects* [17].

Patient comfort

Large-volume treatment at 180–200 rad/fraction, five fractions/week, to 6000–7500 rad generally produces considerable mucositis. Several investigators have reported treatment results following irradiation with schemes that were designed to minimize the acute side effects of therapy.

In 1965, Andrews reported the National Cancer Institute treatment results in 43 patients with head and neck squamous cell carcinoma who received 8000 R to 10,000 R (mode 9000 R) with 2 MV X-rays [5]. The overall treatment time was usually 14 weeks with three fractions administered per week. The use of such a protracted treatment schedule (600 rad/week) is attractive only from the standpoint of acute tolerance; i.e., little or no mucositis is produced. Although a few very early cancers were controlled at the NCI using this schedule, failure to control moderately advanced and advanced cancers was nearly uniform.

At the University of California, San Francisco, in the late 1950s, emphasis was placed on low daily doses for early vocal cord cancer in order to avoid acute mucosal reactions [18]. In general, a dose of 180 rad/fraction was administered to total doses of 5500–7000 rad [19], but in many instances, the daily dose was closer to 160 rad [18]. With these protracted treatment schedules, the local failure rates (T_1, 20%; T_2, 48%) were twice those usually reported.

Split-course irradiation, which was used routinely at the University of Florida between 1969 and 1974, is another means of making the patient more comfortable during the treatment period. By introducing a rest interval during the middle of a treatment course, the patient is relieved of a substantial period of moderately severe or severe mucositis and instead has two shorter periods of milder discomfort. Tumor control by split-course techniques was poor compared to continuous-course schemes [20, 21].

The likely explanation for lower control rates following split-course irradiation or excessively protracted continuous-course techniques is repopulation of clonogenic cells during the treatment course. The time factor is of extreme importance in radiotherapy.

Improvement in therapeutic ratio

During the last decade, hyperfractionation and accelerated fractionation have been used with increasing frequency in an attempt to exploit basic radiobiologic principles to improve the efficacy of radiation therapy. By definition, *hyperfractionated radiotherapy* refers to the delivery of a large number of smaller than conventional fractional doses, in an overall treatment time that is similar to conventional; hyperfractionation is usually accomplished by delivering more than one fraction per day. The total dose is generally slightly higher than that delivered by conventional schemes. If the total dose is not increased over that conventionally utilized, the potential therapeutic advantage of hyperfractionation may be lost. The usual aim is to deliver a dose that will increase the rate of tumor control while keeping the rate of complications at an acceptable level [22].

By definition, *accelerated fractionation* refers to shortening the overall treatment duration, using conventional (180–200 rad) dose fractions. Total dose is similar to or slightly less than conventional. Acceleration may be accomplished in a variety of ways, e.g., by treating a patient six or seven times per week instead of five [23]. Alternatively, it may be accomplished by using multiple fractions per day, 5 days per week. The rationale for such therapies is best explained by considering the important determinants of fractionation response, the so-called 4R's of radiation therapy: repair of sublethal damage, redistribution through the cell cycle, reoxygenation, and regeneration [17].

We have already seen that dose fractionation preferentially spares tissues responsible for late effects relative to those responsible for acute effects. These observed differences in response to fractionation are apparently due to differences in *repair of sublethal damage* between acute- and late-effect tissues [3]; in other words, there are differences in the shapes of the respective cell-survival curves for the two types of tissues. If, as would be expected, rapidly proliferating tumors respond like acutely responding normal tissues, then as one decreases the size of the dose per fraction, one should also see a differential sparing of the tissues responsible for late effects relative to the tumor itself; i.e., the therapeutic ratio should be enhanced. *Hyperfractionation* would theoretically provide a therapeutic gain.

By increasing the number of fractions, one increases the probability that *redistributing tumor cells* (and also actively proliferating normal tissue cells, such as those of skin and mucous membrane) will be irradiated during a sensitive phase of the cell cycle. Since the fibrovascular connective tissues responsible for late radiation damage are relatively nonproliferative, they will be less affected by redistribution between treatments. The result may be less severe late normal-tissue injury for a given rate of tumor control when *hyperfractionation* is used.

Since the *oxygen enhancement ratio* decreases as the dose per fraction is reduced, the extent to which hypoxia limits tumor control may also be less with *hyperfractionated* treatment.

The *regenerative response* of tumors during irradiation is thought to be an important determinant of tumor control in a significant number of patients. *Accelerated fractionation* significantly shortens the overall duration of treatment, thereby reducing the time available for regeneration of clonogenic tumor cells during the treatment course. Accelerated treatment would seem most attractive in the treatment of very rapidly proliferating tumors. Since the ability of acutely responding tissues, such as the skin and mucous membrane, to withstand a course of fractionated treatment depends on their regenerative response during treatment, acute tolerance becomes a limiting factor in attempting to deliver an accelerated course of irradiation without a treatment interruption or without reducing the total dose administered.

Clinical experience with multiple fractions per day

The idea of irradiating head and neck cancers with more than one fraction/day is not new. From 1920–1926, at the Fondation Curie in Paris, France, Coutard [24] routinely treated patients with cancer of the oropharynx, hypopharynx, and larynx twice a day whenever the overall duration of the treatment course was less than 20 days because he thought that the tolerance was better with this approach than with once-a-day treatment. This short-duration, twice-a-day schedule was used only for early cancers. Between 1927 and 1933, Coutard and Baclesse extended the overall treatment time by using markedly reduced doses/fraction, two fractions/day, and stated that with this approach, they were able to cure a number of advanced lesions that up to that time had never been cured [16].

From the 1940s through the 1960s, the vast majority of radiotherapy patients around the world were treated with one fraction/day. In the early 1970s, hyperfractionation was suggested as a possible means of improving the therapeutic ratio [25, 26].

Preliminary results from a number of institutions are summarized below. The results have been grouped according to the strict definitions of hyperfractionation and accelerated fractionation as stated above.

Hyperfractionation

Hyperfractionation schedules reported in the English literature are summarized in Table 1. In addition to using multiple small-dose fractions, all of the schedules offer some additional potential advantage in terms of tumor cell repopulation in that the overall treatment durations are 1–2 weeks shorter than conventional techniques that deliver an equivalent dose. In general, most of the authors have tentatively concluded that their regimens produce acute effects that are equal to or more severe than the acute effects produced by conventional fractionation, equivalent or less severe late effects, and better local-regional control.

Only two trials have treated over 100 patients each. The results from the University of Florida are reported at the end of this paper. The data from the

Table 1. Predominantly hyperfractionated irradiation schedules[a]

Institution (author)	No. of patients	Fraction size (rad)	Treatment schedule	Interfraction interval (hours)	Split course (months)	Total dose (rad)/overall treatment time (weeks)
EORTC[b] (Horiot *et al.* 1985 [27])	272[c]	115	b.i.d.[d] 5 days/wk	4–8	—	8050/7
University of Florida (Parsons *et al.*, 1984)	102	120	b.i.d. 5 days/wk	4–6	—	7440–7920/6½–7
M.D. Anderson Hospital (Meoz *et al.*, 1984 [28])	45	110–120	b.i.d. 5 days/wk	3–6	—	6000–7500/5–6½
University of Minnesota (Medini *et al.*, 1985 [29])	21	110	b.i.d. 5 days/wk	4	—	7480/6½
Reims, France (Panis *et al.*, 1984 [30])	52	110	6 fx/day 5 days/wk	not stated	1	6600/6

[a] The definition of hyperfractionation used in this paper incorporates the following: (1) large number of smaller than conventional fractional doses, (2) overall treatment time similar to conventional, (3) total dose slightly higher than conventional, and (4) more than one fraction administered/day. If all of these conditions were not satisfied by a particular dose strategy, it was not included in this table.

[b] EORTC = European Organization for Research on Treatment of Cancer.

[c] EORTC controlled clinical trial 22791 included 272 patients who were randomized between once-a-day and twice-a-day treatment schemes. The exact number of patients in each subgroup was not published.

[d] b.i.d. = twice a day.

European Organization for Research on Treatment of Cancer (EORTC) are reported below.

Between January 1980 and October 1984, 272 patients with moderately advanced (T2-T3; N0-N1 < 3 cm) squamous cell carcinoma of the oropharynx, exclusive of the base of tongue, were randomly allocated to receive treatment consisting of 7000 rad/35 fractions/7 weeks (200 rad/fraction) vs. 8050 rad/70 fractions/7 weeks (115 rad twice-a-day) under EORTC controlled clinical trial 22791 [27]. Complete follow-up information was available on 254 patients (93%) who received treatment in 25 European institutions. No statistical differences in acute or late effects were observed. Eight percent of the once-a-day patients required a split in the treatment course because of acute mucosal intolerance vs. 12% of the twice-a-day group. The 36-month actuarial local control rate was 72% in the twice-a-day patients vs. 56% in the once-a-day group (p = 0.15). For patients with high (90–100) Karnofsky scores, the difference in local control was more clearly in favor of the twice-a-day group (72% vs. 42%, p = 0.09). There is a 5–10% higher actuarial survival in the twice-a-day group up to 36 months, after which the two curves join together; however, the number of patients at risk for 36 months is small. It must be emphasized that these results are preliminary and further follow-up will be necessary before definitive conclusions can be drawn.

Accelerated fractionation

Relatively few patients have been treated by pure accelerated fractionation regimens because acute mucosal reactions are severe [31–35] (Table 2). Three trials have delivered thrice-a-day treatment for 2 weeks, with total doses limited by acute reactions to approximately 5000 rad. All three of the series reported a number of patients who required hospitalization or who died in the postirradiation period of treatment-related problems. Attempts to increase the dose above the 5000 rad level would require a split in the treatment course, which would largely offset the main potential advantage (shortened overall treatment time) of acceleration.

Knee *et al.* [35] have described an interesting variant of accelerated fractionation in which the basic treatment course (180–200 rad/fraction) and the boost treatment course (120–150 rad/fraction, 3–6h after the basic dose, 2–3 times/week) were administered concomitantly to 53 patients with advanced, recurrent, and/or rapidly progressive squamous cell carcinoma of a variety of head and neck sites. The rationale for this treatment is the same as that for accelerated fractionation in general, but this regimen has the advantage of producing the most severe mucosal reactions in only a limited volume of tissue because only the 'boost' field is treated at an accelerated rate. Considering the advanced stages of disease in the patients treated, the actuarial probability of

Table 2. Predominantly accelerated fractionation schemes[a]

Institution (author)	No. of patients	Fraction size (rad)	Treatment schedule	Interfraction interval (hours)	Split course	Total dose (rad)/overall treatment time
Portsmouth, UK (Resouly and Svboda, 1982)[31]	59	175–230	t.i.d.[b] 5 days/wk	3 minimum	—	5000–5500/1½–2 wk
Parma, Italy (Perracchia and Salti, 1981 [32])	22	200	t.i.d. 5 days/wk	4	—	4800–5400/8–12 days
Amsterdam (Gonzalez et al., 1980 [33])	9	180	t.i.d. 5 days/wk	4	—	4860–5400/11–12 days
Rome (Arcangeli et al., 1979 [34])	6	200	b.i.d.[b] 5 days/wk	5	—	6000–7400/not stated
Rome (Arcangeli et al., 1979 [34])	8	200–150– 150	t.i.d. 5 days/wk	5	—	4650–7400/not stated
M.D. Anderson (Knee et al., 1985 [35])	53	180–200 (basic dose) plus 120–150 (boost dose)	b.i.d.[c]	3–6	—	7000/6 wks (mean)

[a] The definition of accelerated fractionation used in this paper incorporates the following: (1) overall treatment time shorter than conventional, (2) total dose similar to or slightly less than conventional, and (3) more than one fraction administered per day. If all of these conditions were not satisfied by a particular dose strategy, it was not included in this table.

[b] t.i.d. = thrice a day; b.i.d. = twice a day.

[c] Basic dose was administered 5 days per week; boost dose was administered 2–3 days per week.

Table 3. Accelerated, hyperfractionated, split-course fractionation schedules

Institution (author)	No. of patients	Fraction size (rad)	Treatment schedule	Interfraction interval (hours)	Split course (weeks)	Total dose (rad)/overall treatment time (weeks)
Massachusetts General Hospital (Wang *et al.*, 1985 [36])	321	160	b.i.d.[a] 5 days/wk	4 minimum	2	6400–6720/6

[a] b.i.d. = twice a day.

2-year local-regional control was excellent (65%) and the acute tolerance was deemed acceptable.

Accelerated, hyperfractionated, split-course irradiation

Since October 1979, Wang [36] has used a scheme that employs a slightly greater number (40–42 fractions versus 37–40 fractions) of slightly smaller (160 rad versus 180 rad) than conventional fractional doses in an overall treatment time that is accelerated by 1–2 weeks compared to the technique used in the past at Massachusetts General Hospital (Table 3). A 2-week split in the treatment course is mandatory because the mucositis produced is severe. This hybridization of three types of fractionation has produced control results that are superior to those produced at the same institution by once-a-day irradiation. Table 4 summarizes the local control results. For T3-T4 lesions, local control results were significantly better following twice-a-day fractionation. For T1-T2, the results favored twice-a-day fractionation and closely approached statistical significance.

Table 4. Thirty-six month actuarial local control according to disease site and T-stage (Massachusetts General Hospital [36])

	No. of patients (% free of disease)	
	T1-T2	T3-T4
Oral cavity		
Once-a-day[a]	46 (49%)	44 (19%)
Twice-a-day[b]	28 (63%)	33 (57%)
p value	0.06	<0.004
Oropharynx		
Once-a-day	45 (73%)	44 (24%)
Twice-a-day	21 (91%)	53 (57%)
p value	0.081	0.009
Larynx		
Once-a-day	74 (65%)	50 (34%)
Twice-a-day	113 (78%)	73 (63%)
p value	0.14	<0.001

[a] 6500–7000 rad/7.2–8 weeks, 180 rad per fraction, 5 fractions per week.
[b] 6400–6720 rad/6 weeks, 160 rad b.i.d., 10 fractions per week with 2-weeks rest interval after 3840 rad.

Table 5. Other fraction schemes

Institution (author)	No. of patients	Fraction size (rad)	Treatment schedule	Interfraction interval (hours)	Split course (weeks)	Total dose (rad)/overall treatment time (weeks)
EORTC (Horiot et al. 1985 [27])	522[a]	160	t.i.d.[b] 5 days/wk	4	3-5	7200/7-8
Reims, France (Nguyen et al., 1985 [37])	91	90	8 fx/day 5 days/wk	2	2	7200/3½
Radiumhemmet (Backstrom et al., 1973 [26])	17	100	t.i.d. 5 days/wk	4	3-7	8400/9-13
Johannesburg, S. Africa (Nissenbaum et al., 1984 [38])	13	240	b.i.d.[b] 5 days/wk	5-6	3½	4800/5
RTOG[c] (Marcial et al., 1985 [39])	not stated	120	b.i.d. 5 days/wk	not stated	—	6000/5

[a] EORTC (European Organization for Research of Treatment of Cancer) controlled clinical trial 22811 included 522 patients who were randomly allocated to one of three treatment arms as described in the text. The exact number of patients in each arm was not published.
[b] t.i.d. = thrice a day; b.i.d. = twice a day.
[c] RTOG = Radiation Therapy Oncology Group.

Other schemes employing multiple fractions per day

A number of other schemes that defy categorization into the above groupings are shown in Table 5 [26, 27, 37–39]. The number of possibilities is limitless. Some of the schemes have no clear-cut radiobiologic rationale.

The EORTC has conducted a trial using 160 rad thrice daily. The technique has some elements of hyperfractionation (slight decrease in fraction size, total dose and overall treatment time similar to conventional treatment). There is no acceleration of the overall treatment course, and, in fact, the patients are *off* treatment (3–5 weeks split-course) for longer than they are *on* treatment. Between February 1981 and October 1984, 522 patients with T3-T4 or T1-T2 N1 (>3 cm), N2, N3 cancers of a variety of head and neck sites in 15 institutions were randomly allocated under EORTC trial 22811 to one of three treatment arms: (1) 7000 rad/35 fractions/7 weeks; (2) 4800 rad/30 fractions/2 weeks, followed by a 3–5 week rest interval, then 2400 rad/15 fractions/1 week, such that a total dose of 7200 rad was administered on 15 treatment days over 6–8 weeks; (3) as is scheme number 2 above but with the addition of misonidazole [27]. Complete follow-up was available on 498 patients (95%). Preliminary conclusions are as follows. The incidence of severe acute mucosal reactions was significantly greater (p<0.0001) in the thrice-a-day treatment arms. Late complications were also slightly higher in the thrice-a-day arms; all five treatment-related deaths occurred in arms 2 and 3. Three deaths occurred because of hemorrhage secondary to very rapid tumor shrinkage, with insufficient time for normal tissue recovery. Two-year actuarial local control was 32–38% in all three arms. Survival was higher in the two thrice-a-day arms than in arm 1 (40% vs. 26%, p = 0.130). The greater the degree of advancement of neck disease, the greater was the survival benefit following thrice-a-day treatment. All conclusions are very preliminary and will need longer follow-up for verification.

By delivering eight 90 rad fractions per day, Nguyen managed to deliver 7200 rad in 3 ½ weeks with a 2-week split [37]. Extensive bleeding secondary to very rapid tumor shrinkage led to an unacceptable complication rate. This fact, as well as the logistics of treating patients eight times a day, makes this approach unattractive.

Although the technique of Backstrom employs multiple small-dose fractions, it does not strictly fit the definition of hyperfractionation since the 3–7-week split results in considerable protraction of the overall treatment time (9–13 weeks) [26].

The technique of Nissenbaum offers no apparent advantage and, in fact, combines most of the features commonly associated with poor tumor control and increased late effects (low total dose with split-course technique using a reduced number of larger than conventional fractional doses). The reported results were predictably poor [38].

Instead of increasing the total dose of irradiation administered, which is the usual aim of true hyperfractionation schemes, the RTOG (Radiation Therapy

Oncology Group) technique delivered a total dose that is 600–1380 rad (or a 9–19% dose reduction) less than the standard once-a-day RTOG dose of 6600–7380 rad at 180–200 rad fractions. No advantage is taken of the potential therapeutic gain offered by hyperfractionation [39].

University of Florida results

A twice-a-day treatment schedule has been used at the University of Florida to manage moderately advanced and advanced squamous cell carcinomas of the head and neck since March 1978 [40]. Between March 1978 and April 1983, 91 patients received radiation therapy alone to the primary site with neck dissection(s) added in 24; 11 received preoperative irradiation followed by resection of the primary lesion and clinically positive lymph nodes (Table 6). Patients selected for treatment by twice-a-day irradiation generally had unfavorable characteristics such as a large-volume tumor. Most patients with small-volume T2-T3 disease, such as those with superficial lesions of the soft palate that involved a large surface area, were treated by once-a-day techniques. Early (T1-T2) vocal cord cancer has not been treated by twice-a-day techniques at the University of Florida. Only a few patients with nasopharyngeal or nasal cavity/paranasal sinus lesions have been treated by twice-a-day irradiation and are not reported. Most of the early oral cavity cancers seen during this same time period have also been treated by once-a-day techniques. The majority of cancers reported here are therefore oropharyngeal, laryngeal, and hypopharyngeal lesions of moderate or large tumor bulk.

Table 6. Patient distribution according to AJCC stages (University of Florida, 3/78–4/83; analysis 4/85)

	RT ± RND[a] no. of patients[b]	Preoperative RT no. of patients[b]
Stage I	0	0
Stage II	9	0
Stage III	22	3
Stage IVA[c]	18	1
Stage IVB[d]	42	7
	—	—
Total	91	11

[a] RND = radical neck dissection.
[b] 105 primaries in 102 patients. Three patients with simultaneous primaries were staged according to highest stage. Two patients lost to follow-up were excluded.
[c] IVA: T1-T3, N2-N3A disease.
[d] IVB: T4 and/or N3B disease.

A dose of 120 rad was delivered twice daily to the primary site and upper neck nodes with a 4–6-h interfraction interval. Most of the patients were treated with cobalt-60. The low neck and reduced portals to the lymph nodes behind the plane of the spinal cord (posterior electron 'strips') were treated once a day. Treatments were delivered 5 days a week.

When irradiation alone was administered to the primary site (91 patients), the minimum dose was usually 7440–7920 rad/ 62–66 fractions/31–33 treatment days, but for a variety of reasons, doses have varied somewhat. The doses used in 85 patients with oropharyngeal or laryngeal/hypopharyngeal primaries are shown in Table 7. The spinal cord was shielded after 4560 rad/38 fractions/19 days. Further reductions in treatment volume were made whenever possible.

Eleven patients received preoperative radiation (5040–6000 rad/4–5 weeks) followed in 4–6 weeks by resection of the primary lesion plus neck dissection(s).

Acute tolerance

Acute skin and mucous membrane reactions have been more pronounced than those seen with treatment at 180 rad/day. Eleven of 102 patients required a nasogastric feeding tube, usually after 4–6 weeks of therapy; a feeding tube was recommended in two other patients but was refused. Two patients required a split in the treatment course (at 4800 and 6720 rad, respectively) because of acute intolerance. A tracheostomy was necessary at 6960 rad in one patient because of difficulty in handling secretions. Three patients were hospitalized for 7–12 days following irradiation because of dehydration. In most patients, the mucosa was healed within 3–6 weeks following treatment, but in some patients, 2–3 months were required for complete healing.

Table 7. Tumor doses administered according to treatment site (University of Florida, 3/78–4/83; analysis, 4/85)

Dose (rad)	Oropharynx (42 patients)	Larynx/hypopharynx (43 patients)
4800	1	0
6000	0	1
6960	1	1
7440	11	12
7680	9	24
7920	7	5
8160	1	0
7440–7680 + 1000–1500 radium	10	0
7920 + 1000 radium	1	0
8160 + 1500 radium	1	0

Local control

There were 94 primary lesions in 91 patients treated by radiation therapy alone. Thirty-one (94%) of 33 local recurrences were noted within 24 months. Eighteen lesions were excluded from the local control analysis because results of treatment to the primary lesion could not be assessed for a minimum of 2 years. The reasons were death due to intercurrent or metastatic disease (16 patients); death due to unknown cause 2 weeks following completion of radiation (one patient); and, in one patient, resection of the primary site (larynx) due to necrosis (specimen negative for tumor recurrence). There was no clinical evidence of primary tumor recurrence in any of the 18 patients.

Local control results for the remaining 76 lesions are shown according to anatomic site and T-stage in Table 8 and according to dose in Figures 1, 2, and 3. Aside from the fact that none of the four lesions that received less than 7440 rad were controlled, no clear dose-response relationship was apparent.

Local control following preoperative irradiation plus primary resection was obtained in four of five T3 and two of three T4 lesions.

Regional control

Regional control results in patients who had control of disease at the primary site are shown in Table 9.

Table 8. Local control following irradiation alone to the primary site (no. controlled/no. treated)

Primary site	T-stage (AJCC)		
	T2	T3	T4
Gum/retromolar trigone	1/2	n.a.	0/3
Oral tongue/floor of mouth	2/3	n.a.	0/2
Base of tongue	n.a	5/5	2/5
Tonsil	3/5[a]	10/11	1/6[a]
Soft palate	1/1	0/1[a]	n.a.
Pyriform sinus	2/3[a]	0/1	0/2
Pharyngeal wall	1/2	0/1	1/2
Glottic larynx	n.a.	4/6	0/3
Supraglottic larynx	5/5	5/6	0/1
Total	15/21 (71%)	24/31 (77%)	4/24 (17%)

[a] Four failures at ≤6960 rad.
n.a. = no data available.

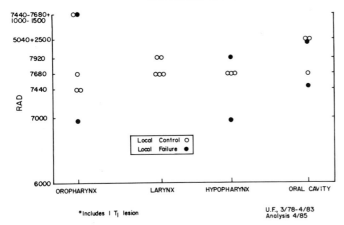

Figure 1. Local control according to tumor site and tumor dose for T2 lesions.

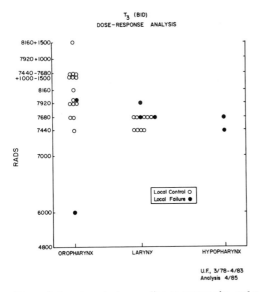

Figure 2. Local control according to tumor site and tumor dose for T3 lesions.

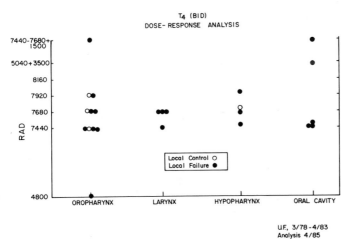

Figure 3. Local control according to tumor site and tumor dose for T4 lesions.

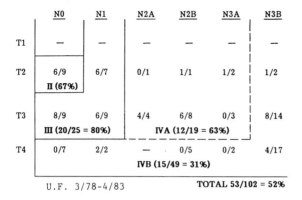

U.F. 3/78-4/83   **TOTAL 53/102 = 52%**

Figure 4. Absolute disease-free survival at 2 years.

Survival

The 2-year absolute survival rate without evidence of disease was 53/102 (52%). Seven (64%) of the 11 patients who received preoperative irradiation to the primary site were alive and free of disease at 2 years. Disease-free survival at two years according to AJCC stage is shown in Figure 4. Stage IV is divided into IVA (favorable) and IVB (unfavorable) [41].

Table 9. Neck control in patients with control of primary disease (no. of heminecks controlled/no. treated)[a]
(University of Florida, 3/78–4/83, analysis 4/85)

Hemineck stage	Radiation therapy alone	Radiation therapy + neck dissection
N0	49/50[b]	—
N1	15/16	6/7
N2A	1/1	4/4
N2B	7/9	9/9
N3A	0/2[c]	2/3
Total	72/78	21/23

[a] One hundred and three of 204 heminecks (102 patients) were excluded from analysis because of failure at the primary site (68 heminecks), death due to intercurrent disease, distant metastases, or complications in <2 years (28), death due to uncontrolled cancer in the contralateral neck (4), death of unknown cause (2), or no treatment to hemineck (1).
[b] 3600 rad (contralateral neck).
[c] Neck dissections were planned in both patients but not performed because of development of distant metastases prior to operation. The doses administered were not considered to be definitive treatment in either patient.

Complications

Complications of irradiation (with or without neck dissection) in 91 patients who received definitive radiation to the primary site consisted of mild (healed spontaneously in less than six months) soft tissue/bone necrosis in eight patients, moderately severe (healed spontaneously in greater than 6 months) soft tissue necroisis in two patients, and three severe complications of irradiation (one chondronecrosis, one bone necrosis, and one esophageal stricture). Complications were dose-related. No transverse myelitis has been observed. Twenty-eight planned neck dissections were performed on 24 patients (four bilateral); there were seven wound infections and one carotid exposure (no carotid ruptures).

Severe complications developed in six of 13 patients who underwent salvage surgery at the primary site with or without neck dissection. One scar contracture was the only complication in three patients who underwent salvage radical neck dissection alone.

Preoperative irradiation plus primary resection and radical neck dissection in 11 patients resulted in two wound infections (one minor) and one permanent gastrostomy.

Conclusions regarding the University of Florida experience

The technique of twice-a-day irradiation used at the University of Florida is similar to that described by Jampolis *et al.* [42]. The technique combines the potential advantages of small-dose fractions with the advantages of a shortened overall treatment time. Twice-a-day irradiation, as reported in our institution, reduces the overall treatment time for advanced cancers by approximately 1 1/2-2 weeks compared to the once-a-day regimen used in the past, e.g., 7500 rad/8–8 1/2 weeks once a day versus 7440–7920 rad/6–6 1/2 weeks twice a day. It is not possible to further diminish the overall treatment time even in rapidly growing tumors because the acute response of the mucosa will not permit it. We have tried to avoid the introduction of a rest interval because this might offset one potential advantage (shortened overall treatment time) of our program. In order to keep acute mucosal tolerance at an acceptable level, the initial treatment volume should be kept fairly 'tight' and two or three field reductions are made as the treatment progresses. Only the initial volume of gross disease receives the final tumor dose. If this policy is not followed, acute intolerance is predictable.

Our preliminary observation was that the acute reactions from our twice-a-day program were roughly equivalent to those produced by 180–200 rad once a day [40]. A larger patient experience now leads us to believe the reactions are more severe. The treatment schedule is just tolerable in the majority of patients, but at least 20% develop significant problems with alimentation requiring nasogastric feeding (11%), treatment interruption (2%), or hospitalization (3%). Two

88

patients treated too recently to be included in the present series have developed aspiration pneumonia in the immediate postirradiation period, resulting in one fatality and requiring intensive medical management in the other. This has prompted us to more liberally recommend gastrostomy prior to treatment for patients with poor nutritional status in whom large volumes of mucosa will be treated to a high dose. We have no data as yet on the results of this approach. From the work of Dutriex, one would predict that the acute effects produced by 120 rad twice daily would be equal to those produced by 240 rad once a day [43]. Since tumors are also acute-effects tissues, their response to 120 rad twice a day may also be similar to their response to 240 rad once a day; at the present time, this concept is unproven.

Patient acceptance of twice-a-day treatment has been good, with very few patients declining treatment with this approach. However, the consequence for the radiation therapy department is an increase from approximately 38–42 treatment visits to 62–66 visits.

The initial results suggest an increase in local control of perhaps 15–20% compared to conventional once-a-day fractionation schemes, and the late effects seem less. There are few subgroups with enough patients to make valid comparisons between the control rates achieved in twice-a-day patients and the control rates achieved following once-a-day irradiation. For T3 squamous cell carcinomas of the base of tongue and tonsillar area treated by continuous-course irradiation with once-a-day fractionation, local control has been obtained in 31/44 patients (70%) [44, 45] vs. 15/16 patients (94%) treated by the twice-a-day technique. The results for T2-T3 lesions of the supraglottic larynx and T3 lesions of the true vocal cord treated by once-a-day continuous-course irradiation were 28/41 (68%) [46, 47] vs. 14/17 (82%) treated by twice-a-day irradiation. Conclusions regarding local control rates should be regarded as preliminary at this time.

The frequency of complications following neck dissection is similar to once-a-day schemes. When salvage surgery has been done for failure at the primary site, the complication rate is similar to that noted after once-a-day therapy.

References

1. Cox, J.D. 1985. Large-dose fractionation (hypofractionation). Cancer 55: 2105–2111.
2. Ellis, F. 1969. Dose, time and fractionation: A clinical hypothesis. Clin. Radiol. 20: 1–7.
3. Thames, H.D., Jr., Withers, H.R., Peters, L.J., Fletcher, G.H. 1982. Changes in early and late radiation responses with altered dose fractionation: Implications for dose-survival relationships. Int. J. Radiat. Oncol. Biol. Phys. 8: 219–226.
4. Withers, H.R., Thames, H.D., Jr., Flow, B.L., Mason, K.A., Hussey, D.H. 1978. The relationship of acute to late skin injury in 2 and 5 fraction/week gamma ray therapy. Int. J. Radiat. Oncol. Biol. Phys. 4: 595–601.
5. Andrews, J.R. 1965. Dose-time relationships in cancer radiotherapy: A clinical radiobiology study of extremes of dose and time. Am. J. Roentgenol. Radium Ther. Nucl. Med. 93: 56–74.

6. Rubenfeld, S. 1953. Experiences with a rapid irradiation technic in oral carcinoma. Radiology 60: 724–731.

7. Atkins, H.L. 1964. Massive dose technique in radiation therapy of inoperable carcinoma of the breast. Am. J. Roentgenol. Radium Ther. Nucl. Med. 91: 80–89.

8. Edelman, A.H., Holtz, S., Powers, W.E. 1965. Rapid radiotherapy for inoperable carcinoma of the breast: Benefits and complications. Am. J. Roentgenol. Radium Ther. Nucl. Med. 93: 585–599.

9. Singh, K. 1978. Two regimes with the same TDF but differing morbidity used in the treatment of stage III carcinoma of the cervix. Br. J. Radiol. 51: 357–362.

10. Bennett M.B. 1978. The treatment of stage III squamous carcinoma of the cervix in air and hyperbaric oxygen (abstr.). Br. J. Radiol. 51: 68.

11. Dische, S., Martin, W.M.C., Anderson, P. 1981. Radiation myelopathy in patients treated for carcinoma of bronchus using a six fraction regime of radiotherapy. Br. J. Radiol. 54: 29–35.

12. Byhardt, R.W., Greenberg, M., Cox, J.D. 1977. Local control of squamous carcinoma of oral cavity and oropharynx with 3 vs. 5 treatment fractions per week. Int. J. Radiat. Oncol. Biol. Phys. 2: 415–420.

13. Kok, G. 1971. The influence of the size of the fraction dose on normal and tumour tissue in ^{60}Co radiation treatment of carcinoma of the larynx and inoperable carcinoma of the breast. Radiol. Clin. Biol. 40: 100–115.

14. Wiernik, G., Bleehen, N.M., Brindle, J., Bullimore, J., Churchill-Davidson, I.F.J., Davidson, J. et al. 1970. Sixth interim progress report of the British Institute of Radiology fractionation study of 3 F/week versus 5 F/week in radiotherapy of the laryngo-pharynx. Br. J. Radiol. 51: 241–250.

15. Handa, K., Edoliya, T.N., Pandey, R.P., Agarwal, Y.C., Sinha, N. 1980. A radiotherapeutic clinical trial of twice per week vs. five times per week in oral cancer. Strahlentherapie 156: 626–631.

16. Coutard, H. 1934. Principles of x-ray therapy of malignant diseases. Lancet 227: 1–8.

17. Withers, H.R. 1984. Biological bases for modifying conventional fractionation regimens in radiotherapy. Strahlentherapie 160: 670–677.

18. Buschke, F., Vaeth, J.M. 1963. Radiation therapy of carcinoma of the vocal cord without mucosal reaction. Am. J. Roentgenol. Radium Ther. Nucl. Med. 89: 29–34.

19. Woodhouse, R.J., Quivey, J.M., Fu, K.K., Sien, P.S., Dedo, H.H., Philips, T.L. 1981. Treatment of carcinoma of the vocal cord: A review of 20 years experience. Laryngoscope 91: 1155–1162.

20. Lindberg, R.D., Fletcher, G.H. 1972. Clinical experiences with altered fractionation. Rev. Interam. Radiol. 7: 15–21.

21. Parsons, J.T., Bova, F.J., Million, R.R. 1980. A re-evaluation of split-course technique for squamous cell carcinoma of the head and neck. Int. J. Radiat. Oncol. Biol. Phys. 6: 1645–1652.

22. Fletcher, G.H. 1983. Keynote address: The scientific basis of the present and future practice of clinical radiotherapy. Int. J. Radiat. Oncol. Biol. Phys. 9: 1073–1082.

23. Lipsett, J.A., Desai, K., Pezner, R., Vora, N., Chong, L.M., Archambeau. J.O. 1984. Acute normal tissue tolerance to 7 day per week accelerated fractionation. Int. J. Radiat. Oncol. Biol. Phys. 10: 1049–1052.

24. Coutard, H. 1932. Roentgen therapy of epitheliomas of the tonsillar region, hypopharynx and larynx from 1920–1926. Am. J. Roentgenol. Radium Ther. 28: 313–331.

25. Withers, H.R. 1972. Cell renewal system concepts and the radiation response. In: Frontiers of Radiation Therapy and Oncology, Vol. 6 (J.M. Vaeth, ed.). Karger, Basel, and Univ. Park Press, Baltimore, pp. 93–107.

26. Backstrom, A., Jakobsson, P.A., Littbrand, B., Wersall, J. 1973. Fractionation scheme with low individual doses in irradiation of carcinoma of the mouth. Acta Radiol. Ther. Phys. Biol. 12: 401–406.

90

27. Horiot, J.C., van den Bogaert, W., de Pauw, M., van Glabbeke, M., Gonzalez, D.G., van der Schueren, E. 1985. EORTC prospective trials of altered fractionation using multiple fractions per day (MFD). Plenary Session Proceedings, XVI International Congress of Radiology, Honolulu, Hawaii, July 8–12, 1985, pp. 95–97.

28. Meoz, R.T., Fletcher, G.H., Peters, L.J., Barkley, H.T., Thames, H.D. 1984. Twice-daily fractionation schemes for advanced head and neck cancer. Int. J. Radiat. Oncol. Biol. Phys. 10: 831–836.

29. Medini, E., Rao, Y., Kim, T., Levitt, S.H. 1985. Radiation therapy for advanced head and neck squamous cell carcinoma using twice-a-day fractionation. Am. J. Clin. Oncol. 8: 65–68.

30. Panis, X., Nguyen, T.D., Froissart, D., Demange, L. 1984. Hyperfractionated radiotherapy with or without misonidazole: Results of a prospective randomized study in stage III-IV squamous cell carcinoma of the head and neck. Int. J. Radiat. Oncol. Biol. Phys. 10: 1845–1849.

31. Resouly, A., Svoboda, V.H.J. 1982. Management of advanced head and neck squamous carcinoma by multiple daily sessions of radiotherapy and surgery. In: Progress in Radio-Oncology II, Baden, Austria, (K.H. Karcher, H.D. Kogelnik, G. Reinartz, eds.). Raven Press, New York, pp. 339–347.

32. Peracchia, G., Salti, C. 1981. Radiotherapy with thrice-a-day fractionation in a short overall time: Clinical experiences. Int. J. Radiat. Oncol. Biol. Phys. 7: 99–104.

33. Gonzalez-Gonzalez, D., Breur, K., van den Schueren, E. 1980. Preliminary results in advances head and neck cancer with radiotherapy by multiple fractions a day. Clin. Radiol. 31: 417–421.

34. Arcangeli, G., Mauro, F., Morelli, D., Nervi, C. 1979. Multiple daily fractionation in radiotherapy: Biological rationale and preliminary clinical experiences. Eur. J. Cancer 15: 1077–1083.

35. Knee, R., Fields, R.S., Peters, L.J. 1985. Concomitant boost radiotherapy for advanced squamous cell carcinoma of the head and neck. Radiother. Oncol. 4: 1–7.

36. Wang, C.C., Blitzer, P.H., Suit, H.D. 1985. Twice-a-day radiation therapy for cancer of the head and neck. Cancer 55: 2100–2104.

37. Nguyen, T.D., Demange, L., Froissart, D., Panis, X., Loirette, M. 1985. Rapid hyperfractionated radiotherapy. Clinical results in 178 advanced squamous cell carcinomas of the head and neck. Cancer 56: 16–19.

38. Nissenbaum, M., Browde, S., Bezwoda, W.R., de Moor, N.G., Derman, D.P. 1984. Treatment of advanced head and neck cancer: Multiple daily dose fractionated radiation therapy and sequential multimodal treatment approach. Med. Pediatr. Oncol. 12: 204–208.

39. Marcial, V.A., Pajak, T.F., Chang, C. 1985. Hyperfractionated photon radiation therapy in the treatment of advanced squamous cell carcinoma of the oral cavity, pharynx, larynx and sinuses, using radiotherapy as the only planned modality: A Radiation Therapy Oncology Group report. (Abstract # 105) Int. J. Radiat. Oncol. Biol. Phys. 11 (suppl. 1): 142.

40. Parsons, J.T., Cassisi, N.J., Million, R.r. 1984. Results of twice-a-day irradiation of squamous cell carcinomas of the head and neck. Int. J. Radiat. Oncol. Biol. Phys. 10: 2041–2051.

41. Mendenhall, W.M., Parsons, J.T., Million, R.R., Cassisl, N.J., Devine, J.W., Greene, B.D. 1984. A favorable subset of AJCC stage IV squamous cell carcinoma of the head and neck. Int. J. Radiat. Oncol. Biol. Phys. 10: 1841–1843.

42. Jampolis, S., Pipard, G., Horiot, J.C., Bolla, M., Le Dorze, C. 1977. Preliminary results using twice-a-day fractionation in the radiotherapeutic management of advanced cancers of the head and neck. A.J.R. 129: 1091–1093.

43. Dutreix, J., Wambersie, A., Bounik, C. 1973. Cellular recovery in human skin reactions: Application to dose fraction number overall time relationship in radiotherapy. Eur. J. Cancer 9: 159–167.

44. Gardner, K.E., Parsons, J.T., Mendenhall, W.M., Million, R.R., Cassisi, N.J. Time-dose relationships for local tumor control and complications following irradiation of squamous cell carcinoma of the base of tongue. Int. J. Radiat. Oncol. Biol. Phys., in press.

45. Mendenhall, W.M., Parsons, J.T., Cassisi, N.J. Million, R.R., Squamous cell carcinoma of the tonsillar area treated with radical irradiation. Submitted for publication.
46. Mendenhall, W.M., Million, R.R., Sharkey, D.E., Cassisi, N.J. 1984. Stage T3 squamous cell carcinoma of the glottic larynx treated with surgery and/or radiation therapy. Int. J. Radiat. Oncol. Biol. Phys. 10: 357–363.
47. Mendenhall, W.M., Million, R.R., Cassisi, N.J. 1984. Squamous cell carcinoma of the supraglottic larynx treated with radical irradiation: Analysis of treatment parameters and results. Int. J. Radiat. Oncol. Biol. Phys. 10: 2223–2230.

7. Brachytherapy – head and neck cancer

DON R. GOFFINET

Introduction

Interstitial implantation of radioactive sources, brachytherapy, is frequently used in the treatment of head and neck cancers. Implanting radioactive isotopes is a means of not only obtaining high localized radiation doses to the tumor bed, but also minimizing normal tissue injury, since the radiation is delivered only to the area of neoplastic involvement. Brachytherapy has been practiced for many years; 226-Radium needles or 222-Radon sources were used initially [1], but it was not until the last decade that interstitial implants have become more popular, due to several factors. The availability of new isotopes, such as 125-Iodine (^{125}I) for permanent implantation and 192-Iridium (^{192}Ir) for removable procedures, has allowed more complex interstitial procedures to be performed, while the latter isotope, by making afterloading possible, has minimized radiation doses to medical personnel [2–4]. Computerized dosimetry has enabled implants to be pre-planned, so that ideal symmetry and proper placement of sources may be determined prior to the procedure, while post-implantation dosimetry not only allows radiation dose rates to be calculated with removable implants, but also provides a method of correlating results and complications with radiation doses [5]. New implant techniques, to be discussed, have also contributed to our ability to perform these procedures effectively and safely. In this chapter, the common radioactive isotopes in use today will be described, as will the techniques of implantation and the results of treatment of selected primary sites and cervical lymph nodes.

Radioactive isotopes

Table 1 lists several radioactive isotopes suitable for brachytherapy. ^{125}I, ^{192}Ir, and ^{137}Cs 137-Cesium are most commonly used at the present time. 125-Iodine seeds, with a long half-life of 60 days and a weak gamma emission (30 Kev), are

C. Jacobs (ed) Cancers of the head and neck.
© *1987, Martinus Nijhoff Publishers, Boston. ISBN 0–89838–825–2. Printed in the Netherlands.*

94

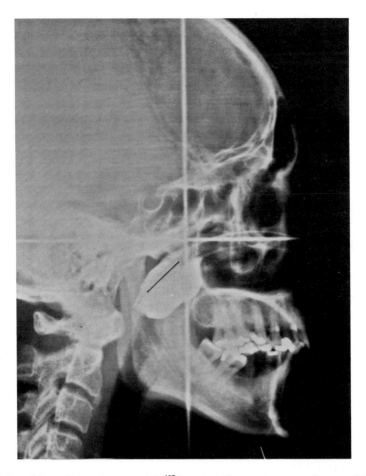

Figure 1. Localizing radiograph, removable ^{137}Cs capsule intracavitary nasopharyngeal boost: the source has been darkened for clarity.

Table 1. Isotopes for brachytherapy

Use	Isotope	Half-life	Energy
Permanent	125-Iodine	60 days	30 Kev
Permanent	222-Radon	3.8 days	1.25 Mev
Permanent	198-Gold	2.7 days	410 Kev
Removable	192-Iridium	74.2 days	340 Kev
Removable	137-Cesium	30 years	660 Kev
Removable	226-Radium	1600 years	1.25 Mev

used primarily for permanent implants. Since the half-life is long, the initial dose rate from ^{125}I is low (7–10 rads per hour), but the total dose to the implant volume after 1 year (six half-lives) may, depending on source strength and spacing, range from 10 to 15 thousand rads. 125-Iodine permanent implants may be used for neoplastic involvement of surgical margins, can be used in the cervical region at the time of radical neck dissection for large lymph node masses, or can be inserted intraoperatively into the pterygoid and/or base skull regions [6–9]. High intensity 125-Iodine seeds, 20–40 mCI/seed, have also been used experimentally as removable implant sources for brain tumors [10], but the most common application of this isotope in the treatment of head and neck cancers has been for permanent implantation, using seeds of approximately 0.5 mCi/activity.

Removable interstitial implants were originally performed with radium needles or capsules, an isotope which could not be easily afterloaded [11]. These procedures now utilize ^{192}Ir seeds, either enclosed in nylon ribbons or in the form of wires. Another isotope used for removable head and neck implantation is ^{137}Cs, which is commonly inserted as an intracavitary capsule. Removable implants have been used for malignancies involving the oral cavity, oropharynx, laryngopharynx, facial skin and lymph nodes [12–15]. Such sites as the nose, nasopharynx (Figure 1), and postoperative cavities (after radical maxillectomy, for example) are implantable via intracavitary routes or by the use of surface applicators or molds (Table 2).

Table 2. Implant sites – head and neck cancer

Permanent – ^{125}I	Removable – ^{192}Ir
1. Neck (and carotid artery)	1. Lip
2. Surgical margins	2. Oral cavity
3. Pterygoids, base skull	Floor of mouth
	Tongue
	Other
	3. Oropharynx
	Tonsil-palate
	Base tongue
	Oropharyngeal walls
	4. Laryngopharynx
	5. Facial skin, nose, pinna, eye
	6. Intracavitary – via molds, plaques, afterloading catheters
	Nasal cavity
	Nasopharynx
	Ear canal
	Post operative (sinuses, etc.)
	7. Interstitial hyperthermia

Primary sites

Oral cavity

Interstitial implants are used either alone or after a course of external beam radiation for oral cavity lesions involving the floor of mouth, tongue, buccal area or, rarely, the retromolar trigone. For T1 lesions or larger but superficial neoplasms, interstitial ^{192}Ir implantation alone, delivering approximately 6000 rads to the tumor volume, is effective treatment and has been the technique of choice in France for many years [16]. Other afterloading techniques, such as trocar-loop and trocar-blind end are also widely used in the treatment of neoplasms involving these sites. With larger floor of mouth neoplasms and with all tongue cancers in a patient with N0 necks, elective cervical irradiation is recommended in addition to interstitial implantation. Pre-implantation irradiation to the primary site of approximately 4500–5000 rads in 5 weeks should precede interstitial implantation, which then delivers another 2500–3000 rads to the tumor bed for larger neoplasms of the oral cavity. Deeply infiltrating, T3 or T4 oral cavity neoplasms, especially those poorly responsive to an initial 5000 rad course of external beam irradiation, may require combined surgical and radiation treatment and may not be suitable for interstitial implant boosts. Skill and judgment are required in selecting patients for interstitial implantation, to minimize such potential risks as mandibular osteoradionecrosis, soft tissue necrosis and ulceration.

Oropharynx

The tonsillo-palatine region, base tongue, and oropharyngeal walls may all be treated by removable 192-Iridium implant boosts. At the Stanford Medical Center since 1975, 50 patients with lesions in these sites (22 with base tongue cancers and 28 with tonsillo-palatine neoplasms) have received such implants.

Base tongue carcinoma
All patients referred to the Stanford Medical Center with newly diagnosed head and neck cancers are seen and examined in a combined modality head and neck tumor board attended by head and neck surgeons, radiation therapists, medical oncologists, dentists, residents, speech pathologists and social workers. These patients are treated and followed by the same multidisciplinary team. Since 1975, 37 operable patients with base tongue carcinomas have been seen, evaluated, and treated at Stanford, 22 by external beam irradiation followed by interstitial implantation, while 15, due to physician preference, underwent primary resection and postoperative irradiation. The AJC stages of these 37 patients, all with squamous carcinomas, are presented in Table 3. Most patients had stage III or

IV neoplasms. The procedures used in the 15 patients treated by surgery varied from partial glossectomy to glossolaryngectomy and all but one of these patients also received a neck dissection (Table 4). The 22 patients treated by radiation therapy and interstitial irradiation received 5000–5500 rads to the primary site, with spinal cord protection after 3800 rads, as well as supplemental low neck irradiation (5000 rads) via a 6 Mev linear accelator at a dose rate of 200 rads per day, five fractions per week, with all fields treated daily.

Two to three weeks after the external beam radiation course, the removable 192-Iridium implant was performed. Prophylactic antibiotics, short course dexamethasone therapy, and a temporary tracheostomy were routinely used. If a persistent cervical lymph node was noted after completion of the external beam radiation course, a radical neck dissection was performed at the time of the ^{192}Ir primary site implant.

Base tongue implantation is a complex procedure, first involving the use of a paired trocar and loop technique through one or both cervical regions at the level of the hyoid bone to ensure adequate irradiation of the pharyngo-epiglottic fold and tonsillo-glossal groove as well as the lateral oropharyngeal wall; by looping this area, the risk of lateral tumor extension from the base tongue to the lateral pharyngeal wall is reduced [13]. Next, multiple trocar pairs are inserted into the base tongue through a submental approach extending anteriorly from the vallecula beyond the circumvallate papillae. After the trocars are positioned, they are

Table 3. Base tongue carcinoma AJC stage – 37 patients

Stage	Surgery – XRT (= 15)	XRT – ^{192}Ir (= 22)
I	o	1
II	2	4
III	9	4
IV	4	13

Table 4. Base tongue carcinoma lymph node therapy – 37 patients

	Surgery – XRT (= 15)	XRT – ^{192}Ir (= 22)
N1, 2, 3	12	14
RND[a]	12	7
Mod. ND[b]	2	0
Neck Failures	8	0
Ipsilateral	5	
Contralateral	3	

[a] RND = radical neck dissection.
[b] Mod. ND = modified neck dissection.

98

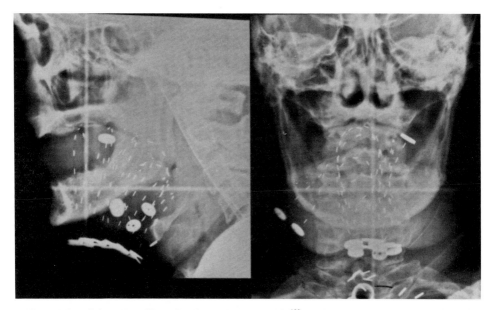

Figure 2. Localizing AP and lateral radiographs, removable ^{192}Ir base tongue and right pharyngo-epiglottic fold implant. Note that ^{192}Ir seeds are placed throughout the base tongue, and extend laterally to the right pharyngeal wall and anteriorly into the oral tongue (T2Nl right base tongue primary cancer).

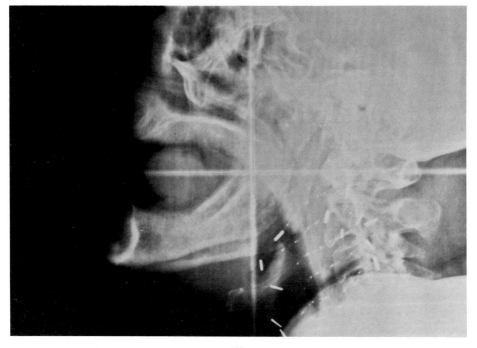

Figure 3. Localizing lateral radiograph, 5 row ^{125}I intraoperative permanent implant.

removed as nylon tubes are pulled into position, forming a 'u-shaped' loop with the free ends emerging through the submental skin. By this multiple pre-planned loop technique, with a spacing of approximately 10 to 15 mm between loops and a distance across each loop of 2.0–2.5 cm, the entire base tongue is implanted as well as the posterior aspect of the oral tongue. If the loop width is insufficient to cover the entire base tongue, additional loops are placed at right angles to also irradiate this area. The ^{192}Ir sources are afterloaded in the Radiation Therapy Division post-operatively. Localizing orthogonal radiographs, which allow computerized dosimetry to be performed, are also obtained at this time (Figure 2). The radiation implant doses delivered in these patients were approximately 2500 rads to a mean volume of 75 cc at 50–75 rads/hour, and 1500 rads to a 1500 cc volume.

The results of treating these patients with base tongue cancers are noted in Table 5. Significantly more patients remain without evidence of disease (NED) in the group treated by irradiation and ^{192}Ir implantation compared to those who received combined surgery and irradiation (77% vs. 27%). There were also twice as many primary site relapses in the surgical group. Significantly fewer neck failures occurred in the 22 irradiated and implanted patients (no relapses vs. eight failures in the surgery-radiation group).

Not only were a higher percentage of patients free of disease in the irradiated and implanted group, but there were also fewer complications and a better functional result in these patients (less sialorrhea, chronic dysphagia and garbled speech). The complications which occured after implantation or surgery are noted in Table 6. The risk of hemorrhage from the lingual artery was approximately 15% in those patients who received irradiation and implantation. The greatest chance of hemorrhage occurring is at the time of implant removal; therefore, either a tracheostomy or endotracheal tube is required during the time of implantation and the cuff must be inflated at the time of source removal to maintain the airway and prevent aspiration if hemorrhage should take place. Three superficial tongue ulcers also occurred in the 22 patients who received radiation therapy

Table 5. Base tongue carcinoma results – 37 patients

	Surgery – XRT (= 15)	XRT – [192]Ir (= 22)	p value
Mean-Fu	37 months	31 months	
NED[a]	4 (27%)	17 (77%)	0.007
Failure			
Tongue	6 (40%)	3 (14%)	n.s.
Neck	8 (53%)	0)	0.0005
Mets[b]	3 (20%)	2 (9%)	n.s.

[a] NED = no evidence of disease.
[b] Mets = metastases.

and implantation, but these all ultimately healed, while a single patient developed mandibular osteoradionecrosis. The combination of external beam irradiation and implantation for base tongue cancers at our institution appears to be at least as effective as resection and postoperative irradiation, while the functional results were superior in the former group.

Tonsillo-palatine implants – 28 patients
The AJC stages of these patients are noted in Table 7. Each of the patients initially received external beam radiation doses to the primary site and neck of approximately 5000 rads in 5 weeks, with a protective spinal cord block inserted after 3800 rads, followed 2–3 weeks later by a ^{192}Ir removable afterloading implant into the site(s) of initial neoplastic involvement. In all patients, the primary site was implanted through an intraoral approach [17]. Curved needles were swaged onto the non-active ends of ^{192}Ir seed-containing nylon ribbons, which were then sewn into the tonsillo-palatine region. The procedures are pre-planned, allowing the ribbons to be inserted into the tumor bed with regular spacing so as to include the area of initial tumor involvement with adequate margins. After the ribbons are sewn into position, the ^{192}Ir seeds are drawn into place by traction on the nylon tubes and secured at the entrance and exit sites by hemostatic clips, at which time excess tubing is trimmed. For all patients with tonsil or tonsillar pillar involvement, the paired trocar and loop technique is then used to implant the tonsillo-glossal groove by a lateral cervical approach similar to that used in the treatment of base tongue carcinoma, incorporating this structure and the adjacent pharyngo-epiglottic fold into the inferior margin of the implant volume. Table 8 lists the results of these procedures in the 28 patients, with a mean follow-up period of 38 months. The primary sites remain controlled in 26 of 28 of these patients (93%). There have been no primary site failures in the 16 individuals with tonsil cancers and only one each in the patients with involvement of either the soft palate or the tonsillar pillars. The one patient with a soft palate cancer who failed locally

Table 6. Base tongue carcinoma complications – 37 patients

Surgery – XRT 9/15 (60%)		XRT – ^{192}Ir 9/22 (41%)	
Dysphagia (tube feedings)	– 6[a]	Tongue ulcer	– 3
Fistula	– 2	Hemorrhage	– 3
Wound infection	– 1	Septicemia	– 1[b]
		ORN	– 1
		Dysphagia	– 1
		(temporary gastrostomy)	

[a] Also impaired speech, sialorrhea, and osteoradionecrosis (1).
[b] Tracheostomy site stenosis.

relapsed on the uvula, which had not been included in the interstitial implant volume. Fifteen of these patients remain alive, while 14 have died, primarily due to the numerous second primary neoplasms which occurred in this group of 28 patients (Table 9). Four of the patients, 14%, have succumbed to second primary malignancies of the esophagus, while three developed other head and neck cancers; miscellaneous neoplasms occurred in three others.

Cervical region

Several brachytherapy techniques (including removable iridium implants, interstitial hyperthermia, or percutaneously or intraoperatively placed 125-Iodine

Table 7. Tonsillo-palatine carcinoma – 28 patients

AJC Stage
I – 4
II – 4
III – 10
IV – 10

Table 8. Tonsillo-palatine carcinoma ^{192}Ir implants – 28 patients (mean follow-up – 38 months).

Primary site	NED[a]
Tonsil 16	13 (81%) – Mets[b] – 1
	Neck – 1
Soft palate – 9	7 (78%) – Neck – 1
	1° – 1
Tonsil pillar – 3	2 (67%) – Neck – 1
Primary controlled: 26/28 (93%)	

[a] NED = no evidence of disease.
[b] Mets = metastases.

Table 9. Tonsillo-palatine carcinoma ^{192}Ir implants – 28 patients

Results			
Alive – 15		Second primaries – 10	
Dead – 13		Esophagus – 4	
Died with	– 4	Head and neck – 3 (floor of mouth 2, tonsil 1)	
2nd primary	– 6	Misc. – 3 (ovary, lung, rectum)	
Intercurrent	– 3		

sources) are used for the treatment of large cervical lymph node masses. At Stanford, we have been interested for several years in the permanent implantation of 125-Iodine sources near or superficial to the carotid artery at the time of resection of large nodal masses. The procedures are performed by sewing # 1 vicryl sutures, which contain regularly spaced and specially inserted ^{125}I seeds, into position over the vessel at the site of tumor removal with pre-planned spacing depending on the desired dose of radiation and the available seed strength. Forty-three patients with massive cervical lymphadenopathy have received such implants; 30 patients were referred following local cervical recurrences, while the 13 other patients with N3 neck masses had no prior treatment. The ^{125}I implant parameters are listed in Table 10. These planar implants, averaging 25–30 cc in volume, have resulted in a local control rate in the implant volume of approximately 80% for both groups (no prior treatment and those with recurrences after prior surgery and/or irradiation). Local control in all head and neck sites was obtained in approximately 50% of the patients. Therefore, increased local control rates have been obtained with combined 125-Iodine seed implants and radical neck dissection compared to neck dissection alone, but these patients with massive cervical lymph node involvement are still at high risk for distant metastases [18].

The complications which occurred after these procedures were primarily ulceration or necrosis of the overlying tissues in approximately 25% of the patients; however, by using ^{125}I seed strengths below 0.50 mCi and implanting volumes less than 25 cc, the risk of ulceration and skin flap loss has been minimized in recent years. If radiation therapy is to be used following ^{125}I seed implantation, the implant volume should be protected by appropriate blocking after approximately 3600 rads have been delivered to that area.

If it is not planned to perform a radical neck dissection, an alternative method of implanting large cervical masses is by the percutaneous use of the trocar and nylon tube ^{192}Ir technique, which can also deliver high radiation doses to the neck via removable sources [19].

Table 10. ^{125}I – suture carrier carotid area implants – 43 patients

Mean	No prior treatment (13 patients)	Prior treatment (surgery and/or XRT) (30 patients)
Implant volume	31.5 cc	25.4 cc
Dose (rads)	16,000	15,600
mCi implanted	19.5	14.5
mCi/seed	0.45	0.41

Dosimetry

At Stanford, implant dosimetry is performed on General Electric treatment planning ([a]) and Vax ([b]) computers. As previously described, a pre-plan program is used routinely for ^{125}I planar implants of the cervical region at the time of radical neck dissection; this program is also used for removable ^{192}Ir implants. Depending on the desired radiation dose, the available radioactive seed strength and the tumor volume, the spacing of the rows of sources is determined by the computer prior to the implant procedure. Post implantation, either at the time of loading the ^{192}Ir seeds or approximately 1 week after the permanent insertion of ^{125}I seeds, orthogonal localizing radiographs are obtained and the seed coordinates are entered into the G.E. computer via a digitizing system. *Iosodose distributions* are obtained in numerous planes through the implant volume. Radiation dose rates or total doses to *volumes* are also calculated, depending on whether the implant is removable or permanent. The volume program, when correlated with the measured implant volume on the orthogonal localizing radiographs, allows isodose contours to be selected to establish the total dose to be delivered for a particular removable implant. This system, which has evolved over many years, has been effective in preventing over or under doses to large portions of the implanted area. When volume data and isodose distributions are both available, the selection of the appropriate radiation dose and the avoidance of over or under dosages, combined with good technique, should ensure the best possible result.

Discussion

Interstitial implantation currently has an important role in the management of head and neck cancers by radiation therapy. High, but relatively safe radiation doses may be delivered to the tumor volume, and although the procedures are complex, the results have been gratifying, especially in cancers involving the oropharynx, oral cavity and the cervical region. It should be stressed that brachytherapy procedures are a team effort and require careful, precise, and skilled technique in the operating room and close cooperation between the surgeon and radiation therapist. Physics support for dosimetry, radiation safety, and localizing procedures is also mandatory. These combined external beam-interstitial implant radiation treatments appear to be as effective as surgery and irradiation and possibly produce even better functional results for patients with squamous carcinomas involving the base tongue.

[a]. General Electric Company, Medical Systems Group, P.O. Box 414, Milwaukee, WI 53201, USA.
[b]. Digital Equipment Corporation, 146 Main Street, Maynard, MA 01754, USA.

104

Other modalities may be used simultaneously with brachytherapy. Since removable implants provide prolonged irradiation of the tumor bed at continuous low dose rates (50 to 100 rads per hour), this may create a favorable situation for concomitant administration of hypoxic cell sensitizing drugs and/or chemotherapeutic agents, but such combined modality treatment is still unproven. In addition, combined interstitial RF or microwave hyperthermia and removable ^{192}Ir head and neck implants have produced excellent short-term tumor regressions. Therefore, interstitial treatment of head and neck cancers has evolved over many years, and at present, with the availability of technical expertise, computerized dosimetry and more useful isotopes and techniques, these procedures not only appear to be effective in producing increased local control rates, but are also relatively safe and complication-free.

References

1. Martin, C.L., Martin, J.A. 1965. Treatment of epithelioma of the lateral oropharynx with low intensity radium needle implants. A.J.R. 93: 7–19.
2. Kim, H., Hilaris, B. 1975. Iodine-125 source in interstitial tumor therapy. A.J.R. 123: 162–169.
3. Vikram, B., Hilaris, B.S., Anderson, L. et al. 1983. Permanent Iodine-125 implants in head and neck cancer. Cancer 51: 1310–1314.
4. Goffinet, D.R., Martinez, A., Pooler, D. et al. 1981. Brachytherapy renaissance. Front. Radiat. Ther. Oncol. 15: 43–57.
5. Sandor, J., Palos, B., Goffinet, D.R. et al. 1979. Dose calculations for planar arrays of ^{192}Ir and ^{125}I seeds for brachytherapy. Appl. Radiol. 8: 41–44.
6. Fee, W.E., Jr., Goffinet, D.R., Fajardo, L.F. et al. 1985. Safety of ^{125}Iodine and ^{192}Iridium implants to the canine carotid artery: preliminary report. Laryngoscope 95: 317–320.
7. Goffinet, D.R., Martinez, A., Fee, W.E. et al. 1983. Intraoperative pterygo-palatine ^{125}I seed implants. Int. J. Radiat. Oncol. Biol. Phys. 9: 103–106.
8. Goffinet, D.R., Martinez, A., Fee, W.E. 1985. ^{125}I vicryl suture implants as a surgical adjuvant in cancer of the head and neck. Int. J. Radiat. Oncol. Biol. Phys. 11: 399–402.
9. Goffinet, D.R., Martinez, A., Pooler, D. 1981. ^{125}I seed implantations as a surgical adjuvant in head and neck cancers. In: Kominierte Chirurgtische und Radiologische Therapie Maligner Tumoren (M. Wannenmacher, ed.). Urban & Schwarzenberg, Munchen, pp. 46-48.
10. Gutin, P.H., Phillips, T.L., Hosobuchi, Y. et al. 1981. Permanent and removable implants for the brachytherapy of brain tumors. Int. J. Radiat. Oncol. Biol. Phys. 7: 1371–1381.
11. Gilbert, F.H., Goffinet, D.R., Dagshaw, M.A. 1975. Carcinoma of the tongue and floor of the mouth: fifteen years' experience with linear accelerator therapy. Cancer 35: 1515–1525.
12. Goffinet, D.R. 1985. Head and neck brachytherapy emphasizing afterloading removable oropharyngeal implants. In: Head and Neck Cancer 1, (P.B. Chreten, M.E. Johns, O.P. Sherd, E.W. Strong, P.W. Ward, B.C. Decker Inc., Philadelphia, pp. 359-364.
13. Goffinet, D.R., Fee, W.E., Jr. Wells, J. et al. 1985. ^{192}Ir pharyngoepiglottic fold interstitial implants. Cancer 55: 941–948.
14. Sealy, R., LeRoux, P.L.M., Hering, E., Buret, E. 1984. The treatment of cancer of the uvula and soft palate with interstitial radioactive wire implants. Int. J. Radiat. Oncol. Biol. Phys. 10: 1951–1955.
15. Syed, A.M.N., Puthawala, A., Fleming, P. et al. 1980. Afterloading interstitial implant in head and neck cancer. Arch. Otolaryngol. 106: 541–546.

16. Pierquin, B., Chassagne, D., Baillet, F., Castro, J.R. 1971. The place of implantation in tongue and floor of the mouth cancer. J.A.M.A. 215: 961–963.
17. Goffinet, D.R., Martinez, A., Palos, B. *et al.* 1977. A method of interstitial tonsillo-palatine implants. Int. J. Radiat. Oncol. Biol. Phys. 2: 155–162.
18. Fee, W.E., Jr., Goffinet, D.R., Paryani, S. *et al.* 1983. Intraoperative Iodine-125 implants: their use in large tumors on the neck attached to the carotid artery. Arch. Otolaryngol. 109: 727–730.
19. Puthawala, A.A., Syed, A.M.N., Neblett, D. *et al.* 1981. The role of afterloading iridium (^{192}Ir) implant in the management of carcinoma of the tongue. Int. J. Radiat. Oncol. Biol. Phys. 7: 407–412.

8. Magnetic resonance imaging of head and neck tumors

KEITH E. KORTMAN, JAMES T. HELSPER, WILSON S. WONG
and WILLIAM G. BRADLEY

Introduction

Effective therapy of head and neck tumors depends on accurate assessment of tumor size, extent, and nodal spread. Physical and endoscopic examination remain the foundation of the clinical staging procedure. They are the most accurate methods of assessing mucosal involvement by tumor. Deep extension of tumor cannot be visualized directly, but can often be inferred by alterations in mucosal contours. Direct or indirect visualization of the vocal cords remains the most effective method of evaluating laryngeal function. In addition, physical examination is the easiest method of evaluating lymphadenopathy, although it is somewhat limited by node location and interobserver variation.

The advent and evolution of X-ray computed tomography (CT) has had a significant impact on the staging process. It allows evaluation of mucosal surfaces which may not be accessible to the endoscopist, and is a more effective method of evaluating submucosal deep extension of tumor. It also permits accurate assessment of bony and cartilagenous structures. In addition, as compared to physical examinination, CT is a more reliable and reproducible method of assessing lymphadenopathy, as it more effectively demonstrates deep nodes, small superficial nodes, necrosis within normal sized nodes, and vascular fixation by metastatic adenopathy.

Magnetic resonance imaging (MRI) is a new imaging modality which, although only recently introduced, is now being used to compliment or supplant CT in the evaluation of head and neck tumors [1, 2]. This method is similar to X-ray CT, in that it produces cross-sectional images of the body with high spatial resolution. However, there are a number of significant differences between the two modalities, with MRI offering a number of significant advantages. It does not require the use of ionizing radiation or contrast injection. Images can be obtained in any of the three orthogonal planes without altering the patient position. There are minimal artifacts from dental fillings or metallic foreign bodies, and there are no beam hardening artifacts from dense bone, such as are seen with CT in the

C. Jacobs (ed) Cancers of the head and neck.
© *1987, Martinus Nijhoff Publishers, Boston. ISBN 0–89838–825–2. Printed in the Netherlands.*

posterior fossa. The contrast resolution of MRI is greater than that of CT, and this property is largely responsible for the greater tissue characterization capability of the former modality.

CT maintains some advantages over MRI, including better spatial resolution and more detailed depiction of bone and calcified cartilage. Many investigators feel that MRI is less sensitive than CT in evaluation of cervical adenopathy. Unlike CT, the time required to generate an MR image is on the order of minutes rather than seconds, and therefore the scans are more subject to degradation by patient motion. In addition, 'dynamic' or phonation scanning cannot be performed. The incidence of claustrophobia is greater with MR than with CT, and occasionally precludes evaluation. Finally, there is a relative limitation of MR scanner availability, and for some patients this factor, combined with the relatively high cost of an MR examination, place significant limitations on the diagnostic workup.

Basic principles of MRI

X-ray CT is based on the principle of differential attenuation of an X-ray beam by orbital electrons. Differences in attenuation (or CT density) are based only on the concentration of electrons within the scanning volume. MRI is based on a more complex interaction between the nuclei of certain chemical species and radio frequency (RF) waves in the presence of an externally applied magnetic field. Clinical imaging is currently largely limited to the study of hydrogen atoms, or protons.

The nucleus of the hydrogen atom is a single, spinning proton. Since spinning, charged particles generate small magnetic fields, the protons behave like small bar magnets. When placed in an external magnetic field, the protons flip slowly back and forth between alignment with (parallel) or against (antiparallel) the field as they undergo random thermal collisions. If the proton is exposed to a radiowave at a particular frequency, it will rapidly flip back and forth, or resonate, between the two alignments. This frequency is determined entirely by the local value of the magnetic field near the proton. Protons in stronger magnetic fields resonate at higher frequencies. During resonance the sample absorbs and re-radiates the radiowaves, which can be detected by an antenna and computer-processed into an MR image [3].

The relationship between the radiofrequency (RF) and the magnetic field strength allows the signal to be spatially localized and an image to be formed. The net magnetic field is made to vary with position by superimposing smaller 'gradient' magnetic fields on the homogeneous main magnetic field. Protons resonating in a position-dependent magnetic field thus have specific frequencies which depend on their exact position in the sample [3].

The strength of the MR signal depends on the hydrogen density and on the chemical environment which is characterized by the 'magnetic relaxation times'

T1 and T2 [4]. Because the MR signal is so much weaker than an X-ray signal, the signal acquisition process must be repeated many times. The amount of recovery which occurs between each repetition is indicated by the T1 relaxation time. The amount of time allowed for this recovery to occur is given by one of the programmable sequence parameters, the repetition time (TR). Following recovery, the next pulsing sequence is initiated with a 90° pulse, after which time the signal then decays with an exponential time constant T2. A portion of this decaying signal can be captured by refocusing the signal with a 180° pulse. The refocused signal is called a 'spin echo'. The time allowed for decay to occur prior to measurement of the spin echo is another programmable sequence parameter, the echo delay time (TE).

Decreasing TR increases the amount of T1-weighting in the image; increasing TR allows differences in proton density to be seen. Increasing TE increases the amount of T2-weighting in the image; decreasing TE (at long TR) results in a proton density image. When the T1 and T2 differences between a lesion and the surrounding normal tissue are known, optimal selection of the sequence parameters TR and TE is possible and contrast between lesion and normal tissue is optimized [5].

Flowing blood has a variable appearance on MR depending on the pulsing sequence and rate and direction of flow. Decreased signal is seen with high velocity and turbulence. Increased signal is noted as unsaturated protons first enter the imaging volume ('flow related enhancement'). Increased signal is also seen on even echo images (when multiple echoes are acquired) during slow laminar flow

Table 1. Signal intensities of normal tissues in the extracranial head and neck

Tissue	Intensity on T1-weighted[a] image	Intensity on T2-weighted[b] image	Basis of intensity pattern
Cortical bone	low	low	decreased proton density
Calcified cartilage	low	low	decreased proton density
Air	very low	very low	decreased proton density
Flowing blood	very low[c]	very low[c]	flow void
Muscle	intermediate low	intermediate low	long T1, short T2
Ligament	intermediate low	intermediate low	long T1, short T2 decreased proton density
Fibro-cartilage	intermediate low	intermediate low	long T1, short T2 decreased proton density
Lymphatic/glandular tissue	intermediate	intermediate high	long T2
Fat/bone marrow	high	intermediate high	short T1

[a] TR = 0.5–1.0 s, TE = 15–40 ms.
[b] TR = 2.0–2.5 s, TE = 50–80 ms.
[c] Exceptions to the pattern are frequently observed due to other flow-related phenomena.

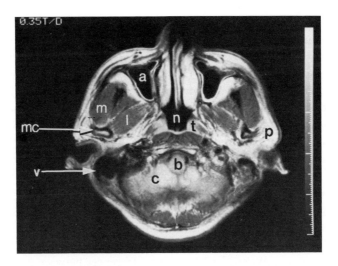

Figure 1. Normal MRI section at the level of the nasopharynx. Local variations in tissue signal intensity reflect differences in proton density and magnetic relaxation times. Air and cortical bone appear dark, reflecting low proton concentration. Vascular structures are also black due to flow-related signal void. Subcutaneous tissues, the parotid glands, and medullary bone appear bright, reflecting their high fat content. Muscular structures have an intermediate/low signal intensity, while lymphoid tissue and brain are intermediate/high in intensity. a = maxillary antrum, m = masseter muscle, l = lateral pterygoid muscle, p = parotid gland, ms = mandibular condyle, v = jugular vein, t = pharyngeal tonsils, n = nasopharyngeal airway, b = brainstem, c = cerebellum.

due to a rephasing phenomenon [6]. Thus, veins and dural sinuses will appear bright on even echo images.

The normal intensity of various anatomic structures will vary depending on the pulsing sequence and sequence parameters utilized, but certain generalizations can be made (Table I). For spin echo imaging, intensity (I) can be expressed by the formula

$$I = H \ f(v) \ [e^{-TR/T1}] \ [1 - e^{-TE/T2}]$$

where H = proton density, f(v) is a function of flow, e is the natural logarithm base, TR is the repetition time, TE is the echo delay time, and T1 and T2 are the longitudinal and transverse relaxation times, respectively.

In keeping with this, any substance with a low concentration of protons will have a low signal intensity. Biologic examples include cortical bone, calcified cartilage, and air within the airway or the paranasal sinuses. Blood vessels will also have a low signal intensity, by virtue of the flow phenomena described above. Muscle, ligamentous structures and fibrocartilage will have an intermediate low signal intensity, reflecting the long T1 and relatively short T2 relaxation times of these structures. Normal lymphathatic and glandular tissues will have an intermediate high signal intensity, due to relatively longer T2 relaxation times. Fat

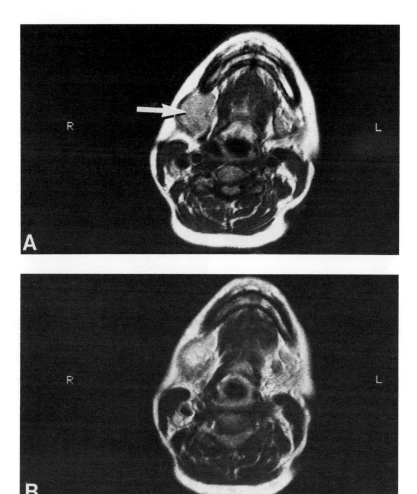

Figure 2. Submandibular gland carcinoma. (A) On a mildly T1-weighted image (TR = 1.0 s, TE = 40 ms), a right submandibular gland mass (arrow) has a signal intensity intermediate between that of muscle and fat. (B) With increased T2-weighted (TR = 2.0 s, TE = 60 ms), the mass increases in intensity.

within fascial planes or marrow cavities will appear bright, as it possesses short T1 and long T2 relaxation times. The normal appearance of various tissues is illustrated in Figure 1.

Pathologic lesions may have a wide range of signal intensities, depending on the composition of the tissue (Table 2). The intensity of solid tumors, both benign and malignant, will be between that of muscle and fat, and will increase with greater T2-weighting of the pulsing sequence (Figure 2). Inflammatory and granulation tissue may have a similar appearance, i.e., it is not possible to distinguish malignancy from infection or acute/subacute postoperative change on

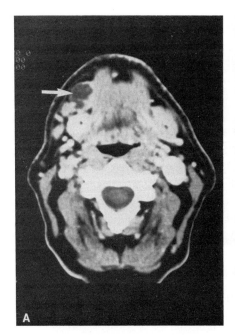
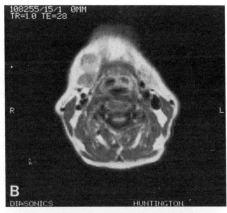
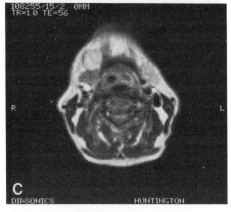

Figure 3. Malignant adenopathy. (A) This patient had an advanced carcinoma of the tongue and extensive right neck adenopathy. This contrast enhanced CT section demonstrates irregular decreased density within a large submandibular node (arrow), indicating malignant invasion and central necrosis. (B) On a mildly T-1-weighted (TR = 1.0 s, TE = 28 ms) image, the node is intermediate in intensity. (C) On a more T2-weighted second echo image (TR = 1.0 s, TE = 56 ms), the intensity of the node increases significantly.

Table 2. Signal intensity of pathologic tissues

Tissue	Intensity on T1-weighted image	Intensity on T2-weighted image	Basis of intensity pattern
Solid neoplasms	intermediate low	intermediate high	long T1, long T2
Granulation tissue	intermediate low	intermediate high	long T1, long T2
Chronic fibrosis	intermediate low	intermediate low	decreased proton dentity
Cyst with pure fluid	low	very high	very long T1, very long T2
Cyst with proteinaceous fluid	intermediate low	high	long T1, long T2
Mucous	intermediate low	high	long T1, long T2
Subacute-subchronic hemorrhage	very high	high	very short T1, long T2

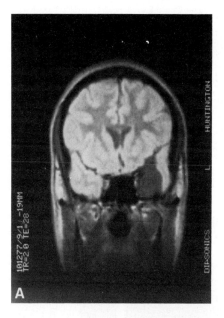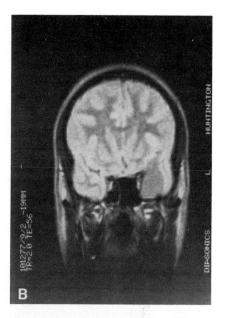

Figure 4. Pure cyst. (A) A left temporal arachnoid cyst appears hypointense on a first echo image (TR = 2.0 s, TE = 28 ms). (B) On a more T2-weighted second echo image TR = 2.0 s, TE = 56 ms), the intensity of the cyst fluid increases significantly. Note the similar signal intensity pattern of intraventricular CSF.

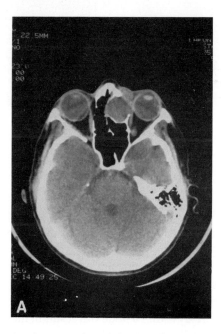

Figure 5. (A) Axial CT section demonstrating a left ethmoid mucocoele extending into the medial canthus.

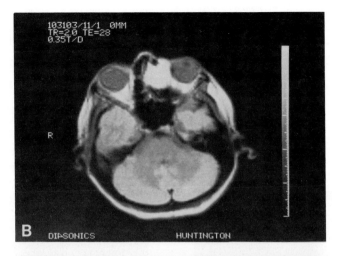

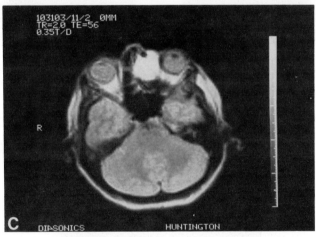

Figure 5. (B) On a corresponding MR image with sequence parameters identical to those used in Figure 4, the lesion is markedly hyperinstense, reflecting the high protein content of inspissated sinus secretions (TR = 2.0 s, TE = 28 ms). (C) The lesion remains hyperintense on the more T2-weighted second echo image (TR = 2.0 s, TE = 56 ms).

the basis of tissue signal intensities alone. Chronic fibrosis will have a low signal intensity on all pulsing sequences.

Measured T1 and T2 values of malignant lymph nodes have been shown to be greater than the values of normal lymphoid tissue *in vitro* [7]. *In vivo*, however, there is sufficient overlap of signal intensity, such that one must largely rely on size criteria. Central necrosis within a node will result in increased signal intensity on T2-weighted images (Figure 3), and when recognized is a fairly reliable indicator of malignancy. Cystic lesions are easily recognized as such on MR

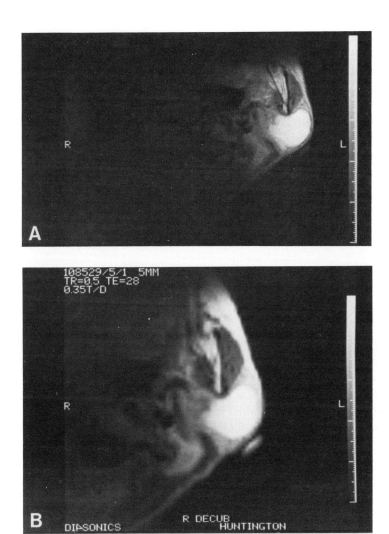

Figure 6. (A) This image was obtained with a radio-frequency coil applied directly to the surface of the parotid gland. An intraparotid hemorrhagic cyst appears markedly hyperintense on this mildly T2-weighted image (TR = 2.0 s, TE = 28 ms). (B) The cyst remains hyperintense on a moderately T1-weighted (TR = 0.5 s, TE = 28 ms) image due to the presence of paramagnetic methemaglobin.

examinations. Cyst fluid with a low protein content (0–10 mg %) has markedly prolonged T1 and T2 relaxation times, appearing dark on T1-weighted images and bright on heavily T2-weighted images (Figure 4). Increased protein content results in T1 shortening and increased intensity on mild to moderate T2-weighted exams (Figure 5). Biologic examples of proteinaceous fluid include inflammatory fluid in the mastoid air cells and mucous within the paranasal sinuses.

Subacute hemorrhage (days to months old) will appear markedly hyperintense on all pulsing sequences secondary to the paramagnetic properties of methemoglobin, a blood breakdown product (Figure 6). Chronic hemorrhage may lead to deposition of hemosiderin, which causes T2 shortening and decreased signal intensity.

To optimize lesion conspicuity, intensity differences between normal and abnormal tissue must be maximized. Tumor and fat are best differentiated on T1-weighted (short TR, short TE) sequences, while tumor and muscle are best distinguished on T2-weighted (long TR, long TE) sequences. Within the temporal bone or paranasal sinuses, tumor can be distinguished from mucous or inflammatory tissue on T2-weighted sequences. In general, an initial MRI examination should include both T1- and T2-weighted sequences.

Clinical imaging

Skull base

CT and MRI are complimentary modalities in the evaluation of skull base lesions [8], although many investigators feel that MRI is the more effective modality overall. CT is superior in demonstrating bone erosion, but may be limited by a number of technical factors. CT definition of soft tissue lesions in the posterior fossa is often limited by beam hardening artifacts. Subtle intra- or extra-cranial extension of a skull base lesion may be difficult to demonstrate on CT, due to the 'partial volume averaging' of bone and soft tissue within the same axial section. Direct coronal CT sections may be acquired by tilting the scanning gantry with the patient's neck hyperextended. This requires a moderate amount of patient cooperation and results in some degree of discomfort. Such an examination is often difficult or impossible in older patients, particularly those with limited neck extension secondary to degenerative disc disease. Even in cooperative patients, spray artifacts from dental fillings may produce significant image degradation.

MRI is not limited by artifacts from beam hardening or dental fillings. Direct coronal and sagittal sections can be obtained with the patient lying supine and comfortably. The bony skull base yields little MR signal, and therefore bone erosion or destruction is not demonstrated directly. However, bone changes can be inferred from the location and extent of the soft tissue abnormality, which is conspicuously shown (Figure 7).

At our institution and others [9], MRI is the modality of choice in the evaluation of suspected acoustic neuromas. Thin slice (3–5 mm), axial sections routinely demonstrate the course and caliber of the 7th and 8th nerves within the internal auditory canal, such that completely intracanalicular tumors, 2–3 mm in size, are easily recognized (Figure 8). Tumor extension into the porus acousticus and

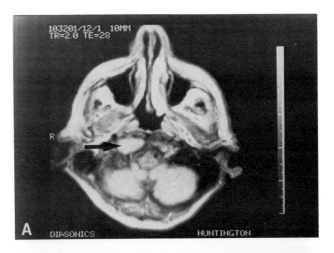

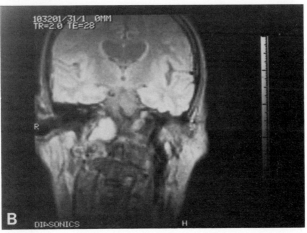

Figure 7. Skull base metastasis. (A) This patient had known metastatic prostate carcinoma and presented with a right twelfth nerve paresis. The transaxial MR image demonstrates an oval soft tissue mass (arrow) involving the right side of the clivus in the expected position of the hypoglossal canal (TR = 2.0 s, TE = 28 ms). (B) The longitudinal extent of the tumor is better appreciated on the direct coronal image (TR = 2.0 s, TE = 28 ms).

cerebellopontine angle cistern is readily identified. Neuromas of other cranial nerves are less common, but can be identified by their characteristic location and secondary fatty atrophy of the muscles innervated by the affected nerve (Figure 9). Both primary and metastatic tumors of the skull base are well demonstrated by MRI. The signal intensity of these lesions is greater than that of normal muscle or brain on T2-weighted images, but nonspecific with respect to tumor type. Coronal and/or sagittal scans are often helpful in demonstrating intracranial extension (Figure 10).

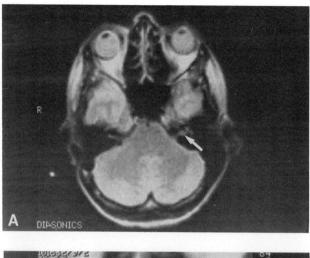

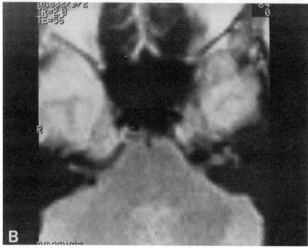

Figure 8. Intracanalicular acoustic neuroma. (A) An axial MR image demonstrates a three mm bulbous mass (arrow) involving the 8th nerve within the internal auditory canal (TR = 2.0 s, TE = 56 ms). (B) Magnified image.

Glomus tumors appear as irregular high intensity masses in characteristic locations, most frequently the jugular foramen or middle ear (Figure 11). Jugular vein occlusion and/or slow flow may result in alterations of normal flow-related intensity patterns, as low intensity flow void is replaced by high intensity thrombus or paradoxical high signal on even-numbered spin echos. Normal variations in flow patterns may mimic these changes, and a specific diagnosis relies on

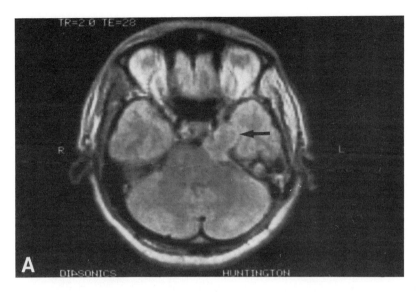

Figure 9. Fifth nerve neuroma. (A) A lobulated isointense mass (arrow) can be seen within the cavernous sinus and the region of Meckel's cave (TR = 2.0 s, TE = 28 ms).

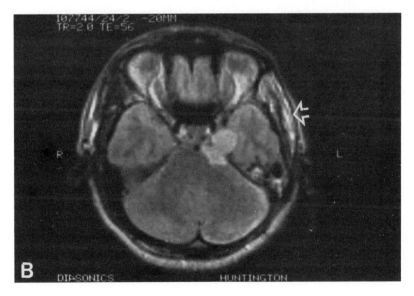

Figure 9. Fifth nerve neuroma. (B) The mass appears hyperintense on a more T2-weighted second echo image TR = 2.0 s, TE = 56 ms). Note the asymmetric high intensity within the left temporalis muscle (open arrow). This is due to fatty atrophy.

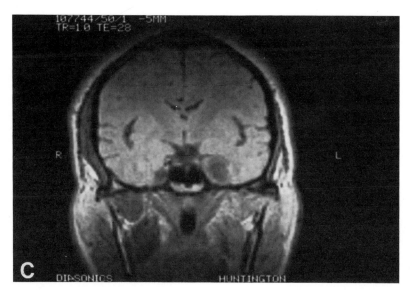

Figure 9. Fifth nerve neuroma. (C) On a mildly T1-weighted coronal image, the mass (arrow) appears hypointense. The left sided muscles of mastication are all more intense than those on the right, again secondary to fatty atrophy of structures innervated by the fifth nerve.

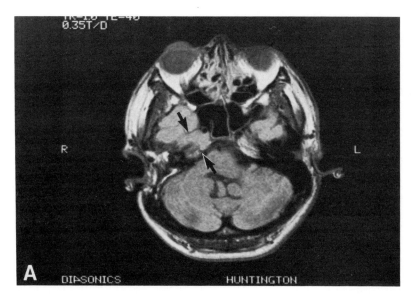

Figure 10. Chondrosarcoma of the skull base. (A) This patient presented with right facial pain and numbness. A mildly T1-weighted axial image demonstrates an expansile and destructive mass (arrowheads) in the right petrous apex, extending into the temporal fossa (TR = 1.0 s, TE = 40 ms).

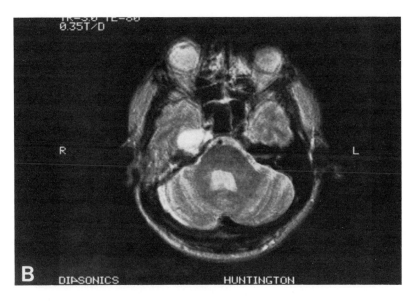

Figure 10. Chondrosarcoma of the skull base. (B) A heavily T2-weighted mass, although slightly degraded by motion, more conspicuously demonstrates the mass, which now appears moderately hyperintense (TR = 3.0 s, TE = 80 ms).

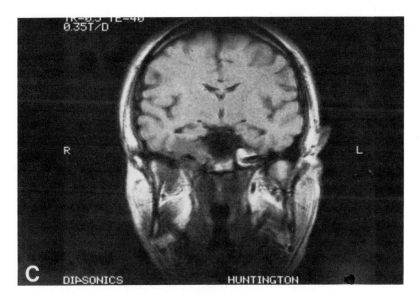

Figure 10. Chondrosarcoma of the skull base. (C) A moderately T1-weighted coronal image effectively demonstrates the tumor's intracranial extent (TR = 0.5 s, TE = 40 ms).

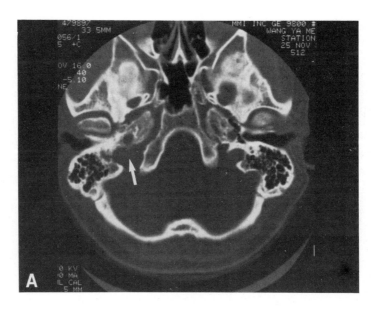

Figure 11. Glomus jugulare tumor. (A) This patient presented with pulsatile tinnitus. The axial CT section with bone window settings demonstrates irregular erosion of the right jugular fossa (arrow).

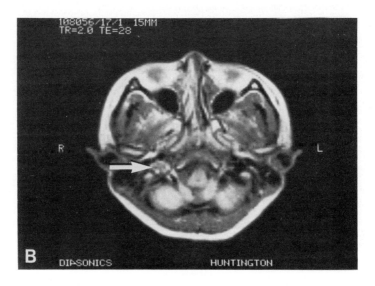

Figure 11. Glomus jugulare tumor. (B) On a corresponding MR image, the mass (arrow) appears heterogeneous with an intensity similar to brain parenchyma (TR = 2.0 s, TE = 28 ms).

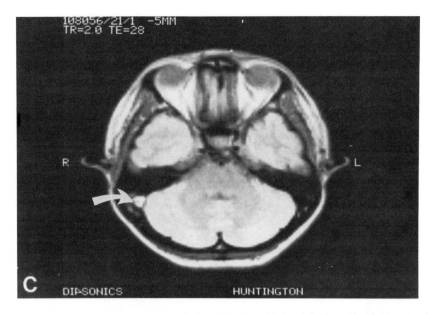

Figure 11. Glomus jugulare tumor. (C) Occlusion of the sigmoid sinus is indicated by high intraluminal signal intensity (curved arrow) (TR = 2.0 s, TE = 28 ms).

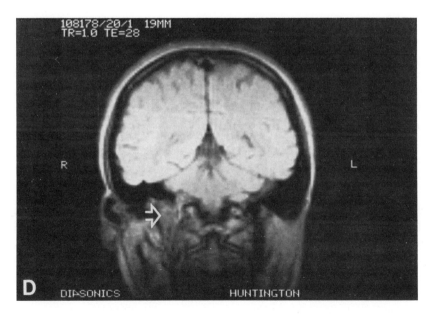

Figure 11. Glomus jugulare tumor. (D) On a direct coronal section, the tumor (open arrow) can be seen extending longitudinally within the jugular canal. Note the patent low intensity jugular vein on the left side (TR = 1.0 s, TE = 28 ms).

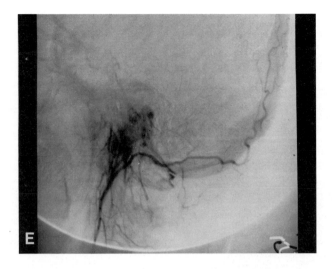

Figure 11. Glomus jugulare tumor. (E) An external carotid arteriogram demonstrates the vascular nature of the lesion.

demonstration of a soft tissue mass with bone destruction and/or confirmation by angiography.

Temporal bone pathology often produces hearing loss. Conductive hearing loss is best evaluated by high resolution CT, as congenital and inflammatory abnormalities of the middle and inner ear are optimally demonstrated by thin slice 'bone-target' sections. Because of the efficiency of MRI in demonstrating acoustic neuromas, it is the modality of choice in evaluation of sensorineural hearing loss.

Nasopharynx

In evaluation of suspected nasopharyngeal carcinoma, the goals of imaging are to define the degree of submucosal infiltration and the extent of metastatic spread to lymph nodes. Deep extension can be demonstrated by CT, but this modality may be limited by artifacts from adjacent bone or dental fillings. Furthermore, tumor and muscle appear isodense on CT, and may be difficult to differentiate. Retropharyngeal nodes are difficult to separate from the adjacent prevertebral musculature.

MRI is ideally suited to the evaluation of the nasopharynx [10]. It yields high contrast between tumor, pharyngeal musculature, and fat in the parapharyngeal

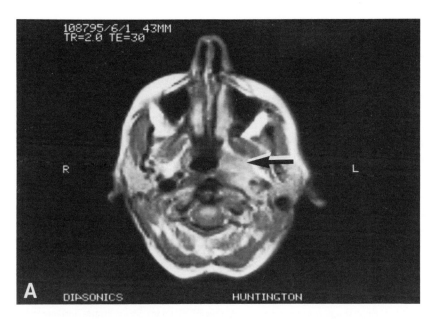

Figure 12. Nasopharyngeal carcinoma. (A) This woman presented with left pharyngeal pain and cranial nerve dysfunction. A mildly T2-weighted axial image demonstrates a mass (arrow) in the left nasopharynx extending laterally into the parapharyngeal space (TR = 2.0 s, TE = 30 ms).

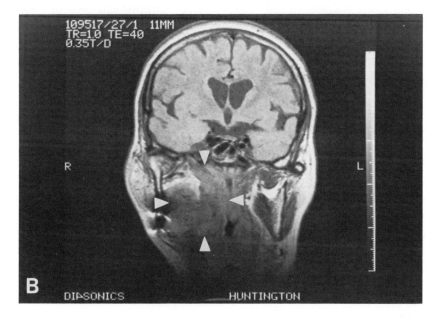

Figure 12. Nasopharyngeal carcinoma. (B) A different patient with a very large right-sided nasopharyngeal carcinoma. A T1-weighted (TR = 1.0 s, TE = 40 ms) coronal section effectively demonstrates the longitudinal extent of the mass (arrowheads). Low intensity artifacts along the right mandible are due to surgical clips.

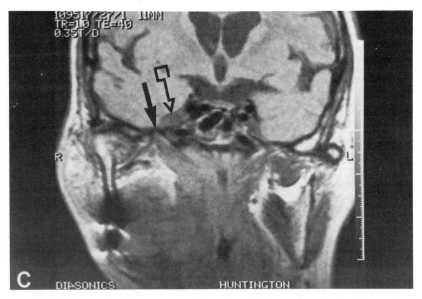

Figure 12. Nasopharyngeal carcinoma. (C) A magnified image demonstrates intracranial tumor extension through the foramen rotundum (closed arrow) and into the cavernous sinus (boxed arrow).

space (Figure 12). Extension of nasopharyngeal malignancies beyond the pharyngobasilar fascia is conspicuously demonstrated. Superior extension of tumor to the skull base is readily identified on coronal images, as is intracranial tumor spread. High intensity retropharyngeal nodes can be easily distinguished from the low intensity of adjacent prevertebral musculature. Tumors arising in the parapharangeal space or infratemporal fossa are also well demonstrated (Figure 13).

Oropharynx, tongue, and floor of mouth

Here, as in other regions of the upper aerodigestive tract, the role of imaging is not to make a specific diagnosis. This is most frequently accomplished by thin needle biopsy in the office or clinic. The goals of imaging are to determine the extent of the primary tumor and the presence of associated adenopathy. MRI and CT compliment each other in the evaluation of oral cavity lesions, and both are utilized routinely at our institution. Both modalities are effective in showing the extent of lesions in the oropharynx and floor of mouth (Figure 14), although CT better demonstrates tumor involvement of the mandible. Tongue tumors are most conspicuously demonstrated on T2-weighted MR images (Figure 15). With respect to surgical planning, tumor extension across the midline of the tongue and the status of the lingual arteries and hypoglossal nerves are readily assessed. Coronal MR sections will demonstrate inferior extension into the hypopharynx and supraglottic larynx. CT is superior in demonstrating cervical adenopathy.

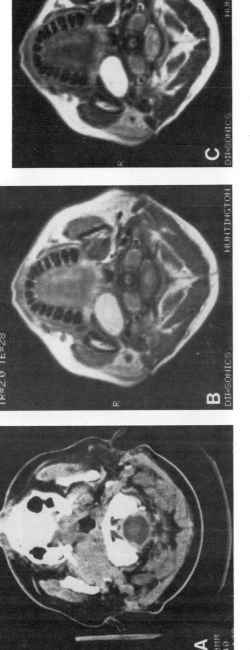
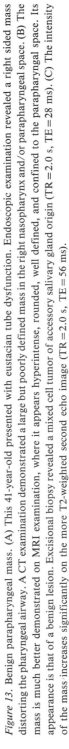

Figure 13. Benign parapharyngeal mass. (A) This 41-year-old presented with eustacian tube dysfunction. Endoscopic examination revealed a right sided mass distorting the pharyngeal airway. A CT examination demonstrated a large but poorly defined mass in the right nasopharynx and/or parapharyngeal space. (B) The mass is much better demonstrated on MRI examination, where it appears hyperintense, rounded, well defined, and confined to the parapharyngeal space. Its appearance is that of a benign lesion. Excisional biopsy revealed a mixed cell tumor of accessory salivary gland origin (TR = 2.0 s, TE = 28 ms). (C) The intensity of the mass increases significantly on the more T2-weighted second echo image (TR = 2.0 s, TE = 56 ms).

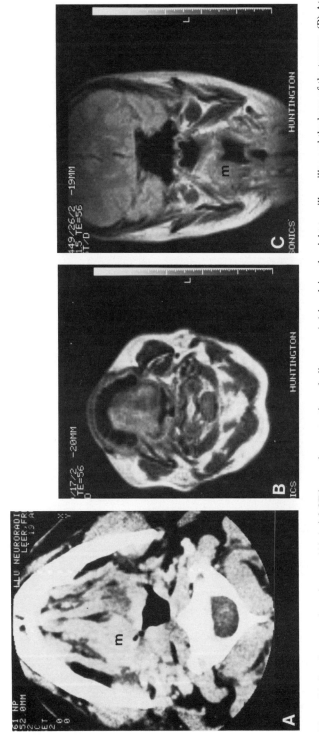

Figure 14. Oropharyngeal carcinoma. (A) Axial CT image demonstrating a bulky mass (m) involving the right tonsillar pillar and the base of the tongue. (B) At a sligthly higher level, an MR image demonstrates hyperintense tumor extension into the right side of the mobile tongue (TR = 1.0 s, TE = 56 ms). (C) Longitudinal extension of the mass (m) along the posterior pharyngeal wall is well demonstrated on this coronal section (TR = 1.5 s, TE = 56 ms).

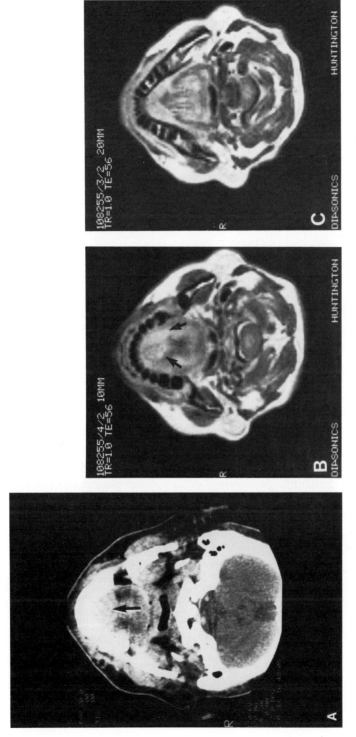

Figure 15. Tongue carcinoma. (A) This patient presented with an ulcerated mass in the anterior tongue. A contrast enhanced CT suggested a hyperdense lesion anteriorly (arrow), but the image was degraded by beam hardening artifact. (B) The extent of the tumor (arrowheads) within the mobile tongue is much more clearly demonstrated on the corresponding MR image (TR = 1.0 s, TE = 56 ms). (C) Slightly more inferior section demonstrating involvement of the myohyoid muscles.

Hypopharynx and larynx

CT has an established role in the evaluation of hypopharyngeal and laryngeal malignancies. It accurately demonstrates submucosal extension, cartilaginous involvement, and cervical adenopathy. Two properties of CT make it particularly effective in this region. The first is the ability to do thin section (3–5 mm) imaging while preserving a high level of signal to noise. Thus, small contiguous structures such as the true and false vocal cords can be depicted on separate CT sections, and involvement of these structures by contiguous tumor can be readily demonstrated. This thin slice capability has obvious implications in surgical planning, i.e., total laryngectomy vs. conservation procedure. A second advantage is the short CT scan time (3–5 s/slice), minimizing artifacts related to patient motion. Patients with laryngeal malignancies often have copious airway secretions, and may need to swallow or cough frequently. With few exceptions, such movement does not significantly degrade the CT examination.

MRI is more limited in both regards. A decrease in slice thickness below 5 mm leads to significant reduction in signal-to-noise and resolving capability. To some degree, this may be offset by an application of surface coils, i.e., RF coils applied to the surface of the neck which allow more detailed examination of superficial structures [11, 12]. Surface coil technology is evolving rapidly, but currently optimized MR spatial resolution remains less than that achieved by CT.

Patient motion is a more significant problem. CT images are obtained slice by slice, with time alloted between slices for cooling of the X-ray tube. Consecutive MR images are obtained simultaneously, i.e., the time required to obtain an entire sequence of slices is also the time required to produce a single image. While overall CT and MR imaging times are comparable (10–30 min), the time required to produce a single image is orders of magnitude greater with MR than with CT. For this reason, coughing, swallowing, or any other patient motion leads to significant degradation of the MR images.

While MR accurately depicts tumor invasion of marrow fat within the laryngeal cartilages, tumor involvement of densely calcified cartilage is much more evident on CT. As previously mentioned, CT is also more effective in the demonstration of cervical adenopathy.

For these reasons, at our institution, CT remains the modality of choice in the evaluation of laryngeal or hypopharyngeal malignancies, with MRI used as an adjunct study when indicated. Direct coronal MR images accurately demonstrate infra-, supra-, or transglottic tumor extension, (Figure 16) and sagittal images can be used to assess the pre-epiglottic space and anterior commissure.

Benign neck lesions can be effectively evaluated with either modality. Sagittal MR images are particularly effective in the evaluation of midline lesions, such as thyroglossal duct cysts (Figure 17).

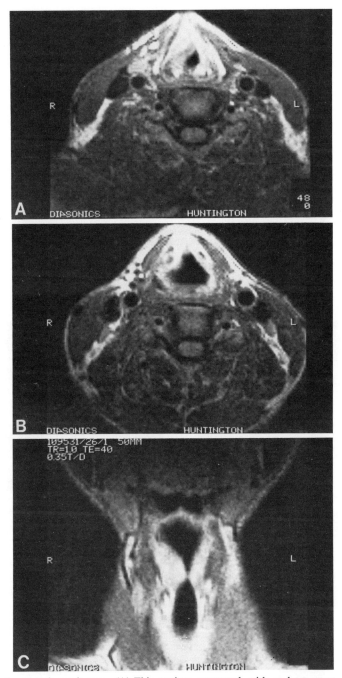

Figure 16. Laryngeal carcinoma. (A) This patient presented with a hoarseness. Endoscopic examination revealed a right glottic mass and a mild vocal cord paresis. An axial image at the level of the cords and obtained with a surface coil demonstrated a relatively bulky mass involving the right true cord and extending through the anterior commissure across the midline (TR = 0.5 s, TE = 40 ms). (B) At a slightly higher level superior tumor extension is manifested as thickening of the right aryepiglottic fold. (C) A direct coronal section verified supraglottic tumor extension (TR = 1.0 s, TE = 40 ms).

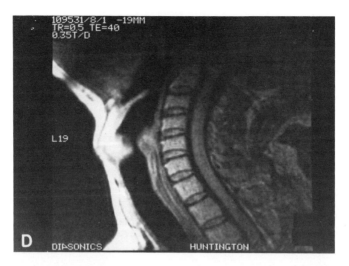

Figure 16. Laryngeal carcinoma. (D) The anterior commissure involvement is graphically depicted on this midline sagittal image (TR = 0.5 s, TE = 40 ms).

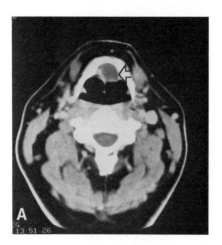 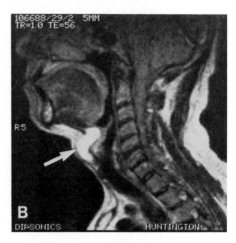

Figure 17. Thyroglossal duct cyst. (A) A CT section at the level of the hyoid bone reveals a low density midline mass (open arrow), the location and appearance of which are typical of a thyroglossal duct cyt. (B) The longitudinal course of the cyst (closed arrow) is graphically demonstrated on the sagittal MR image (TR = 1.0 s, TE = 56 ms).

Salivary glands

More than 75% of salivary gland tumors occur in the parotid gland. Unlike other head and neck regions, where squamous cell carcinomas predominate, salivary gland pathology is varied. A tissue diagnosis is usually obtained via fine needle biopsy. The role of imaging prior to biopsy or surgical excision is to determine

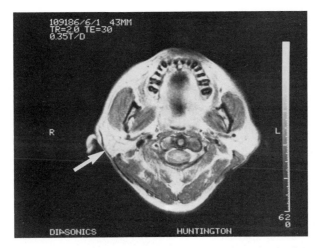

Figure 18. Normal facial nerve. Within the high intensity right parotid gland (arrow), the lower intensity facial nerve can be seen coursing from posteromedial to anterolateral, giving off several branches into the substance of the gland (TR = 2.0 s, TE = 30 ms).

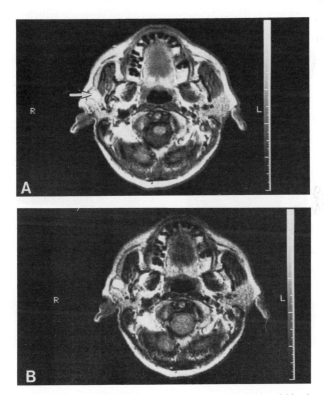

Figure 19. (A) A slightly hyperintense rounded mass (arrow) can be seen within the anterior aspect of the superficial lobe of the right parotid gland (TR = 1.0 s, TE = 40 ms). (B) The contrast between mass and normal gland increases on the more T2-weighted second echo image (TR = 1.0 s, TE = 80 ms).

the exact location and extent of tumor, i.e., intra- vs. extra-parotid, superficial vs. deep lobe. Both CT and MRI are effective in demonstrating these lesions. MRI may have a slight advantage in its ability to determine tumor location with respect to the facial nerve, which can be frequently recognized as a linear or branching low intensity structure within the higher intensity substance of the parotid gland (Figure 18). With CT, the plane of the facial nerve is approximated by the location of the enhancing retromandibular vein, and therefore tumors between the vein and the nerve may be falsely localized to the superficial lobe. MR signal intensities of various salivary gland tumors overlap, but mixed cell tumors appear more intense than other lesions on T2-weighted images (Figure 19).

Paranasal sinuses

In the evaluation of mass lesions within the paranasal sinuses, MRI and CT play complimentary roles. Nearly all soft tissue lesions within a sinus will have similar CT densities, and therefore it is difficult to differentiate inflammatory or obstructive change from tumor. This distinction can often be made with MRI (Figure 20).

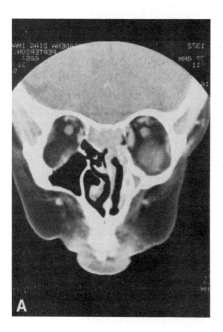 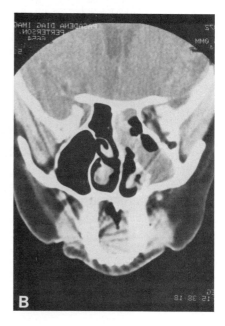

Figure 20. Sinus carcinoma. (A) This patient presented with facial pain and bloody sinus discharge. A direct coronal CT section demonstrates abnormal soft tissue density within the left and right ethmoid air cells and the left nasal cavity. (B) On a more posterior section, abnormal soft tissue density is seen within the left sphenoid sinus and extending inferiorly through the sinus floor and ostium of the left maxillary sinus into the maxillary antrum.

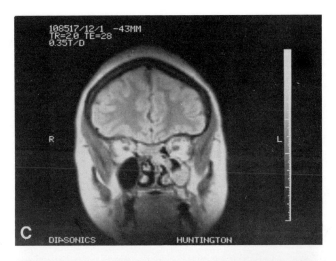

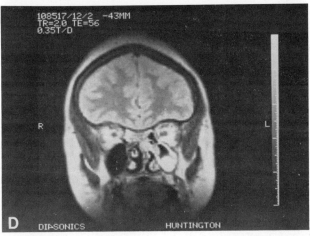

Figure 20. Sinus carcinoma. (C) At a level between A and B, a coronal MR image demonstrates similar findings (TR = 2.0 s, TE = 28 ms). (D) With increased T2-weighting (TR = 2.0 s, TE = 56 ms), hyperintense sinus secretions within the inferolateral aspect of the antrum can be distinguished from less intense tumor at the ostium. Excisional biopsy revealed an adenocarcinoma.

CT more effectively demonstrates expansion, erosion, or destruction of the bony walls of the sinus. Tumor extension into an adjacent sinus, the nasal cavity, or the orbit is readily demonstrated with either modality. Because of its greater contrast resolution, intracranial extension of a sinus lesion is better demonstrated by MRI than by CT.

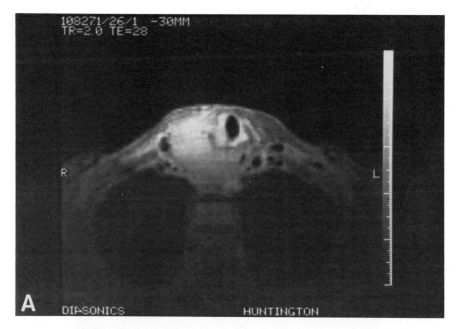

Figure 21. Thyroid carcinoma. (A) This patient presented with a bulky neck mass. An axial MR image at the subglottic level demonstrates a large mass extending primarily from the right lobe at the thyroid and displacing the subglottic airway (surface coil, TR = 2.0 s, TE = 28 ms).

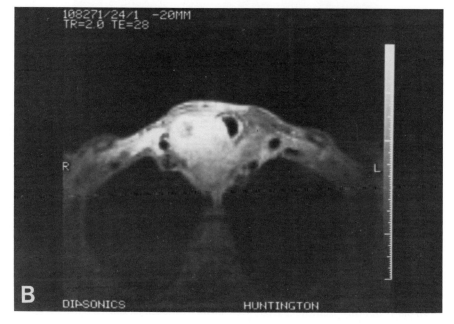

Figure 21. Thyroid carcinoma. (B) A more inferior section demonstrating invasion of the subglottic trachea and posterior extension across the midline (TR = 2.0 s, TE = 28 ms).

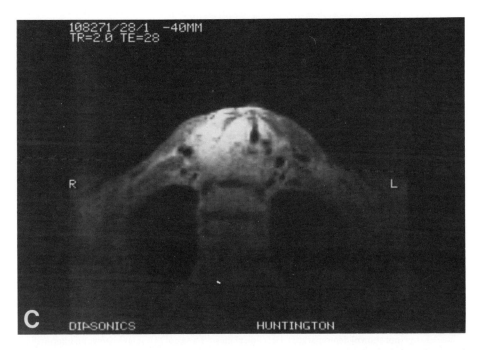

Figure 21. Thyroid carcinoma. (C) Superiorly, the mass extends into the right glottis and paralaryngeal soft tissues (TR = 2.0 s, TE = 28 ms).

Thyroid and parathyroid glands

Currently, suspected thyroid or parathyroid masses are best evaluated by a combination of radionuclide scintigraphy and ultrasound. CT and MRI have limited roles, with the possible exception of malignant tumor staging. Extension of a thyroid malignancy outside the gland can be demonstrated by either modality (Figure 21), but intrathoracic extension is better depicted by MRI. Cervical adenopathy is more apparent on CT. Small parathyroid adenomas are more easily resolved with CT than with MRI.

Thoracic inlet

Lesions at the thoracic inlet are difficult to evaluate with CT secondary to attenuation of the X-ray beam by overlying shoulders. MRI is not limited in this regard, and yields a natural high contrast between fat (high intensity), blood vessels (low intensity), and soft tissue structures or lesions (medium intensity). Thus, patients with symptoms with airway obstruction, vascular compromise, or brachial plexopathy are best studied with MRI (Figure 22).

138

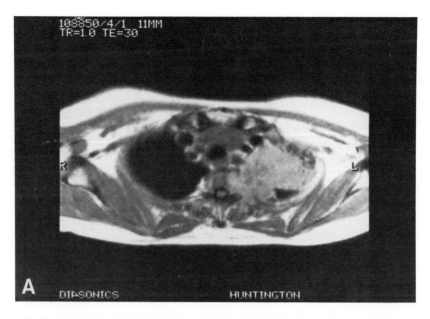

Figure 22. Pancoast tumor. (A) This patient presented with shoulder pain and a Horner's syndrome. A chest X-ray (not shown) demonstrated a left apical mass. The axial MR image shows an intermediate intensity mass occupying the lung apex, extending into the superior mediastinum and eroding a thoracic vertebal body (TR = 1.0 s, TE = 30 ms).

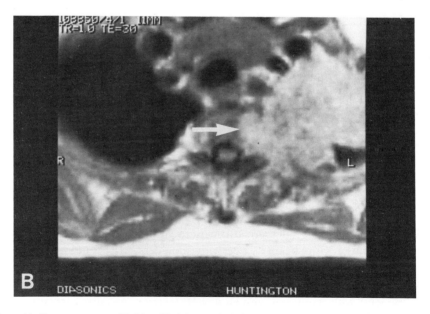

Figure 22. Pancoast tumor. (B) Magnified image depicting vertebral body erosion (arrow).

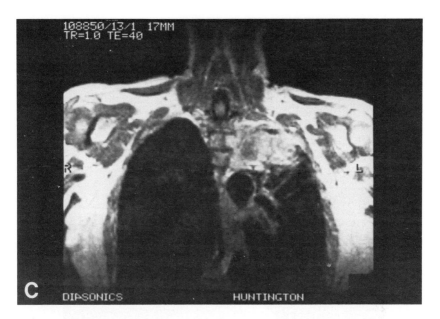

Figure 22. Pancoast's tumor. (C) A direct coronal image graphically demonstrates the relation of the mass to the spinal column, the superior mediastinum, and the subjecent low intensity aortic knob (TR = 1.0 s, TE = 40 ms).

Cervical adenopathy

There is some controversy regarding the relative effectiveness of MRI and CT in the evaluation of cervical adenopathy [13]. In our experience, the greater contrast resolution of MRI does not compensate for its lesser spatial resolution as compared with CT. Spatial resolution may be increased with the use of surface coils (Figure 23), but in most cases the entire neck cannot be studied effectively in a cost- and time-efficient manner. Vascular encasement or fixation by metastatic adenopathy may be better appreciated with MRI because of the natural contrast of flowing blood and tumor. For these reasons, we feel CT is the initial modality of choice in the evaluation of cervical adenopathy, with MRI effective as an adjunct procedure when vascular fixation is suspected.

Recent developments and future trends

There has been a striking and progressive increase in MR image quality within the last few years. Continued improvements in computer software are anticipated, and will lead to even greater diagnostic effectiveness and clinical application. The expected availability of paramagnetic contrast material will have a major impact,

140

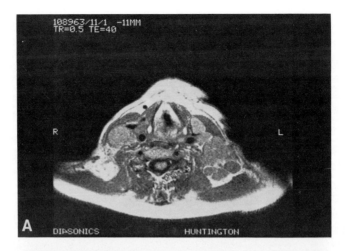

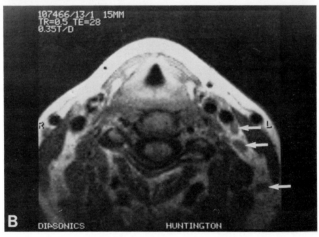

Figure 23. Cervical adenopathy. (A) An axial MR image demonstrates multiple one to three cm medium intensity masses in the soft tissues of the neck. Excisional biopsy revealed lymphoma (TR = 0.5 s, TE = 40 ms). (B) Surface coil image in another patient. Several 3 to 5 mm nodes can be seen within the left posterior triangle (arrows) (TR = 0.5 s, TE = 28 ms).

particularly in imaging of the brain and extracranial head and neck. Finally, increased user experience and the conduction of carefully controlled comparison studies will undoubtedly increase the efficacy of this modality in the evaluation of patients with head and neck tumors.

Summary

In recent years and months, MRI has been shown effective in the evaluation of a number of head and neck lesions. While additional controlled and comparison studies are needed, MRI appears to be the consensus examination of choice in the work-up of lesions at the skull base and within the nasopharynx. In other areas, such as the oropharynx, salivary glands, and the paranasal sinuses, MRI appears to be comparable or complimentary to CT. In the evaluation of laryngeal tumors and cervical adenopathy, the role of MRI is yet to be defined, but one would predict a progressive increase in its efficacy with evolving technical advances.

Magnetic resonance at HMRI

The Huntington Medical Research Institutes houses four magnetic resonance units: a Diasonics 0.35 Tesla whole body imager, a 4.7 Tesla Chemical Shift Imager capable of both imaging and spectroscopy, and two Bruker 'wide bore' spectrometers operating at 180 and 260 megahertz.

The 'wide bore' units are used primarily for metabolic studies on cardiac ischemia. Phosphorus spectra are observed in working rabbit heart preparations perfused with a fluocarbon blood substitute. The 4.7 Tesla unit is used to study muscle and tumors in human limbs, and heart and brain in canines.

The Diasonics imager was placed in service in May of 1983. As of January 1987 over 9000 patients had been examined using the instrument. Sixty-nine percent of the patients have had brain examinations and 19% had have spine examinations. Of the remaining 12%, many have undergone imaging for suspected head and neck malignancies, often in conjunction with high resolution CT studies.

Continuing imaging research is directed at improving knowledge about the physical and chemical bases of image appearence in various disease states, and improving sensitivity, specificity and imaging speed by optimizing radiofrequency pulse sequences, coil design and use of image-enhancing contrast agents. Several protocols are being utilized to more accurately determine the effectiveness of MRI in head and neck tumor staging.

References

1. Stark, D.D., Moss, A.A., Gamsu, G., Clark, O.H., Gooding, G.A.W., Webb, W.R. 1984. Magnetic resonance imaging of the neck, Part I: normal anatomy. Radiology 150: 447–454.
2. Stark, D.D., Moss, A.A., Gamsu, G., Clark, O.H., Gooding, G.A.W., Webb, W.R. 1984. Magnetic resonance imaging of the neck, Part II: pathologic findings. Radiology 150: 455–461.
3. Bradley, W.G., Crooks, L.E., Newton, T.H. 1983. Physical principles of NMR. In: Advanced Imaging Techniques, Vol. II (T.H. Newton, D.G. Potts, eds.). Clavadel Press, San Francisco, Chapter 3.
4. Bradley, W.G. 1984. Effect of magnetic relaxation times on magnetic resonance image interpretation. Noninvas. Med. Imag. 1: 193–204.
5. Crooks, L.E., Ortendahl, D.A., Kaufman, L. et al. 1983. Clinical efficacy of NMR imaging. Radiology 146: 123–128.
6. Waluch, V., Bradley, W.G. 1984. NMR Even echo rephasing in slow laminar flow. J. Comput. Assist. Tomogr. 8: 594–598.
7. Dooms, G.C., Hricak, H., Moseley, M.E., Bottles, K., Fisher, M., Higgins, C.B. 1985. Characterization of lymphadenopathy by magnetic resonance relaxation times: preliminary results. Radiology 155: 691–697.
8. Hans, J.C., Huss, R.G., Benson, J.E. et al. 1985. MR imaging of the skull-base. J. Comput. Assist. Tomogr. 5: 944–952.

142

9. New, P.F.J., Bachow, P.D., Wismer, G.L. *et al*. 1985. MR imaging of the acoustic nerves in small acoustic neuromas at 0.6 T: Prospective study. A.J.N.R. 2: 175–170.
10. Dillon, W.P., Mills, C.M., Kjos, B., DeGroot, J., Brant-Zawadski, M. 1984. Magnetic resonance imaging of the nasopharynx. Radiology 152: 731–738.
11. Lufkin, R.B., Hanafee, W.N.. 1985. Application of surface coils to MR anatomy of larynx. A.J.N.R. 6: 491–497.
12. Lufkin, R.B., Hanafee, W.N., Wortham, D. *et al*. 1985. Larynx and hypopharynx: MR image with surface coils. Radiology 158: 747–757.
13. Dooms, G.C., Hricak, H., Crooks, L.E., Higgins, C.B. 1984. Magnetic resonance imaging of the lymph nodes: Comparison with CT. Radiology 153: 179–728.

9. Timing of chemotherapy as part of multi-modality treatment in patients with advanced head and neck cancer

MUHYI AL-SARRAF

Introduction

Patients with locally advanced (stage III and IV) squamous cancer of the head and neck have had poor prognosis in spite of standard therapy [1–10]. For those patients with operable and resectable disease the accepted conventional treatments are:
1. surgery alone;
2. pre-operative radiotherapy followed by surgery;
3. surgery followed by radiotherapy;
4. radiotherapy alone.
The overall survival results reported for radical surgery for primary and regional disease, with or without the addition of radiation (pre-op or post-op), in resectable head and neck cancers are the same. No randomized trials have ever been reported showing statistical differences in survival between these modes of treatment. Selected patient reports from some institutions favor the combined approach of surgery and radiation therapy over surgery alone, especially in relationship to the disease-free survival [1–7].

Most investigators agree that the results of radiotherapy alone in patients with locally advanced but resectable head and neck cancer are inferior to the results obtained with surgery with or without radiotherapy [3, 4].

In 1977, Vandenbrouch et al. [5] reported on the results of a randomized trial of pre-operative versus post-operative irradiation in treatment of tumors of the hypopharynx, suggesting the superiority of post-operative treatment in disease-free relapse rate and overall survival. A large randomized study conducted by the Radiation Therapy Oncology Group (RTOG) did not confirm such conclusions [6, 7] although in certain subgroups, the results of post-operative radiotherapy were superior to pre-operative treatment.

It is accepted by most investigators that surgery followed by radiotherapy is the standard treatment for patients with resectable and operable cancer of the head and neck for three major reasons: (1) the higher incidence of surgical

C. Jacobs (ed) Cancers of the head and neck.
© 1987, Martinus Nijhoff Publishers, Boston. ISBN 0–89838–825–2. Printed in the Netherlands.

complications in the pre-irradiated patients; (2) about 20% of the patients may refuse planned radical surgery, especially those with good response to pre-operative radiation treatment; and (3) the possibility that the exact extent of surgery may vary in patients with the same site and T & N stage of cancer treated after pre-operative radiotherapy vs. those treated before radiation.

However, the combination of radical surgery and post-operative radiotherapy have not produced adequate tumor control in the majority of the patients with locally advanced disease [1–10]. The incidence of loco-regional failure can be as high as 60%, and distant metastases developed in 10 to 50% of the cases.

In patients with unresectable cancer and/or an inoperable disease, radiotherapy alone is the accepted conventional treatment. It was reported that the degree of response of these patients to such treatment is the most important factor that determines the overall survival [14]. Inspite of initial good response to irradiation, most of these patients are dead within 36 months with a high incidence of local and/or regional lymph node failure.

Because of the continued poor results with the 'standard' definitive treatment in patients with locally advanced squamous cell cancer of the head and neck, many attempts to improve upon such results have been studied and reported [15]. The most recent and perhaps most promising of these clinical trials is the use of chemotherapy as part of combined modality treatment for patients with head and neck cancer.

Until recently, systemic chemotherapy, single agents or combinations had been employed for palliation purposes only for those patients with recurrent disease or distant metastases occurring after primary treatment (surgery or radiotherapy). With the introduction of more active agents(s) (e.g. Cisplatin) and the finding of a high overall response rate with better complete response when induction Cisplatin-based combination was given as the initial treatment, the value of combination chemotherapy as part of the combined modality therapy is being intensely evaluated [15].

The best chemotherapy combination

Before testing the value of chemotherapy as part of other definitive treatments for patients with head and neck cancer, it is important to identify and utilize the best chemotherapy regimen.

At the time of surgical resection, the surgeon removes all the gross tumor with a healthy margin. He then obtains multiple frozen biopsies, and if all are negative, he will reconstruct the space created. This is considered adequate resection.

The radiotherapist usually delivers the highest possible tolerable dose with a port to cover all known disease areas and possible drainage lymph nodes. This is considered adequate radiotherapy.

As medical oncologists, we have to be allowed to utilize the best and most adequate chemotherapy, especially when there is a question of the value of this modality of treatment as an adjunct to the other definitive therapies.

So, the question is how do we define the best and most adequate chemotherapy? In Table 1 some of the elements used in selecting the best chemotherapy for randomized trials are defined. One of the most important factors in selecting chemotherapy is the incidence of clinical complete response achieved by such treatment. In utilizing Cisplatin-based combinations, the reported incidence of

Table 1. Definition of the best chemotherapy

A. *Effectiveness*
  1. Incidence of clinical complete response
  2. Incidence of histological complete response after resection or 'adequate' biopsy
B. *Administration*
  1. The number of courses needed to induce clinical complete response
  2. The number of courses that need to be given after achievement of clinical complete response
  3. Overall total number of courses
  4. Total dose of the more 'toxic' agent(s)
  5. Frequency and duration of such chemotherapy
C. *Safety*
  1. Incidence of acute side effects
    a. Nausea and/or vomiting
    b. Myelosuppression
    c. Renal impairment
    d. Hair loss
    e. Other GI side effects
  2. Incidence of subacute side effects
    a. Peripheral neuorpathy
  3. Incidence of chronic side effects
    a. Deafness
    b. Renal impairment
    c. Pulmonary failure
    d. Second primary cancer
D. *Tolerance*
  1. Patient acceptance
  2. Incidence of patient exclusion
  3. Delay of definitive therapy, surgery and/or radiotherapy
  4. Acceptance by the multimodality team
E. *Cost*
  1. Inpatient vs. outpatient administration
  2. The need for central I.V. line
  3. Laboratory tests needed
  4. Supportive care needed
  5. Days in hospital and days lost from work
  6. Duration of each treatment course

---

clinical complete response (CR) to induction varies from one report to another and ranges from 0 to 54% [15]. It seems important, therefore, to identify factors that might influence the incidence of CR, and some of them are:

1. number of courses of chemotherapy given;
2. type of combination utilized;
3. stage of disease:
   a. Stage III vs. stage IV,
   b. $T_4N_0M_0$ vs. $T_4N_3M_o$;
4. performance status;
5. other
   a. tumor differentiation,
   b. site of primary tumor,
   c. intensity of chemotherapy,
   d. sequential chemotherapy with two non-cross resistant combinations.

The factors that influence the incidence of clinical CR to inital chemotherapy may also influence the incidence of histological CR after surgical resection or 'adequate' multiple biopsies [16–19]. The most important factors that might influence the incidence of histological CR are the N stage (No) and number and type of chemotherapy courses given.

At Wayne State University, three sequential pilots with induction chemotherapy between 1979 and 1982 (two courses of Cisplatin, Oncovin and bleomycin COB [20, 21], two courses of Cisplatin and 96-h 5-fluorouracil (5-FU) infusion [22, 23] or three courses of Cisplatin and 120-h 5-FU infusion [24] produced overall clinical CRs of 29%, 19% and 54% respectively. For patients with clinical CR who underwent surgical resection, the histological CRs were 1/10, 2/2 and 10/20 respectively with each chemotherapy [16].

The type of induction chemotherapy did influence the overall survival of these patients regardless of the subsequent definitive therapy [12, 18, 24–26].

Also, patients achieving clinical complete response to the initial chemotherapy had significantly superior survival to those patients with less than CR to treatment regardless of the subsequent definitive therapy [16, 29]. More importantly, those CR patients who were found to have no histological disease after surgical resection had statistically superior survival when compared to those clinical CRs who had residual disease at surgery [16].

It is very important to mention that the time when clinical CR was achieved in relation to the number of courses of chemotherapy was critical in determining the incidence of histological CR and possible influence on overall survival. A clinical CR occurring after one course of chemotherapy when additional courses were planned, was a more favorable prognostic factor than clinical CR occurring at the end of the last planned course of chemotherapy.

Another important factor that influenced the incidence of CR after initial chemotherapy and the overall survival was the stage of disease (stage III vs. stage IV) and especially the actual T & N of the disease (Tables 2, 3 and Figure 1).

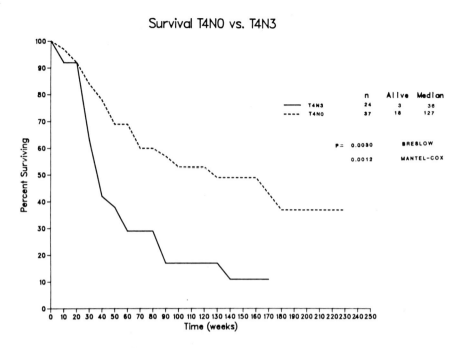

Survival T4N0 vs. T4N3

	n	Alive	Median
——— T4N3	24	3	36
- - - T4N0	37	18	127

P= 0.0030   BRESLOW

0.0012   MANTEL-COX

Figure 1. Overall survival in weeks for patients with stage T_4N_0 vs. T_4N_3.

Table 2. Incidence of complete response to three courses of Cisplatin and 120-h 5-FU infusion by stage of disease

	Stage III	Stage IV
CR	13	35
PR	2	33
NR	2	3
CR/total	13/17	35/71
	(76%)	(49%)

Table 3. Incidence of complete response to three courses of Cisplatin and 120-h 5-FU infusion by T & N stage

	$T_4N_0M_0$	$T_4N_3M_0$
CR	12	3
PR	2	11
NR	2	0
CR/total	12/16	3/14
	(75%)	(21%)

In stage III disease the clinical CR to three courses of Cisplatin and 5-FU infusion was 76% (13/17) vs. 49% for stage IV disease. The clinical CR to the same chemotherapy for T_4N_0 disease was 75% vs. 21% for T_4N_3. Overall survival for patients with $T_4N_0M_0$ stage of this disease was statistically significant as compared to overall survival of patients with $T_4N_3M_0$ cancer, regardless of response to initial chemotherapy and subsequent definitive treatment (Figure 1).

It is worth mentioning that T_4 or N_3 disease is very poorly defined by the AJC and UICC system, and many subgroups of the disease could be identified that might influence the CR rate to initial chemotherapy and the overall survival of these patients.

Despite about 10 years of trials with induction chemotherapy, we do not know what is the best chemotherapy regimen available at the present time, and we do not have the research yet to determine the best chemotherapy possible.

Another possibility of effective modality is combining chemotherapy and radiotherapy simultaneously [15, 28]. This is especially true with the combination of Cisplatin and radiotherapy. This combination is active with a clinical CR of about 70% on the cooperative group level (RTOG), and the side effects are reversible and acceptable [28, 29]. The effectiveness of this combination for patients with inoperable, locally advanced head and neck cancer opened another avenue of utilizing this combination the pre-operative [30] or post-operative (in progress) set up.

When to include chemotherapy in multipodality treatment

At what stage of drug development and at what level of antitumor activity should we introduce these agents into multipodality treatment and begin testing their value?

We believe we have to have clinical complete response rate that is as high as possible. Additional courses given before definitive therapy may enable us to obtain the highest rate of true histological complete response and to influence patient survival and the quality of survival. This must be done without jeopardizing or delaying definitive treatments like surgery or radiotherapy.

At the same time, because of poor results (particularly overall survival), the high incidence of loco-regional failure, and the possibility of systemic metastases after our present 'definitive' treatments, it is becoming a moral and ethnical issue whether to withhold combination chemotherapy with its modest clinical activities (up to 50% CR) from multimodality therapy.

As was mentioned earlier, we are in the 10th year of clinical trials, and we still do not know the best chemotherapy regimen which will produce the expected impact as part of other definitive treatments in patients with locally advanced head and neck cancer.

The number of additional years needed to reach this regimen is unknown, and it depends on many factors including resources, new agent(s), safer agent(s), investigators and institutional committment. Besides all pilot studies from single institutions have to be tested and accepted by other institutions and on the national level by cooperative multi-institution group.

In 1978, with activation of the Head and Neck Contract Program, sponsored by the National Cancer Institute, one course of Cisplatin and bleomycin was used as initial therapy as part of the experimental arms to be followed by surgery and post-operative radiotherapy. This chemotherapy produced about a 50% overall response and only a 5% clinical complete response [31].

In 1979, Southwest Oncology Group (SWOG) activated a randomized trial to test two courses of Cisplatin, Oncovin and bleomycin in patients with inoperable locally advanced head and neck cancer to be followed by radiotherapy vs. radiotherapy alone. The overall response rate to this combination was about 80% and clinical CR about 20–30%.

In 1983, the Radiation Therapy Oncology Group (RTOG) activated a randomized trial in patients with resectable cancer to test the efficacy of three courses of Cisplatin and 5-FU infusion as part of combined modality therapy. This protocol is now active nationwide by the mechanism of the Head and Neck Cancer Intergroup (protocol # 0034). This combination produced 90% overall response, up to 50% clinical CR, and up to 50% of those clinical CRs are histological CR.

The problem that we have to study in future trials is the value of chemotherapy; if no real advantage can be obtained, is this due to the fact that chemotherapy may not have a place in the combined modality settings, or have we not found the most active and effective chemotherapy? The latter possibility means we still have a long road ahead of us in order to continue to improve on the activity and the safety of our chemotherapy.

Timing and sequence of chemotherapy as part of multimodality treatment

The next question that needs to be answered after achieving the best chemotherapy is the timing and sequence of such treatment as part of multimodality therapy. Many strategies can be designed for further trial:
1. induction, before definitive treatment;
2. post-surgery chemotherapy;
3. post-radiotherapy chemotherapy;
4. chemotherapy combined with simultanous radiation;
5. combination of the above.
Since 1975, when chemotherapy was added to the multimodality treatments for locally advanced head and neck cancer, all pilot studies conducted gave chemotherapy before definitive therapy of surgery and/or radiotherapy. This was done for one obvious reason to test the effectiveness of such agents on measurable gross disease. This is the only way to test chemotherapy in previously untreated patients.

The use of chemotherapy as the initial treatment will continue for the near future, at least until we find the best chemotherapy regimen. In order to test the actual value on disease-free survival and overall survival and as part of the multimodality treatment, the timing and the sequence of these therapies need to be established to obtain the best results possible, especially in patients with resectable cancer.

Some problems occurred with induction chemotherapy in patients with resectable and operable, locally advanced head and neck cancer. In these patients surgery is accepted as the most important part of the multimodality therapy at the present time. With improvement in incidence of clinical CR to pre-operative radiotherapy or initial good response (CR) with the induction chemotherapy many problems have arisen.

Patients refusal of surgery or further therapy

In patients treated with pre-operative radiotherapy, only 20% will refuse the planned surgical resection, particularly those who achieve a complete response.

The refusal of planned surgery after induction chemotherapy is even higher and is now approaching 30–35% of the patients. Of those patients who achieve clinical CR after induction chemotherapy, more than 50% may refuse surgical resection, and some patients may even refuse any further therapy. It may create a major problem in the overall results of the multimodality therapy if the most important modality of treatment is refused. Also this will create a major difficulty in randomized trials when trying to test the efficacy of induction chemotherapy as part of multi-modality therapy vs. standard therapy (surgery and post-op radiotherapy). In the experimental arm, 30% of the patients might not have the planned surgical resection.

Is the planned surgery after induction chemotherapy the same as pre-planned?

The decision as to the extent of the radical surgical resection for patients with locally advanced resectable cancer of the head and neck is made after completion of triple endoscopy and other evaluations. Those patients scheduled for surgery first, without pre-operative treatment, have the adequate resection as planned. In those patients with the same stage and site of malignant disease but with good response to induction chemotherapy (especially a CR), the extent of surgery, the definition of negative margin, and the results of frozen section biopsies may not be the same, even if performed by the same surgeon.

Another major question is why should one expect following three courses of induction chemotherapy and achievement of good response followed by planned surgery significant improvement in cure rate vs. radical surgery and removal of all gross tumor with negative margins without pre-operative therapy? At the end of both treatment arms, patients have no evidence of disease.

The effectiveness of chemotherapy is measured by the incidence of response, especially, CR in patients with advanced disease. It is expected to have the same, if not better, effect when the same chemotherapy is used with the same number of courses on minimal residual disease achieved after surgical resection.

Because of all of the above reasons and other possible factors, we initiated a pilot study for resectable disease in which three courses of Cisplatin and a 120-h 5-FU infusion were given after surgery and before radiotherapy [32]. Following the demonstration of the feasibility with this type of multimodality treatment, two pilots were activated at the same time by us in the RTOG in 1981. One utilized induction chemotherapy followed by surgery and post-operative radiotherapy. The second pilot utilized the same chemotherapy after surgery and before radiotherapy. The side effects of chemotherapy were the same, regardless of the sequence of chemotherapy in relation to the definitive treatment. Survival favored chemotherapy in the middle 'sandwich', despite a greater number of patients with stage IV and poorer performance status in this group [33].

Late in 1983, RTOG activated a randomized trial to compare surgery followed by radiotherapy vs. surgery followed by chemotherapy and then followed by radiation therapy. In 1985 this important study was accepted and activated by the Head and Neck Intergroup. The randomization occurred after surgery, and those patients with positive margins were excluded. Because of this, pathological stage and surgery were equal in both arms.

We did not include maintenance chemotherapy because of the difficulty in accomplishing such therapy with the Head and Neck Contract Group, and the difficulty faced by many cooperative groups in trying to activate such a study with poor accrual.

There are many other possible designs of timing and sequence of chemotherapy as part of multimodality therapy. These will be part of further investigations.

Regardless of the optimal sequence of chemotherapy as part of the multimodality approach, and because of the need for more effective and safe chemotherapy, induction chemotherapy is the only way to test the effectiveness of chemotherapy in previously untreated patients before it can be utilized in randomized trials.

The objective for continuing trials with induction chemotherapy, aside from determining safety and tolerance levels, is to increase the incidence of clinical CR and histological CR based on surgical resection or 'adequate' biopsy [34, 35].

Other trials are underway at the institutional level to minimize the surgical resection [19, 20, 36], and on the national level a trial is being carried out by the V.A. laryngeal cancer group. This study randomizes resectable stage III and IV laryngeal cancer patients to surgery and radiotherapy vs. induction chemotherapy with Cisplatin and 5-FU infusion. Then the good responders receive total radio-

152

therapy, while patients with poor or no response will have surgery and post-operative radiotherapy.

This is an important phase of combined modality therapy development for locally advanced head and neck cancer, especially since we feel we have not reached to our best possible chemotherapy combination.

Summary and further challenge

The results of definitive therapy for patients with locally advanced head and neck cancer are poor and not acceptable. For resectable disease, surgery is still the most important modality, and little further improvement can be done on 'adequate' radical surgery. On the other hand, because of the morbidity of such a procedure and the functional and cosmetic effect, the aims for less or delay of surgery is the challenge of the future, provided we do not jeopardize patients' quality of life or overall survival.

Radiotherapy is an important component for treatment of these patients, and many attempts are underway to improve on its effectiveness. These include: radiosensitizers, radioprotectors, hyperfractionation, hyperthermia, neutron, etc.

Chemotherapy is an effective anti-tumor modality, producing excellent overall response and up to 50% complete clinical response. Chemotherapy research is underway to improve on the results of this antitumor property, especially the rate of clinical and histological CR. And so chemotherapy may have a greater promise in improving results of our treatment in cancer of the head and neck. The value of chemotherapy as part of multimodality treatment and as a possible means to reduce surgical morbidity and mutilation are being investigated. The challenges of the future are: (1) to identify the best chemotherapy possible, (2) to further test the timing and sequence of such chemotherapy as part of other therapy for head and neck cancer, (3) to investigate the value of our best chemotherapy with the proper doses, courses, frequency, and timing for these patients, and (4) to continue our work to lessen or delay 'radical resection', which may cause considerable morbidity and affect the quality of life of these patients.

References

1. Cachin, Y., Eschwage, F. 1975. Combination of radiotherapy and surgery in the treatment of head and neck cancer. Cancer Treat. Rev. 2: 177–191.
2. Fletcher, G.H., Jesse, R.H. 1977. The place of irradiation in the management of the primary lesion in head and neck cancer. Cancer 39: 862–867.
3. Hintz, B., Charyulu, K., Chandler, J.R. et al. 1979. Randomized study of control of the primary tumor and survival using pre-operative radiation, radiation alone or surgery alone in head and neck carcinomas. J. Surg. Oncol. 12: 75–85.

4. Schuller, D.E., McGuirt, W.F., Krause, C.J., McCabe, B.F., Pflung, B.K. 1979. Symposium: Adjuvant cancer therapy of head and neck tumors. Increased survival with surgery alone vs. combined therapy. Laryngoscope 89: 582–594.

5. Vandenbrouck, C., Sancho, H., LeFur, R., Richard, J.M., Cachin, Y. 1977. Results of a randomized clinical trial of pre-operative irradiation vs. post-operative in treatment of tumors of the hypopharynx. Cancer 39: 1445–1449.

6. Snow, J.B., Gelber, R.D., Kramer, S. *et al.* 1980. Randomized pre-operative and post-operative radiation therapy for patients with carcinoma of the head and neck. Preliminary report. Laryngoscope 90: 930–945.

7. Kramer, S., Gelber, R.D., Snow, J.B., Davis, L.W., Marcial, V.A., Lowry, L.D. 1985. Pre-operative vs. post-operative radiation therapy for patients with carcinoma of the head and neck. Progress report. Head Neck Surg. 3: 255.

8. Vikram, B., Strong, E.W., Shah, H.P., Spiro, R. 1984. Failure at the primary site following multimodality treatment in advance head and neck cancer. Head Neck Surg. 6: 720–723.

9. Vikram, B., Strong, E.W., Shah, J.P., Spiro, R. 1984. Failure in the neck following multimodality treatment for advanced head and neck cancer. Head Neck Surg. 6: 724–729.

10. Vikram, B., Strong, E.W., Shah, J.P., Spiro, R. Failure at distant sites following multimodality treatment for advanced head and neck cancer. Head Neck Surg. 6: 730–733.

11. Probert, J.C., Thompson, R.W., Bagshaw, M.A. 1974. Patterns of spread of distant metastases in head and neck cancer. Cancer 33: 127–133.

12. O'Brien, P., Carlson, R., Steubner, F., Stanley, C. 1971. Distant metastases in epidermoid cell carcinoma of the head and neck. Cancer 27: 304–307.

13. Papal, J.R. 1984. Distant metastases from head and neck cancer. Cancer 53: 342–345.

14. Fazekos, J.T., Sommer, C., Kramer, S. 1983. Tumor regression and other prognosticators in advanced head and neck cancers. Int. J. Radiat. Oncol. Biol. Phys. 9: 957–959.

15. Al-Sarraf, M. 1984. Chemotherapy strategies in squamous cell carcinoma of the head and neck. CRC Crit. Rev. Oncol. Hematol. 1: 323–355.

16. Al-Kourainy, K., Crissman, J., Ensley, J., Kish, J., Simpson, W., Cummings, G., Al-Sarraf, M. 1985. Achievement of superior survival of histologically negative vs. histologically positive clinically complete responders to cis-platinum (CACP) combinations in patients with locally advanced head and neck cancer. Proc. Am. Soc. Cancer Res. 26: 164.

17. Amrein, P., Weitzman, S. 1985. 24-Hour infusion Cisplatin (CP) and 5 day infusion 5-fluorouracil (5-FU) in squamous cell carcinoma of the head and neck (SCC H & N). Proc. Am. Soc. Clin. Oncol. 4: 133.

18. Kies, M.S., Lester, E.P., Gordon, L.I., Blough, R.R., Gongol, J., Taylor, S.G. IV. 1985. Cisplatin and infusion 5-fluorouracil (5-FU) in Stage III and IV squamous cancer of the head and neck. Proc. Am. Soc. Clin. Oncol. 4: 139.

19. Jacobs, C., Goffinet, D., Fee, W., Goffinet, L., Hopp, M. 1985. Chemotherapy as a substitute for surgery in the treatment of advanced operable head and neck cancer. An NCOG Pilot. Proc. Am. Soc. Clin. Oncol. 4: 137.

20. Al-Sarraf, M., Binns, P., Vaishampayan, G., Loh, J., Weaver, A. 1979. The adjuvant use of cis-platinum, Oncovin and bleomycin (COB) prior to surgery and/or radiotherapy in untreated epidermoid cancer of the head and neck. In: Adjuvant Therapy of Cancer II. S.E. Jones, S.E. Salmon, eds.). Grune & Stratton, Inc., New York, pp. 421-428.

21. Al-Sarraf, M., Drelichman, A., Jacobs, J., Kinzie, J., Hoschner, J., Loh, J.J.K., Weaver, A. 1981. Adjuvant chemotherapy with cis-platinum, oncovin, and bleomycin followed by surgery and/or radiotherapy in patients with advanced previously untreated head and neck cancer. Final Report. In: Adjuvant Therapy of Cancer III. (S.E. Jones, S.E. Salmon, eds.). Grune & Stratton Inc. New York, pp. 145-152.

22. Al-Sarraf, M., Drelichman, A., Peppard, S., Hoschner, J., Kinzie, J., Loh, J., Weaver, A. 1981. Adjuvant cis-platinum and 5-fluorouracil 96 hour infusion in previously untreated epidermoid

cancers of the head and neck. Proc. Am. Soc. Clin. Oncol. and Am. Assoc. Cancer Res. 22: 428.

23. Kish, J., Drelichman, A., Jacobs, J., Hoschner, J., Kinzie, J., Loh, J., Weaver, A., Al-Sarraf, M. 1982. Clinical trial of cis-platinum and 5-FU infusion as initial treatment for advanced squamous carcinoma of the head and neck. Cancer Treat. Rep. 66: 471–474.

24. Weaver, A., Fleming, S., Ensley, J., Kish, J.A., Jacobs, J., Kinzie, J., Crissman, J., Al-Sarraf, M. 1984. Superior complete clinical response and survival rates with initial bolus cis-platinum and 120 hour 5-FU infusion before definitive therapy in patients with locally advanced head and neck cancer. Am. J. Surg. 148: 525–529.

25. Rooney, M., Stanley, R., Weaver, A. et al. 1983. Superior results in complete response rate and overall survival in patients with advanced head and neck cancer treated with three courses of 120 hour 5-FU infusion and cis-platinum. Proc. Am. Soc. Clin. Oncol. 2: 159.

26. Rooney, M., Kish, J., Jacobs, J. et al. 1985. Improved complete response rate and survival in advanced head and neck cancer after 3 course induction therapy with 120 hour 5-FU infusion and cis-platinum. Cancer 55: 1123–1128.

27. Kies, M.S., Gordon, G.I., Hauck, W.W. et al. 1985. Analysis of complete responders after initial treatment with chemotherapy in head and neck cancer. Otolaryngol. Head Neck Surg. 93: 199–205.

28. Al-Sarraf, M., Marcial, V., Mowry, P., Green, M., Laramore, G., Pajak, T. 1985. Superior local control with combination of high dose cis-platinum and radiotherapy. An RTOG Study. Proc. Am. Assoc. Cancer Res. 26:169.

29. Al-Sarraf, M., Jacobs, J., Kinzie, J., Marcial, V., Velez-Garcia, E., Glick, J., Fu, K. 1983. Combined modality therapy utilizing single high intermittent dose of cis-platinum and radiation in patients with advanced head and neck cancer. Proc. Am. Soc. Clin. Oncol. 2: 159.

30. Slotman, G.J., Glicksman, A.S., Doolittle, C.H. et al. 1985. Preliminary experience with pre-operative synchronous cis-platinum (DDP) and radiation therapy (RT) in stage III and IV head and neck cancer. Proc. Am. Soc. Clin. Oncol. 4: 148.

31. Baker, S.R., Makuch, R.W., Wolf, G. 1981. Pre-operative cisplatin and bleomycin therapy in head and neck squamous carcinoma. Prognostic factors for tumor response. Arch. Otolaryngol. 107: 683–689.

32. Al-Sarraf, M., Kinzie, J., Jacobs, J., Loh, J.J.K., Weaver, A. 1982. New way of giving chemotherapy as part of multi-disciplinary treatment for patients with head and neck cancers. Preliminary Report. Proc. Am. Assoc. Cancer Res. 23: 134.

33. Al-Sarraf, M., Pajak, T., Laramore, G. 1985. Timing of chemotherapy as part of definitive treatment for patients with advanced head and neck cancer. An RTOG Study. Proc. Am. Soc. Clin. Oncol. 4: 141.

34. Ensley, J., Kish, J., Jacobs, J., Weaver, A., Kinzie, J., Crissman, J., Al-Sarraf, M. 1985. The use of a five course, alternating combination chemotherapy induction regimen in advanced squamous cell cancer of the head and neck (SCC of H & N). Proc. Am. Soc. Clin. Oncol. 4: 143.

35. Greenberg, B., Ahman, F., Garewal, H., Koopmann, C., Coulthand, S., Berzes, H., Alberts, D. 1985. Neo-adjuvant therapy for advanced head and neck cancer with allopurinol-modulated high dose 5-flurouracil (5-FU) and cis-platinum (CP). Proc. Am. Soc. Clin. Oncol. 4: 146.

36. Ensley, H.F., Jacobs, J.R., Weaver, A., Kinzie, J., Crissman, J., Kish, J., Cummings, G., Al-Sarraf, M. 1984. The correlation between response to cis-platinum combination chemotherapy and subsequent radiotherapy in previously untreated patients with advanced squamous cell cancers of the head and neck. Cancer 54: 811–814.

10. Immunology of the lymph node

DAVID E. SCHULLER

Introduction

A considerable body of information exists in the medical literature about neck nodes in patients with head and neck malignancies. Much of this literature discusses the frequency of nodal involvement with metastases. This literature has clearly documented that the cervical lymphatic system plays a potential role in altering the behavior of head and neck malignancies and also needs to be an important consideration in the development of therapeutic programs. A wealth of clinical data exists, and thorough anatomic reports have been published [1]. But the literature has recently changed some what in that it now contains discussions of this cancer and its impact on the immune system [2–11].

As the body of information expands concerning the role of the cervical lymphatic system in the immunologic reaction to cancer, it is anticipated that this will have an impact on the objectives of cancer treatment. This chapter will initially review the anatomical make-up of the cervical lymphatic system and how it is altered by cancer. This information will provide a basis for a more specific discussion of the immunoactivity of patients with head and neck cancer, especially as it relates to the cervical lymphatic system.

Anatomy of cervical lymphatic system

The smallest vessels within the cervical lymphatic system are the capillaries. These capillaries are similar to blood capillaries in that they contain only endothelium; however, blood capillaries are larger. Lymphatic capillaries are capable of containing a considerable amount of lymphatic fluid. The capillaries join to ultimately become collecting vessels. These are multi-layered vessels that contain numerous valves.

Normal nodes in the neck are usually 1–2 cm in diameter. There are also nodes which are not identifiable without the use of magnification. In addition to these

C. Jacobs (ed) Cancers of the head and neck.
© *1987, Martinus Nijhoff Publishers, Boston. ISBN 0–89838–825–2. Printed in the Netherlands.*

156

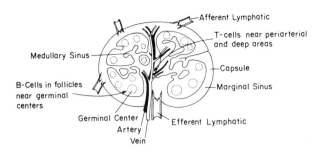

Figure 1. The normal cervical lymph node which is not involved with cancer usually has recognizable anatomic architecture that shows the location of T and B cells.

small nodes, there are even smaller aggregates of lymphocytes called nodules, and these are usually 2 mm or less in diameter. It is the nodes and nodules which are connected with the vessels of the lymphatic system. There are other collections of lymphoid tissue, such as in the nasopharynx and the gastrointestinal tract which are not connected with the nodes and nodules and their collecting vessels.

The individual node has a somewhat consistent architecture. There are usually single or multiple afferent and efferent vessels. The outer layer of the node is referred to as the capsule (Figure 1). The marginal sinus is located in the periphery adjacent to the capsule, and the medullary sinuses are located in the central portion. There are germinal centers and follicles throughout a lymph node. B-lymphocytes seem to be concentrated in the follicles near the germinal centers. This is in contrast to the T-lymphocytes which appear near the periarterial regions [12].

The collecting vessels joining all the lymph nodes ultimately fuse to form collecting trunks. These will eventually drain into the venous system at the point of junction of the internal jugular with the subclavian vein. Although the thoracic duct is the largest communication of the lymphatic with the venous system, it is important to recognize that there is a similar but not as large connection on the right side of the neck.

Neoplastic involvement of neck nodes

Neck nodes are frequently involved with metastatic squamous carcinoma. This involvement alters the patient's prognosis. The critical point important to the understanding of the nodal involvement is to recognize how neoplasm anatomically becomes involved. Anatomic studies have documented the continuity of lymphatic channels from primary tumor sites to the neck nodes. This anatomic fact lead to the impression that cancer involvement of the neck nodes was secondary to contiguous growth of the primary tumor within the lumen of the lymphatic vessels. This contiguous growth ultimately involved the nodes. However, Ottavianai [13] demonstrated that nodal involvement is not via contiguous growth, but rather as emboli of groups of tumor cells.

These tumor emboli appear to become trapped by the reticulum fibers of the marginal sinuses. The emboli become trapped after they have entered the node from the afferent channels. Subsequent growth causes alteration in lymphatic flow through the involved nodes. If this growth is extensive enough, it can alter lymphatic pressure throughout the cervical lymphatic system which has an impact on the propagation of cancer cells to other nodal chains that normally would not receive lymphatic fluid according to normal anatomic descriptions.

A substantial component of the body's lymphatic system is anatomically confined to the neck. There are estimates that approximately 800 nodes exist in the average human, and 300 (37.5%) are in the cervical lymphatic system [14].

Immunoreactivity to head and neck cancer

Numerous reports have been published discussing the systemic immuno-competence of patients with head and neck cancer. There currently is no single diagnostic study which consistently and reliably presents an accurate description of the immunoreactivity. This explains the multitude of tests now utilized to assess immunoreactivity.

It is important to recognize that the patient population most frequently involved with head and neck cancer are generally exposed to extrinsic factors that in themselves are immunodepressing factors. The elderly patient, who has been using cigarettes and alcohol for long periods of time, with a compromised nutritional status, has essentially subjected himself to a series of factors that have been documented to all be immunosuppressive.

It is also necessary to recognize that current conventional forms of cancer treatment are also immunosuppressive. Radiation therapy has been proven to be immunosuppressive [15–18]. Chemotherapy is also immunosuppressive [19]. General anesthetics in surgery can also reduce immunoreactivity [20, 21].

All of these statements concerning the measurement of the immune response are based on assessments of the *systemic* immunity. It has not been until recently that the actual immune activity of the neck nodes has been addressed. If the regional nodes are capable of reacting immunologically, then this information could be important to the therapeutic program. Clearly the current practice of eradicating the entire regional nodal system with either surgery and/or radiation therapy would potentially be detrimental to the patient's prognosis. These concerns provide the stimuli for developing a better understanding of the potential immunologic capabilities of neck nodes.

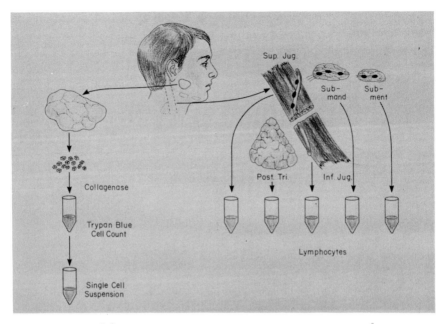

Figure 2. A schematic illustration of the preparation of single cell suspensions of tumor cells and lymphocytes arising from each of the five major nodal groups.

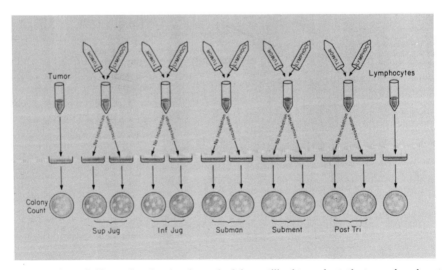

Figure 3. A schematic illustration showing the methodology utilized to evaluate the tumor-lymphocyte interaction. Colony counts were obtained for single cell suspensions of tumor only, tumor-lymphocyte mixture for both pre-incubated and non-incubated for each of the neck nodal groups, and lymphocytes only.

Immunoreactivity of the cervical lymphatic system

The previous section documented the wealth of information that has been published characterizing the immune system's reaction to head and neck cancer in humans. All of this literature has attempted to study it by measuring the immune capabilities of the person as a single unit. The presumption is that what is being assessed by measuring skin test reaction or T-lymphocyte stimulation to mitogens, for example, is an accurate reflection of the ability to deal with the antigenic stimulus of tumor. Until recently there has been little discussion of what may be occurring immunologically as a result of the tumor stimulation of the neck nodes. This *regional* immune response has the potential of being a more accurate characterization of the body's true response to tumor rather than a nonspecific assessment of immunoreactivity. But there was a problem in that no mechanisms existed to study the immunoreactivity of the neck nodes.

The clonogenic assay, as described by Hamburger and Salmon [22], is a technique which is a means of permitting tumor cell growth in soft agar so that it can be utilized for chemosensitivity testing. However, this methodology can also be utilized to study tumor-lymphocyte dynamics. It was precisely this experimental design which has permitted an evaluation of T-lymphocytes extracted from metastatic and non-metastatic neck nodes in patients with head and neck carcinoma, which in turn has provided the opportunity to assess regional immunoreactivity.

The experimental design involves the preparation of single cell suspensions of both tumor cells and lymphocytes obtained from different anatomic regions of a neck specimen following radical neck dissection (Figure 2). After these single cell suspensions are prepared, the tumor cells and lymphocytes can be mixed and plated on soft agar (Figure 3). Suspensions in soft agar of tumor cells only and another suspension of lymphocytes only serve as controls. The number of tumor colonies counted in the tumor-lymphocyte mixtures when compared with the tumor only soft agar suspensions would provide a basis for assessing the immune impact of the lymphocytes on subsequent tumor growth.

The criteria for what represented an acceptable colony were the same that have been reported by others [22–24]. A colony was not considered acceptable unless it contained at least thirty cells or was at least 60 mm in diameter using a Nikon inverted phase-contrast microscope (40 ×). Figure 4 represents the appearance of a tumor bolus in the tumor only control soft agar dish. Figure 5 represents the appearance of lymphocyte control in soft agar. The tumor lymphocyte mixture appears as shown in Figure 6. Inhibition or stimulation of tumor growth is defined as a ratio comparing the number of colonies in the tumor-lymphocyte mixture as the numerator and the number of colonies from the agar dishes containing tumor only as the denominator. Extensive investigations have been performed to document that what miscroscopically appeared to be tumor cells in soft agar when mixed with lymphocytes was not artifact [25].

160

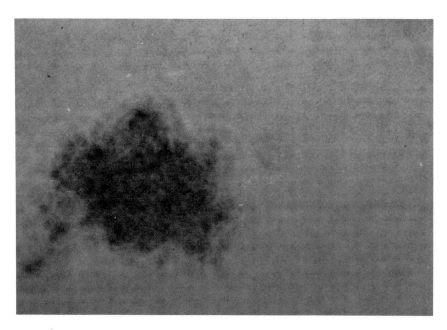

Figure 4. Soft agar dish which demonstrates tumor bolus with no lymphocytes (original magnification × 1582).

Figure 5. Photomicrograph showing soft agar dish where lymphocytes only have been suspended (original magnification × 1582).

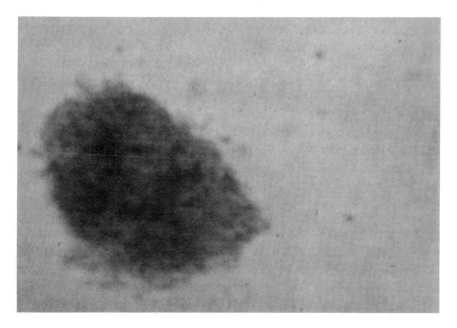

Figure 6. Soft agar dish which shows tumor-lymphocyte mixture. The tumor bolus is surrounded by the small dot-like structures which are the lymphocytes (original magnification × 1582).

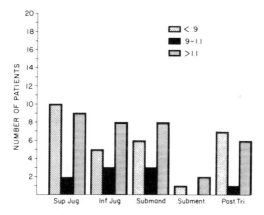

Figure 7. Distribution of patients whose tumor-lymphocyte interactinon was grouped according to those demonstrating apparent inhibition (<0.9), little change (0.9–1.1), or stimulation (>1.1) in that group of patients whose tumor-lymphocyte mixture was immediately suspended in soft agar.

The soft agar experiments studying tumor-lymphocyte mixtures demonstrated that there were times when tumor inhibition occurred. There was also evidence of minimal impact on tumor cell growth. But it was also not uncommon to see evidence of stimulation of growth occurring when lymphocytes were mixed with tumor cells (Figure 7). This figure clearly demonstrates that some type of dynamic interaction is occurring with the lymphocytes from neck nodes and head and neck cancer. It is rare for such a mixture not to have an impact on tumor cell growth.

This demonstration that cells derived from regional lymph nodes have an impact on tumor growth is not unique to head and neck neoplasms. Fisher and co-workers [26–30] used an animal model to demonstrate regional nodal immune capabilities. They were able to prove that immunity could not develop in the absence of regional nodes in this animal system. In fact, later studies by this group [31] demonstrated a decrease in the systemic immunity with the removal of the regional lymph nodes which resulted in an increased frequency of tumor occurrence when the animal was then challenged with tumor cells. Fisher and co-workers also extended this work to humans with breast or colon cancers. They demonstrated that regional nodes were immunoactive in patients with and also without metastases to these nodes.

One of the fascinating reports by Fisher suggests that a difference exists in the immune capabilities of axillary lymph nodes in women with breast cancer depending on the anatomic position of the node within the axilla [32]. However, the immunocapabilities of lymphocytes derived from neck nodes from different regions within the neck in patients with head and neck cancers all appear to have similar immune capabilities.

There has been some questions as to whether recurrent cancer is a reflecton or possibly a cause of an altered immune state. However, there is information [25] that regional nodal immunoreactivity exists in both patients with previously untreated cancer and/or in patients with recurrent disease. In this same study, Schuller noted no difference in immunoreactivity in patients who have disease in contrast to those who are free of disease.

The other question involves whether or not there is a relationship between what is noted with *regional* immunoactivity when compared to the battery of tests assessing the *systemic* response. There is some information in the literature that many of the usual assessments of systemic immune competence, such as total lymphocyte count, helper/suppressor ratio, immunoglobulins, skin testing, and lymphoblast transformation, can be normal even in patients with advanced stage head and neck cancers.

Reports of comparisons between serum and neck node T and B cell populations from patients with head and neck cancer have been published. The proportions of nodal T and B cells and even T cell subpopulations were similar to those seen in the serum. Some trends have been noted regarding the relationship of some of the T-cell sub-populations. Although not statistically significant, Schuller's study [25] found a trend toward lower serum helper/suppressor ratios being associated with tumor/lymphocyte growth patterns in soft agar, and these were consistent with increased tumor growth. One disparity between the serum and node T cell sub-populations does exist. The absolute value of the helper/suppressor ratio in nodes from patients with head and neck cancers is significantly higher than that recorded from the same patient's serum.

The current American Joint Committee Staging system for neck nodes in head and neck cancer represents an attempt to provide prognostic information. This system is heavily weighted towards the significance of the numbers and/or size of metastatic nodes. However, the clinical usefulness of numbers and size of metastatic nodes in terms of their prognostic accuracy is currently being challenged [33, 34]. The information obtained from tumor growth patterns in soft agar have not shown any relationship to currently existing factors utilizing the staging of nodal disease.

Immunomodulation

If indeed the T-lymphocytes from neck nodes in patients with head and neck cancer have an impact on tumor growth, the next logical hypothesis would be that these lymphocytes could be modulated to enhance their reaction to tumor. A study by Schuller and co-workers [35] has demonstrated that non-specific immune stimulants, such as bacillus Calmette-Guerin (BCG) or N-acetylmuramyldipeptide (MDP), are capable of altering the immune capabilities of the lymphocytes from neck nodes after a period of incubation. Results from experiments with a similar design using soft agar and tumor-lymphocyte mixtures demonstrated the ability of non-specific immunomodulators to enhance the amount of tumor growth inhibition seen when compared to the controls of tumor only and tumor-lymphocyte mixtures without immunostimulation.

Histologic immune staging

Means of assessing the regional immune capabilities of neck nodes have been undertaken by others [36] using different approaches. Berlinger [36] noted differences in the nodal architecture and was able to correlate them with survival in a group of head and neck cancer patients. Patients with marked histiocytic response oftentimes had a more favorable prognosis. This work actually reinforces an earlier report by Black *et al.* [37] who noted a relationship to the histopathologic structure of lymph nodes in patients with breast cancer. But it has been difficult to standardize these histologic parameters.

Treatment implications

Current conventional treatment programs for most malignancies, including head and neck neoplasms, involve the non-specific treatment of tumor-containing tissue. Whether it is surgery, radiation therapy, or chemotherapy, or any combinations of the above, they all involve the treatment of not only tumor but also non-tumor containing tissue. The surgeon for example intentionally resects a cuff of normal tissue about the primary tumor in an effort to completely remove the tumor. The nodal disease in patients with squamous cancer is oftentimes treated by intentionally sacrificing critically important structures as a means of increasing the chances of total tumor removal. Critical to the discussion of whether or not this non-specific approach is advisable or desirable is the determination of whether neck nodes act as a passive filtration system or if they clearly have the potential to aid in the destruction of neoplasm. There is strong evidence to suggest that T-lymphocytes from neck nodes in patients with squamous cancer are capable of mounting an effective response designed at destroying tumor. These observations support the notion that specific treatment programs that eradicate only tumor-containing tissue might increase the patient's chance of utilizing his immune system to help with the tumor destruction. Currently, such specificity is not available. However, observations regarding the immunocapabilities of regional neck nodes confirm the advisability of pursuing highly specific treatment programs that preserve the non-involved nodal architecture which may then be immunostimulated to eradicate any microscopic residual disease.

Summary

The neck nodes in patients with head and neck cancer are frequently involved with metastatic disease. This involvement dramatically alters the patient's prognosis. There is evidence that T-lymphocytes derived from neck nodes in head and neck cancer patients are capable of reacting immunologically to tumor. It is this immune capability that supports the continued pursuit of new cancer treatment programs that are more specific and result in the treatment of tumor-containing tissue rather than eradication of both tumor and non-tumor-containing tissue with conventional therapy.

References

1. Rouviere, H. 1930. Anatomy of the Human Lymphatic System, Translated by M.J. Tobias from the Original Work Anatomie Des Lymphatiques De L'Homme. Edwards Brothers, inc., Ann Arbor, MI.
2. Krause, C.J., Nysather, J.O. 1977. Current concepts of tumor immunology. II. Tumor immunodetection. Ann. Otol. Rhinol. Laryngol. 86: 871–874.
3. Beltz, W.R., Levy, N.L. 1975. Multiplicity of the tumor-directed immune response. Arch. Otolaryngol. 101: 660–663.
4. Brookes, G.B., Clifford, P. 1981. Nutritional status and general immune competence in patients with head and neck cancer. J.R. Soc. Med. 74: 132–139.
5. Browder, J.P., Chretien, P.B. 1977. Immune reactivity in head and neck squamous cell carcinoma and relevance to the design of immunotherapy trials. Sem. Oncol. 4: 431–439.

6. Koperstzych, S. 1976. Cell-mediated immunity in patient with carcinoma. Coorelation between clinical stage and immunocompetence. Cancer 28: 1149–1154.

7. Olivari, A. 1976. Cell-mediated immune response in head and neck cancer patients. J. Surg. Oncol. 8: 287–294.

8. Parker, R. 1975. On the immunology of head and neck cancer – A prognostic index. J. Laryngol. Otol. 89: 687–695.

9. Eilber, F.R., Morton, D.L., Ketcham, A.S. 1974. Immunologic abnormalities in head and neck cancer. AM. J. Surg. 118: 534–538.

10. Taylor, S.G., Stafford, P.C., 1982. Antigen specificity of squamous cancers of the head and neck based on tumor site using the slide leukocyte adherence inhibition assay. J. Surg. Oncol. 20: 41–45.

11. Krause, C.J. 1979. Characteristics of tumor associated antigens in squamous cell carcinoma. Laryngoscope 89: 1105–1120.

12. Johns, M.D. 1979. Immunological considerations of head and neck cancer. In: Tumors of the Head and Neck, Clinical and Pathological Considerations (J.G. Batsakis, ed.). Williams and Wilkins Co., Baltimore, M.D., pp. 501–502.

13. Ottavianai, G. 1954. L'uso del neoprene Nelle Iniezone Dei Vasi Linfatici. Anteneo Parmense 25: 109–116.

14. Hellstrom, K.E., Hellstrom, I. 1971. Immunologic defenses against cancer. In: Immunobiology (R.A. Good, D.W. Fisher, eds.). Sinauer Associates, Inc., Stanford, CT.

15. Goswitz, F.A., Andrew, G.A., Krisely, R.M.P. 1963. Effects of local irradiation on the peripheral blood and bone marrow. Blood 21: 605.

16. Thomas, J.W., Cory, P., Lewis, H.S. et al. 1971. Effect of therapeutic irradiation on lymphocyte transformation in lung cancer. Cancer 27: 1046.

17. Cosimi, A.B., Brunstetter, F.H., Hemmerer, W.T. 1973. Cellular immune competence of breast cancer patients receiving immunotherapy. Arch. Surg. 107: 531–535.

18. Jenkins, V.K., Griffiths, C.M., Ray, P. et al. 1980. Radiotherapy and head and neck cancer. Arch. Otolaryngol. 106: 414–418.

19. Roth, J.A., Eilber, F.R., Morten, D.L. 1970. Effect of adriamycin and high dose methotrexate on in vivo and in vitro cell-mediated immunity in cancer patients. Cancer 41: 814.

20. Jubert, A.V., Lee, E.T., Hersh, E.M. et al. 1973. Effects of surgery, anesthesia, and intraoperative blood loss in immunocompetence. J. Surg. Res. 15: 399.

21. Lundy, J., Raaf, J.H., Deakins, S. et al. 1975. The acute and chronic effects of alcohol on the human immune system. Surg. Gynecol. Obstet. 141: 212.

22. Hamburger, A.W., Salmon, S.E. 1977. Primary bioassay of human tumor stem cells. Science 197: 461–463.

23. VonHoff, D.O., Casper, J., Bradley, E. et al. 1980. Direct cloning of human neuroblastoma cells on soft agar culture. Cancer Res. 40: 3591–3597.

24. Hamburger, A., Salmon, S.E. 1977. Primary Bioassay of human myeloma stem cells. J. Clin. Invest. 60: 846–854.

25. Schuller, D.E. 1984. An assessment of neck node immunoreactivity in head and neck cancer. Laryngoscope Suppl. # 35 Vol. 97, # 11 Part 2.

26. Fisher, E.R., Fisher, B. 1977. Role of regional lymph nodes. In: Secondary spread in Breast Cancer (B.A. Stoll, ed.). Heinemann Medical and Year Book Medical.

27. Fisher, B., Wolmark, N., Coyle, J. et al. 1975. Studies concerning the regional lymph node in cancer. VIII. Effect of two asynchronous tumor foci on lymph node cytoxicity. Cancer 36: 521–527.

28. Fisher, B., Saffer, E, Fisher, E.R. 1974. Studies concerning the regional lymph node in cancer. IV. Tumor inhibition by regional node cells. Cancer 33: 631–636.

29. Fisher, E.R., Riebord, H.E., Fisher, E.R. 1973. Studies concerning the regional lymph node in cancer. V. Histologic and ultrastructural findings in regional and nonregional nodes. Lab. Invest. 28: 126–132.

30. Fisher, E.R., Saffer, E., Fisher, B. 1913. Studies concerning the regional lymph node in cancer. VI. Correlation of lymphocytes transformation of regional node celles and some histopathologic discriminants. Cancer 32: 104–111.

31. Fisher, B, Fisher, E.R. 1972. Studies concerning the regional lymph node in cancer. II. Maintenance of immunity. Cancer 29: 1496–1501.

32. Fisher, B., Saffer, E.A., Fisher, E.R. 1974. Studies concerning the regional lymph node in cancer. VII. Thymidine uptake by cells from nodes of breast cancer patients relative to axillary location and histopathologic discriminants. Cancer 33: 271–279.

33. Sessions, D.G. 1976. Surgical pathology of cancer of the larynx and hypopharynx. Laryngoscope 86: 814–821.

34. Schuller, D.E., McGuirt, W.F., McCabe, B.F. *et al.* 1980. The prognostic significance of metastatic cervical lymph nodes. Laryngoscope 90: 557–570.

35. Schuller, D.E., Libby, D.H., Rinehart, J.J., Milo, G.G., Koolemans-Beynen, A. 1985. Immunomodulation of nodal lymphocytes in head and neck cancer. Arch. Otolaryngol. Vol. 111, July.

36. Berlinger, N.T., Tsakraklides, V., Pollak, K. *et al.* 1976. Prognostic significance of lymph node histology in patients with squamous cell carcinoma of the larynx, pharynx, or oral cavity. Laryngoscope 86: 792–803.

37. Black, M.M., Kerpe, S., Speer, F.D. 1953. Lymph node structure in patients with cancer of the breast. Am. J. Pathol. 29: 505–521.

11. Nasopharyngeal carcinoma: relationship to Epstein-Barr virus and treatment with interferon

JOSEPH M. CONNORS and CHARLOTTE JACOBS

Introduction – Nasopharyngeal carcinoma

Nasopharyngeal carcinoma (NPC) is a unique epithelial neoplasm which accounts for 85% of malignancies of the nasopharynx [1]. It has several special characteristics, including its geographical and ethnic distribution and its relationship to Epstein-Barr virus (EBV), the causative agent of infectious mononucleosis. Although relatively rare in the overall population of North America with an incidence of 4 per million, it is 25 times more common in Chinese Americans [1] and also has an increased frequency in Alaskan natives [2]. Worldwide it is an important tumor because of its wide distribution and high incidence in certain areas such as Southern China [3], North Africa [4, 5] and Southeast Asia [5]. It occurs about twice as often in males and reaches its peak incidence in the fourth through sixth decades [1].

Nasopharyngeal carcinoma has been associated with environmental exposure to smoke and cooking fumes and with inflammatory conditions of the ear, nose, and throat [6], but a consistently identified set of high risk factors has not emerged. It is more frequent in persons with HLA-A2 haplotype with fewer than two B locus antigens, indicating, along with the geographical and ethnic distributions, the likelihood of a genetic contribution to susceptibility. Additional background characteristics and the biological and pathologic findings typical of this disease have recently been reviewed [7].

Nasopharyngeal carcinoma typically spreads locally and metastasizes first to the cervical lymph nodes. Local invasion of the base of the skull may be present in 5 to 25% of patients on presentation [8, 9], and cervical lymph node metastases are detectable in 60 to 85% [8–10]; both findings are associated with poor prognosis. The best treatment results have been obtained with radiation therapy to both the primary site (6000 to 7000 rads in 6 to 7 weeks) and the neck lymph nodes (usually 4000 to 5000 rads depending upon extent of involvement). Single institution series have produced long-term disease-free survivals of 40 to 60% using these radiation techniques [8–10]. Despite this progress, however, 50 to 60%

C. Jacobs (ed) Cancers of the head and neck.
© *1987, Martinus Nijhoff Publishers, Boston. ISBN 0–89838–825–2. Printed in the Netherlands.*

of patients with NPC either present with advanced disease or relapse either inside maximally treated radiation fields or in distant sites, usually bone, liver or lung. Although NPC is responsive to chemotherapy [11], results reported to date have been disappointing and indicate that there is only a limited palliative role for available systemic agents.

Nasopharyngeal carcinoma and Epstein-Barr virus

Epstein-Barr virus (EBV), a large DNA human virus, is the causative agent of infectious mononucleosis and has been closely associated with two human neoplasms: Burkitt's lymphoma [12] and nasopharyngeal carcinoma (NPC). The association between EBV and NPC has been extensively documented and is summarized in Table 1. A definite picture linking EBV to NPC emerges from

Table 1. Evidence of association between Epstein-Barr virus (EBV) and nasopharyngeal carcinoma (NPC)

Evidence (references)

Viral
  NPC cells uniquely contain EBV nuclear antigen [13–15]
  NPC cells contain EBV DNA [13, 15–18]
  EBV can be recovered from NPC cells [19]

Serologic
  IgA anti-EBV-VCA is increased in NPC patients [4, 14, 15, 17, 20–27]
  IgA anti-EBV-EAD is increased in NPC patients [15, 20, 24, 25, 27]
  IgA anti-EBV-VCA distinguishes NPC from other neoplasms [4, 16, 22, 24, 26–30]
  IgA anti-EBV-VCA is a useful screening tool for NPC [4, 16, 26, 28–32]
  ↑ IgA anti-EBV-VCA precedes NPC presentation [32, 33]
  ↑ IgA anti-EBV-VCA precedes relapse of NPC [20, 28, 32]
  ↑ IgA anti-EBV-VCA level correlates with ↑ tumor burden [16, 20, 27]
  ↑ IgA anti-EBV-VCA level correlates with ↓ prognosis [27, 28]
  ↑ Anti-EBV-DNAase antibody levels correlate with ↓ prognosis [34]
  Effective NPC treatment decreases IgA anti-EBV-VCA levels [20, 26–28, 32]
  NPC patients have salivary IgA anti-EBV-VCA [35]
  NPC family members have IgA anti-EBV-VCA [36]
  NPC health care workers have IgA anti-EBV-VCA [36]

Cell mediated immunity
  ↑ ADCC against EBV containing cells correlates with ↑ tumor burden and ↓ prognosis [37–39]
  NPC patients have selectively decreased EBV specific T-cell activity [21]

DNA = deoxyribonucleic acid; IgA = immunoglobulin A; VCA = viral capsid antigen; EAD = early antigen diffuse type; ADCC = antibody dependent cellular cytotoxity.

these data. The viral genome and associated nuclear antigen (EBNA) are found in neoplastic cells from patients with NPC but not from patients with other carcinomas or lymphomas. The transmitable virus can be recovered from these cells. Immunoglobulin type A antibodies against the virus, which are relatively specific for NPC, are found in elevated levels in NPC patients and can be used as screening or diagnostic tools to identify NPC patients. The titres of these antibodies rise preceding clinical presentation or relapse. In addition the level of the titres correlates directly with presence of cervical metastases, increased tumor burden, and prognosis. Health care workers and family members in contact with NPC patients have heightened antibody responses. T-cell mediated immunity to EBV is selectivity deficient in NPC patients, and decreased antibody dependent cellular cytoxicity for EBV-containing cells correlates with high tumor burden and unfavorable prognosis. These latter data are consistent with active immune regulation and may indicate a potential use for immune modulators in treatment. Although not proof of causation, this unique association between EBV and NPC implies an important role for virus-host interaction in the natural history of the disease.

Interferon

The interferons (IFN) make up a family of related complex glycoproteins and proteins with cell growth and expression-regulating properties. There are three major species each of which is produced by a different type of cell: alpha IFN by leukocytes, beta IFN by fibroblasts and gamma IFN by T-cell lymphocytes. IFN has been shown to have anti-viral activity against the following viruses which have been associated with malignancy: hepatitis B [40], papovavirus [41], Varicella-zoster [42, 43], Herpes simplex [44] and EBV [45].

A detailed rationale for the use of IFN as an anti-neoplastic agent has been outlined by Borden [46]. Kirkwood and Ernstoff have reviewed the actual use of IFN for the treatment of human neoplasms [47]. They described the antineoplastic activity of IFN for a range of diseases including breast carcinoma, ovarian carcinoma, renal cell adenocarcinoma, melanoma, carcinoid, hairy cell leukemia, non-Hodgkin's lymphoma, myeloma and mycoses fungoides. Of particular relevance to NPC may be the reports of responses to IFN in two groups of patients. Patients with uterine cervical carcinoma, a papova- and herpes-virus associated neoplasm, have been reported to respond to topical IFN [48]. Also, patients with juvenile laryngeal papillomatosis, a papovavirus-associated tumor of the upper airways, have responded to systematically administered IFN [49].

Three observations provide a rationale for testing the usefulness of IFN in the treatment of NPC: (a) NPC is associated with EBV, and IFN is known to have general anti-viral and specific anti-EBV activity [45]; (b) IFN has anti-neoplastic properties possibly independent of its anti-viral activity; (c) the natural history of NPC correlates with measurable changes in serologic and cell-mediated types of immunity directed against EBV, and IFN is a known immunomodulator and potentional immunopotentiator. Finally, the lack of currently available effective systemic treatments for NPC indicates a need to explore new types of therapy.

Interferon treatment of nasopharyngeal carcinoma

Preliminary studies

In 1980 Treuner and his co-workers reported the results of IFN treatment in a 16-year old boy with locally advanced, chemotherapy refractory NPC [50]. Over a 5-month treatment course with beta IFN the child had complete resolution of disease, accompanied, interestingly, by normalization of anti-EBV serologic studies and the eventual development of an anti-IFN antibody which was completely neutralizing for beta IFN [51, 52]. In 1980, Howarth and Merigan treated an adolescent who had regionally recurrent NPC with both alpha and beta IFN without benefit [53]. In 1983, Matheson and co-workers reported a partial response in a patient with locally recurrent NPC using a combination of intralesional and intravenous beta IFN [54].

Table 2. Patient characteristics and treatment outcomes

Age	KPS[a]	Disease site	Days of IFN	Outcome
28	60	Bone, lung, liver	22	Progression
60	40	Brain	23	Progression
33	60	Nasopharynx, bone, liver	30	Progression
53	60	Nasopharynx, bone, liver	3	Progression
55	100	Nasopharynx	28	Progression
52	60	Lymph nodes, adrenals	13	Stable, declined further treatment
40	90	Nasopharynx, sinuses	30	Stable
27	100	Lung	21	Stable, withdrawn due to neutropenia
53	80	Bone, neck mass	30	<50% reduction
75	60	Lung	30	<50% reduction
63	50	Nasopharynx, palate, tonsil	30	90% reduction
21	80	Bone	30	>50% reduction

[a] Karnofsky performance status.

Clinical trials

Between 1980 and 1983 we tested the use of alpha IFN in a phase II trial for patients with recurrent or metastatic NPC. The results in the first 12 patients have been reported in detail [53] and are summarized here.

Human alpha IFN with a specific activity of 10 reference units per milligram protein and a concentration of 4×10^6 reference units per millilitre was given at at dose of 10×10^6 units IM daily for 30 days to patients with locally recurrent or metastatic NPC who had relapsed after initial high-dose radiation therapy. The toxicities encountered were typical of IFN and consisted of universal fatigue, fever, anorexia and myalgias and asymptomatic modest rises in serum liver enzyme activity (50%) or reversible moderate bone marrow suppression (thrombocytopenia – 16%, leukopenia – 25%). No toxicity unique to NPC patients emerged, although one patient withdrew because of myalgia, and another had the IFN discontinued because of persistent leukopenia.

Clinical characteristics, sites of disease, number of days of treatment and outcome for the 12 NPC patients treated with IFN are shown in Table 2. Four patients developed measurable tumor response: two had less than a 50% reduction and two had objective partial (> 50%) response. Maintenance IFN preserved the partial responses for 1 and 6 months, respectively. These results indicate a definite, albeit moderate, response rate using acceptable doses of impure IFN over a relatively short period and confirm the activity of IFN in NPC.

Treuner and his co-workers have now reported the results of treatment of a total of six children, ages 9 to 16 years, with advanced NPC, using beta IFN [55]. In addition to the previously reported complete remission [50] which has now lasted 2 ½ years, they have seen stable disease in three. Martens reported the results of treatment with beta IFN of seven adult patients with poor prognosis NPC. Three were treated adjuvantly after radiation and had progression of tumor noted

Table 3. Results of phase II clinical trials testing IFN for NPC

Interferon	No. of patients	Response[a]				
		CR	PR	MR/Stable	Rate (CR + PR)	Reference
Alpha	12	0	2	3	17%	53
Beta	6	1	0	2	17%	55
Beta	4	0	1	1	25%	56
Beta	3	0	0	2	0	57

[a] Responses: CR = complete response, PR = partial response, MR = measurable but < 50%.

at 7, 10 and 28 months. Four were treated for locoregional persistence or recurrence (three patients) or distant metastases (one patient). One had a 90% tumor regression lasting 6 months, one had stable disease for 2 months and two had progression. Finally, Furukawa treated three adult Japanese patients with beta IFN [57]. In two the disease remained stable, and in one it progressed. The summarized results from these four series [54, 55–57] are shown in Table 3. Only patients with evaluable disease are included, and the three adjuvant patients [56] are omitted. Combining the 25 reported patients, one arrives at an overall response rate of 16%. No substantive difference between alpha and beta IFN has been demonstrated. Likewise, there was no difference between pediatric and adult patients. Since in all other respects the disease is similar in children and adults [58], this lack of difference is not surprising. Dosing and schedule varied so widely among the studies that they cannot be evaluated.

In three of the clinical trials summarized above, serial measurements of anti-EBV serologic tests ware performed [53, 55, 57]. Only two patients had a change in titre. In one patient, the anti-EBV-VCA titre rose with progressive disease [53], and in the patient with a complete response the serologic titres all fell to normal [55]. In the alpha IFN trial [53], six patients were checked for oropharyngeal excretion of EBV [59, 60] before, during and after IFN. No virus was detected.

Conclusion

The rationale for testing IFN in patients with NPC is compelling. This neoplasm is associated with a virus, has a course which correlates well with immunologic changes, and has no effective systemic therapy available today for recurrent or metastatic disease. A modest but definite responsiveness of the tumor to IFN has been demonstrated in four separate clinical trials, consistent with a response rate of approximately 15–20%. One prolonged complete remission has been reported. Lack of a higher response rate may be related to several factors: short trial duration, impure IFN preparations, suboptimal IFN doses, compromised patient performance status at treatment initiation or heavy pre-treatment with chemotherapy or radiation. Observation of a definite response rate under these conditions should prompt further investigation of IFN in the treatment of NPC patients. It seems quite possible that better opportunities for increased efficacy may occur earlier in the course of the disease. Perhaps intervention at a time when virus-host interaction may be still important would be more rewarding. Such opportunities may be present in the setting of detection of high-risk patients found in screening programs using anti-EBV-VCA levels or when radiation has rendered the patient free of detectable disease. Certainly, a neoplasm with the worldwide importance of NPC deserves thorough investigation of any potentially helpful treatment, such as IFN, at several different stages in its clinical evolution.

References

1. Levine, P.H., Connelly, R.R., Easton, J.M. 1980. Demographic patterns for nasopharyngeal carcinoma in the United States. Int. J. Cancer 26: 741–748.
2. Lanier, A. 1977. Survey of cancer incidence in Alaskan natives. Nat. Cancer Inst. Monog. 47: 87–88.
3. Clifford, P. 1970. A review on the epidemiology of nasopharyngeal carcinoma. Int. J. Cancer 5: 287–309.
4. Malik, M.O.A., Banatvala, J., Hutt, M.S.R., Abu-Sim, A.Y., Hidaytallah, A., El-Hadi, A.E. 1979. Epstein-Barr virus antibodies in Sudanese patients with nasopharyngeal carcinoma: a preliminary report. J.N.C.I. 62: 221–224.
5. Muir, C.S. 1971. Nasopharyngeal carcinoma in non-Chinese populations with special reference to southeast Asia and Africa. Int. J. Cancer 8: 351–363.
6. Henderson, B.E., Louie, E., Jing, S.J., Buell, P., Gardner, M.E. 1976. Risk factors associated with nasopharyngeal carcinoma. N. Engl. J. Med. 295: 1101–1106.
7. Fedder, M., Gonzalez, M.F., 1985. Nasopharyngeal carcinoma: brief review. A. J. Med. 79: 365–369.
8. Baker, S.R., Wolfe, R.A. 1982. Prognostic factors of nasopharyngeal malignancy. Cancer 42: 163–169.
9. Mesic, J.B., Fletcher, G.H., Goepfert, H. 1981. Megavoltage irradiation of epithelial tumors of the nasopharynx. Int. J. Rad.iat. Oncol. Biol. Ohys. 7: 447–453.
10. Hoppe, R.T., Goffinet, D.R., Bagshaw, M.A. 1946. Carcinoma of the nasopharynx. Cancer 37: 2605–2612.
11. Decker, D.A., Drelichman, A., Al-Sarraf, M., Crissman, J., Reed, M.L. 1983. Chemotherapy for nasopharyngeal carcinoma. Cancer 52: 602–605.
12. Heule, W., Heule, G., Lennette, E.T. 1979. The Epstein-Barr virus. Sci. Am. 241: 48–49.
13. Huang, D.P., Ho, H.C., Henle, W., Henle, G., Saw, D., Lui, M. 1970. Presence of EBNA in nasopharyngeal carcinoma and control patient tissues related to EBV serology. Int. J. Cancer 22: 266–274.
14. Lanier, A., Bender, T., Talbot, M. *et al.* 1980. Epstein-Barr virus DNA in tumor tissue from native Alaskan patients with nasopharyngeal carcinoma. Lancet 2: 1095.
15. Lanier, A.P., Bornkamm, G.W., Henle, W. *et al.* 1981. Association of Epstein-Barr virus with nasopharyngeal carcinoma in Alaskan native patients: serum antibodies and tissue EBNA and DNA. Int. J. Cancer 28: 301–305.
16. Ringborn, U., Henle, W., Henle, G. *et al.* 1983. Epstein-Barr virus specific serodiagnostic tests in carcinomas of the head and neck. Cancer 52: 1237–1243.
17. Andersson-Anvret, M., Forsby, N., Klein, G., Henle, W., Biorklund, A. 1979. Relationship between the Epstein-Barr virus genome and nasopharyngeal carcinoma in caucasian patients. Int. J. Cancer 23: 762–767.
18. Desgranges, C., Pi, G.H., Bornkamm, G.W., Legrand, C., Zeng, Y., De-The, G. 1983. Presence of EBV-DNA sequences in nasopharyngeal cells of individuals without IgA-VCA antibodies. Int. J. Cancer 32: 543–545.
19. Tumper, P.A., Epstein, M.A., Giovanella, B.C., Finerty, D. 1977. Isolation of infectious EB virus from the epithelial tumor cells of nasopharyngeal carcinoma. Int. J. Cancer 20: 655–662.
20. Henle, W., Ho, J.H.C., Henle, G, Chau, J.W.C., Kwan, H.C. 1977. Nasopharyngeal carcinoma: significance of changes in Epstein-Barr virus related antibody patterns following therapy. Int. J. Cancer 20: 663–672.
21. Moss, D.J., Chan, S.H., Burrows, S.R. *et al.* 1983. Epstein-Barr virus specific T-cell response in nasopharyngeal carcinoma patients. Int. J. Cancer 32: 301–305.
22. Ho, H.L., Kwan, H.C., Wu, P., Chan, S.K., Ng, M.H., Saw, D. 1978. Epstein-Barr antibodies in suspected nasopharyngeal carcinoma. Lancet 2: 1094–1095.

23. Ho, H.C., Ng, M.H., Kwan, H.C. 1978. Factors affecting serum IgA antibody to Epstein-Barr viral capsid antigens in nasopharyngeal carcinoma. Br. J. Cancer 37: 356–362.

24. Desgranges, C., De-The, G. 1979. Epstein-Barr virus specific IgA serum antibodies in nasopharyngeal and other respiratory carcinomas. Int. J. Cancer 24: 555–559.

25. Naegele, R.F., Champion, J., Murphy, D., Henle, G., Henle, W. 1982. Nasopharyngeal carcinoma in American children: Epstein-Barr virus specific antibody titers and prognosis. Int. J. Cancer 29: 209–212.

26. Tamada, A., Makimoto, K., Yamabe, H. et al. 1984. Titers of Epstein-Barr virus related antibodies in nasopharyngeal carcinoma in Japan. Cancer 53: 430–440.

27. Henle, G., Henle, W. 1976. Epstein-Barr virus specific IgA serum antibodies as an outstanding feature of nasopharyngeal carcinoma. Int. J. Cancer 17: 1–7.

28. Pearson, G.R., Weiland, L.H., Neel, H.B. et al. 1983. Application of Epstein-Barr virus (EBV) serology to the diagnosis of North American nasopharyngeal carcinoma. Cancer 51: 260–268.

29. Coates, H.L., Pearson, G.R., Neel, H.B., Weiland, L.H., Devine, K.D. 1978. An immunologic basis for detection of occult primary malignancies of the head and neck. Cancer 41: 912–918.

30. Ho, H.C., Ng, M.H., Kwan, H.C., Chau, J.W.C. 1976. Epstein-Barr virus specific IgA and IgG serum antibodies in nasopharyngeal carcinoma. Br. J. Cancer 34: 655–660.

31. Zeng, Y., Zhang, L.G., Li, H.Y., et al. 1982. Serological mass survey for early detection of nasopharyngeal carcinoma in Wuzhou City, China. Int. J. Cancer 39: 139–141.

32. Lanier, A.P., Henle, W., Bender, T.R., Henle, G., Talbot, M. 1980. Epstein-Barr virus specific antibody titers in seven Alaskan natives before and after diagnosis of nasopharyngeal carcinoma. Int. J. Cancer 26: 133–137.

33. Ho, H.C., Kwan, H.C., Ng, M.H., De-The, G. 1978. Serum IgA antibodies to Epstein-Barr virus capsid antigen preceding symptoms of nasopharyngeal carcinoma. Lancet 1: 436.

34. Tan, R.S., Cheng, Y.C., Naegele, R.F., Henle, W., Glaser, R., Champion, J. 1982. Antibody responses to Epstein-Barr virus specific DNase in relation to the prognosis of juvenile patients with nasopharyngeal carcinoma. Int. J. Cancer 30: 561–565.

35. Desgranges, C., Li, J.Y., De-The, G. 1977. EBV specific secretory IgA in saliva of NPC patients. Presence of secretory piece in epithelial malignant cells. Int. J. Cancer 20: 881–886.

36. Ho, H.C., Kwan, H.C., Poon, Y.F., Tse, K.C., Ng, L.H. 1978. Epstein-Barr virus infection in staff treating patients with nasopharyngeal carcinoma. Lancet 1: 710–711.

37. Pearson, G.R., Neel, H.B., Weiland, L.H. et al. Antibody dependent cellular cytotoxicity and disease course in North American patients with nasopharyngeal carcinoma: a prospective study. Int. J. Cancer 33: 777–782.

38. Chan, S.H., Levin, P.H., De-The, G.B. et al. 1979. A comparison of the prognostic value of antibody dependent lymphocyte cytotoxicity and other EBV antibody assays in Chinese patients with nasopharyngeal carcinoma. Int. J. Cancer 23: 181–185.

39. Pearson, G.R., Johansson, B., Klein, G. 1978. Antibody dependent cellular cytotoxicity against Epstein-Barr virus associated antigens in African patients with nasopharyngeal carcinoma. Int. J. Cancer 22: 120–125.

40. Greenberg, H.B., Pollard, R.B., Lutwick, L.I., Gregory, P.B., Robinson, W.S., Merigan, T.C. 1976. Effect of human leukocyte interferon on hepatitis B virus infection in patients with chronic active hepatitis. N. Engl. J. Med. 295: 517–522.

41. Oxman, M.W. 1973. Interferon, tumors and tumor viruses. In: Interferon and Interferon Inducers (N.B. Finter, ed.). American Elsevier Publishing Co., New York, pp. 391–479.

42. Arvin, A.M., Kushner, J.H., Feldman, S., Baehner, R.L., Hammond, D., Merigan, T.C. 1982. Human leukocyte interferon for the treatment of varicella in children with cancer. N. Engl. J. Med. 306: 761–765.

43. Merigen, T.C., Rand, K.H., Pollard, R.B. et al. 1978. Human leukocyte interferon for the treatment of herpes zoster in patients with cancer. N. Engl. J. Med. 298: 981–987.

44. Rasmussen, L., Farley, L.B. 1975. Inhibition of herpesvirus replication by human interferon. Infect. Immun. 12: 104–108.
45. Cheeseman, S.H., Henle, W., Rubin, R. 1980. Epstein-Barr virus infection in renal transplant recipients. Ann. Intern. Med. 93: 39–42.
46. Borden, E.C.. 1979. Interferons: rationale for clinical trials in neoplastic disease. Ann. Intern. Med. 91: 472–479.
47. Kirkwood, J.M., Ernstoff, M.S. 1984. Interferons in the treatment of human cancer. J. Clin. Oncol. 2: 336–352.
48. Krasic, J., Kirkmajer, V., Knezevic, M. et al. 1981. Influence of human leukocyte interferon on squamous cell carcinoma of the uterine cervix. Clinical, histological and histochemical observations III. J. Cancer Res. Clin. Oncol. 101: 309–315.
49. Haglund, S., Lundquist, P.G., Cantell, K. et al. 1981. Interferon therapy in juvenile laryngeal papillomatosis. Arch. Otolaryngol. 107: 327–332.
50. Treuner, J., Niethammer, D., Dannecker, G., Hogmann, R., Neef, V., Hofschneider, P.H. 1980. Successful treatment of nasopharyngeal carcinoma with interferon. Lancet 1: 817–818.
51. Vallbracht, A., Treuner, J., Flehmig, K., Joester, E., Biethammer, D. 1981. Interferon neutralizing antibodies in a patient treated with human fibroblast interferon. Nature 289: 496–497.
52. Vallbracht A., Treuner, J., Manncke, K.H., Niethammer, D., 1982. Autoantibodies against human beta interferon following treatment with interferon. J. Interferon Res. 2: 107–110.
53. Connors, J.M., Andiman, W.A., Howarth, C.B. et al. 1985. Treatment of nasopharyngeal carcinoma with human leukocyte interferon. J. Clin. Oncol. 3: 813–817.
54. Matheson, D.S., Tan, Y.H., Green, B., McPherson, T.A. 1983. Effect of fibroblast derived interferon administration on immune responsiveness in a patient with nasopharyngeal carcinoma. J. Interferon Res. 3: 437–441.
55. Treuner, J., Niethammer, D., 1984. Behandlung des nasopharynxkarzinoms mit Interferon. Strahlentherapie 160, special issue 78: 184–187.
56. Mertens, R., Karstens, J.H., Ammon, J., Classen, H.W., Mittermayer, C. 1984. Bisherige Erfahrungen der Interferontherapie an 7 Patienten mit nasopharynxkarzinom. Strahlentherapie 160, special issue 78: 188–193.
57. Furukawa, M., 1984. Treatment and clinical results of nasopharyngeal carcinoma (NPC) with interferon (IFN-beta) and its effects on Epstein-Barr virus (EBV) serology. Otolaryngology (Tokyo) 56: 899–903.
58. Jenkin, R.D., Anderson, J.R., Jereb, B. et al. 1981. Nasopharyngeal carcinoma – a retrospective review of patients less than thirty years of age: A report from Childrens Cancer Study Group. Cancer 47: 360–366.
59. Strauch, B., Siegel, N., Andrews, L., Miller, G. 1974. Oropharyngeal excretion of Epstein-Barr virus by renal transplant recipients and other patients treated with immunosuppressive drugs. Lancet 1: 234–237.
60. Chang, R.S., Lewis, J.P., Reynolds, R.D. et al., 1978. Oropharyngeal excretion of Epstein-Barr virus by patients with lymphoproliferative disorders and by recipients of renal homografts. Ann. Intern. Med. 88: 34–40.

12. The use of retinoids in head and neck cancer

REUBEN LOTAN, STIMSON P. SCHANTZ and WAUN KI HONG

The natural history of head and neck cancer

Squamous cell carcinoma (SCC) of the head and neck, which occurs in this country most commonly between the ages of 40 and 70 years, accounts for 5% of all tumors and affects approximately 26,000 persons each year [1]. More than 90% of patients with head and neck cancer will have a history of tobacco consumption [2–4]. The estimated age-standardized mortality rate for laryngeal cancer is 0.96 deaths per 100,000 person years, less than one-twentieth of the heavy smoker [3]. Evidence from multiple independent investigations indicates that tobacco usage is linearly related to the development of head and neck cancer [4–7]. Areas within the upper aerodigestive tract at risk for the development of SCC relate to the manner in which tobacco is consumed [7]. Moore and Catlin have postulated that the relationship of tobacco usage to the site of head and neck cancer depends on prolonged contact of concentrated carcinogens suspended in saliva and subsequent 'pooling' in mucous reservoirs [8]. Such a hypothesis accounts for the observation that in this country 75% of cancers in the oral cavity originate in a horseshoe-shaped area consisting of only 20% of the surface area of the entire oral mucosa. This region extends from the anterior floor of the mouth backward along both lingual-alveolar sulci to include the lateral margin of the mobile tongue and the anterior tonsillar pillar-retromolar trigone complex. It is the wide area of exposure to carcinogenic compounds that accounts for the 'field cancerization' concept first related by Slaughter et al. [9]. According to this concept, mucosal abnormalities exist over a broad area of oral, pharyngeal, and laryngeal epithelia and are not merely confined to the site of neoplastic transformation that is clinically or histopathologically apparent. This hypothesis provides an explanation for the high development rate of multiple primary cancers throughout the upper aerodigestive tract. Tobacco-induced alterations have been documented by histopathologic analyses, cellular biochemical analyses, and genetic transformation. A tobacco-related polycyclic hydrocarbon carcinogen, benzo [a]pyrene, when dispersed in saline and administered to hams-

C. Jacobs (ed) Cancers of the head and neck.
© *1987, Martinus Nijhoff Publishers, Boston. ISBN 0–89838–825–2. Printed in the Netherlands.*

ters by repeated tracheal installations yielded incidences of tumors, mostly SCC, up to 100%. A sequence of changes from normal columnar, to mucous-producing bronchial epithelium, to areas of squamous metaplasia, and to squamous tumors developed [10]. These changes were identical to mucosal alterations in human subjects with a history of smoking [11].

Besides the strong association of tobacco abuse among the population of head and neck cancer patients, a positive history of excessive alcohol ingestion is commonly reported in these persons. However, despite this association, there is no clearly established evidence that implicates alcohol as the sole carcinogen in either humans or animals [12, 13]. Indeed, studies have demonstrated that among nonsmokers, no increase in head and neck cancer has been observed in those who are alcoholics [12]. Because of its effect, however, alcohol can be viewed as a cocarcinogen that may possibly augment the carcinogenic potential of more fundamental etiologic factors [14, 15]. Among smokers, there exists a linear dose response between levels of alcohol consumption and cancer risk [14]. Thus, the effects of alcohol are an important consideration in the etiology of the disease.

The effects of alcohol as a cancer-promoting agent may be indirect, i.e., cancer-potentiating factors may result from processes occurring in parallel to alcohol consumption. Perhpas the most widely studied relevant process may be the role of nutritional defiency. Alcoholics are characteristically nutritionally depleted [12]. The increased risk of head and neck cancer may not relate to direct effects of alcohol, but may result from the associated impaired nutrient absorption [16]. Indeed, studies have shown that alcoholic patients who developed head and neck cancer had lower serum albumin and vitamin levels than did other alcoholics without cancer, which supports the role of malnutrition [16].

The incidence of head and neck cancer is substantially lower than the proportion of smokers and alcohol users. Hence, additional factors must be involved in the causation of these cancers. Recent reports presented evidence incriminating viral agents in the cause of head and neck cancers. Epstein-Barr virus [17], papilloma virus [18], and herpes virus [19] have been found in head and neck neoplasms. Seroepidemiological evidence suggests that herpes simplex type I may act as an initiator in the development of head and neck cancer [19]. The ability of viruses to exist in a latent form within the host cells and the capability of certain tumor promoters to activate such viruses may be important factors in head and neck carcinogenesis.

There exists another major consideration in the pathogenesis and progression of head and neck cancer, namely, the role of immune responses. Factors associated with the development of the disease, i.e., tobacco, alcohol, chronic viral infections, age, and malnutrition can all be characterized as immunosuppressive [20]. Our understanding of the significance of this deficient immune response is rudimentary and in some instances, contradictory. Yet, a dominant theme throughout the literature on the immunology of head and neck cancer exists. The presence of impaired host response in these patients, whether it be measured by delayed-type hypersensitivity to skin test recall antigens, *in vitro* blastogenesis response to mitogens, or reduced circulating T-cell populations, will portend a worse prognosis [20].

It is unfortunate that the incidence of head and neck cancer seems to be increasing. The effectiveness of surgery or radiotherapy or both to control locoregional disease is well established, especially in early-stage disease [21]. Despite improved local control rates by surgery or radiotherapy or both, the overall survival rate has not improved in the past two decades [22]. Local recurrence and distant metastases are still major problems. A high rate of local recurrence at the primary site was observed in patients presenting with advanced stages such as T_3 or T_4. Further, recent investigations indicate that up to 40% of patients with T_3 or T_4 tumor develop distant metastases [22]. Because of the high recurrence rate, there have been numerous clinical trials of chemotherapy in an adjuvant setting in the past 10 years, but no impact on survival has yet been made [23].

Further, a patient with SCC of the head and neck region is at increased risk for developing an additional second primary neoplasm [24–30]. Many patients treated at an early stage and presumably cured will develop a second metachronous primary neoplasm in the aerodigestive tract. The site of the second primary neoplasm varies from 10% in the larynx to 40% in the oropharynx [26]. This patient is more likely to die of the second cancer than of the initial primary tumor; therefore, no improvement in survival has been made in the last two decades. The pathogenesis of second primary tumors and recurrence at primary sites after a long disease-free interval is not well understood. It has been suggested that field cancerization is related to diffuse mucosal membrane diathesis as condemned mucosa after exposure to carcinogens or as possible submucosal metastases from the original tumor [28]. Recent investigations indicate that premalignant lesions are seen in normal-appearing epithelium adjacent to SCC [31]. This premalignant lesion will progress in severity and result in frank malignancy ultimately, either as a local recurrence or as a metachronous second primary tumor [28, 31]. Hence, there is a need for suppressing this progression to malignancy.

Retinoids, a group of metabolites and synthetic analogs of vitamin A (retinol), are excellent candidates for this purpose since these compounds are capable of modulating the growth and differentiation of preneoplastic cells and malignant carcinoma cells [32, 33], as well as enhancing host antitumor immune responses [34–36]. This chapter will review the background and present a rationale for using retinoids as adjuvant and chemopreventive agents in the treatment of head and neck squamous cell carcinoma (HNSCC) in humans.

Vitamin A: retinoids and the differentiation and growth of normal epithelial cells

Vitamin A deficiency in rodents leads to squamous metaplasia [37]. It is thought that in the absence of vitamin A, basal cells proliferate and express an abnormal pattern of differentiation into squamous keratinizing cells instead of into columnar, mucous, and ciliated cells [38–42]. Vitamin A and certain retinoids are capable of reversing these effects of vitamin A deficiency both *in vivo* [43] and in organ culture [42, 44, 45]. Indeed, cytokinetic and ultrastructural changes that accompany this reversal indicate that retinoids, such as β-all trans retinoic acid, inhibit basal cell proliferation, stimulate mucous cell proliferation, and redirect differentiation into mucous and ciliated cells instead of into squamous cells, thereby restoring normal epithelial morphology [46]. Excess of vitamin A or of retinoids also abrogates epithelial cell differentiation *in vivo* and in organ culture by inhibiting keratinization and inducing mucous metaplasia in epidermal cells. This effect is reversed after removal of the retinoid [47–49].

Advances in techniques for the *in vitro* growth of epithelial cells, such as keratinocytes, have made it possible to investigate the effects of retinoids under more controlled conditions. Extensive studies with normal murine and human keratinocytes have further demonstrated the remarkable ability of retinoids to modulate squamous differentiation. Thus, treatment of keratinocytes with retinoids increases desquamation of superficial cells [50, 51] and results in a morphological conversion to a secretory epithelium [52, 53]. The underlying biochemical changes induced by retinoids include a reduction in the formation of cornified envelopes [54–56] and a decrease in the transcription of the genes coding for keratins of M_r 67 Kd and 56.5 Kd and a concurrent stimulated transcription of the genes for keratins of M_r 52 Kd and 40 Kd [57, 58]. Specific changes have also been observed in cell surface components such as an increased expression of pemphigoid antigen [59], stimulated incorporation of monosaccharides into glycoproteins [60, 61], and a reduced cell surface binding of certain lectins [62]. In addition to influencing spontaneous keratinization, retinoids also inhibit the terminal differentiation of keratinocytes exposed to Ca^{2+} or phorbol ester tumor promoters [63, 64].

The proliferation of keratinocytes from different tissues is modulated differentially by retinoids. Thus, retinoids have been found to either inhibit [53] or stimulate [65–67] the growth of some cells, or they have not affected the growth of other cells [50, 68].

Most of the above-mentioned studies employed epidermal cells; however, it is quite plausible to assume that similar effects might be exerted by retinoids on other epithelial cells such as those of the upper aerodigestive tract.

Vitamin A and retinoids as inhibitors of epithelial cancer development and growth

The incidence of spontaneous [69] or carcinogen-induced [70] carcinomas in vitamin A-deficient animals was higher than in control ones. These observations suggested a relationship between retinoids and cancer development. It is interesting that the metaplasia that appears in epithelia during vitamin A deficiency is similar to the preneoplastic lesions caused by chemical carcinogens. Since vitamin A and retinoids can reverse the abnormal differentiation in vitamin A-deficient animals or in organ cultures, attempts were made to reverse the effects of carcinogens by retinoids. Such studies have demonstrated that retinoids can block and reverse hyperplastic changes induced by chemical carcinogens in prostate organ cultures [71]. Subsequent investigations have shown that various retinoids are able to suppress the development of carcinomas in different epithelial tissues of rodents exposed to certain chemical carcinogens [72]. It is noteworthy that Saffioti *et al.* demonstrated that vitamin A derivatives were able to prevent hydrocarbon-induced trachebronchial squamous metaplasia in the hamster, which provided initial evidence for the support of retinoids in the control of tobacco-induced cancers [73].

Pertinent to the therapeutic application of retinoids against tobacco-induced neoplasias is the issue of genetic alterations. Tobacco derived hydrocarbons will affect chromosomal stability [74]. The induction of chromosomal abnormalities may begin with the binding of carcinogen metabolites to cellular DNA [75]. Genta *et al.* have demonstrated that retinoid deficiency enhances this binding [75]. In their experiments, four times as much benzo [a]pyrene metabolites bound to tracheal DNA from animals fed a diet deficient of vitamin A as compared with normal animals. Thus, vitamin A derivatives may affect the binding of tobacco-derived hydrocarbons to epithelial DNA of the upper aerodigestive mucosa.

When retinoids were administered to rats exposed to carcinogens only after the removal of a palpable mammary tumor, a time when several preneoplastic lesions are present, there was a significant decrease in the incidence of new tumors [76]. These studies also indicated that the retinoid effects were reversible. Although the exact mechanism of action of retinoids is not known, it is thought that they inhibit the promotion stage of carcinogenesis and suppress the progression of preneoplastic lesions to carcinomas. These effects might result from retinoid-induced inhibition of the proliferation of preneoplastic cells or, alternatively, from redirecting the abberant differentiation of preneoplastic cells to a normal pathway.

Retinoids can reduce the growth rate and lower the saturation density of various cultured human and rodent adenocarcinomas and SCC [33, 77–83]. The synthesis and secretion of high M_r glycoproteins (mucins) was stimulated by treatment of bronchial adenocarcinomas and SCC [81]. In contrast, the synthesis of a M_r 67 Kd keratin by carcinoma cells was suppressed [84].

The results of these extensive studies strongly suggest that retinoids should be

182

useful and effective agents for suppression and prevention of carcinogenesis, tumor progression, and for inhibition of tumor growth.

Effect of retinoids on premalignant lesions and cancer in humans

The results of a number of investigations support the use of retinoids in humans. Retinoids can inhibit the growth of a number of dysplastic skin lesions, basal cell carcinoma and SCC of the skin, and mycosis fungoides [85–90]. A recent study reported that retinoids show antitumor activity against recurrent HNSCC [91].

Retinoids have been used in various types of premalignant lesions [92, 93]. A phase I trial of retinoids in patients with myelodysplastic syndrome reported improvement of hematologic parameters [94]. Local application of retinoids in patients with cervical dysplasia resulted in reversal of dysplasia in several cases with limited side effects [95]. Recent investigations show the ability of retinoids to reverse metaplastic lesions in the lungs of heavy smokers [96].

Reversal of premalignant oral leukoplakia by retinoids: a double-blind randomized trial

A number of nonrandomized clinical trials with oral leukoplakia patients have demonstrated that these premalignant lesions can be reversed by treatment with 13-cis retinoic acid [92, 93]. These reports have recently been confirmed in a controlled, double-blind randomized trial [97]. A total of 44 patients were accrued

Table 1. Clinical response to 13-cis retinoic acid in oral leukoplakia

Patients	Treatment		
	13-cRA[a]	Placebo	P value
Number			
Total	24	20	
Response			
Progression	0	4	
Stable lesions	6	12	
Partial response	14	2	
Complete response	2	0	
Partial + complete	16 (67%)	2 (10%)	0.002

[a] 13-cRA = 13-cis retinoic acid.

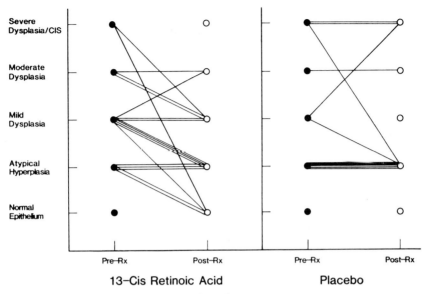

Figure 1. Histologic response of oral leukoplakia patients.

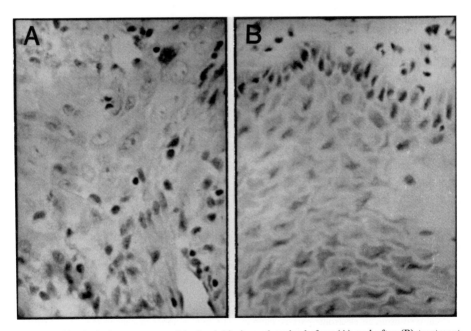

Figure 2. Histological appearance of leukoplakia in oral cavity before (A) and after (B) treatment with 13-cis retinoic acid. A patient with oral leukoplakia was treated with 13-cis retinoic acid (2 mg/kg/day) by mouth for 3 months. Note that the severe degree of dysplasia before treatment was reversed to normal-appearing epithelium at the site of the lesion after treatment.

and all were evaluated for response to treatment. 13-Cis-retinoic acid (1 to 2 mg/kg) was given orally each day for 3 months, with 6 months follow-up, for a total duration of 9 months. A major objective response occurred in 67% (16/24) of patients in the 13-cis retinoic acid group vs 10% (2/20) in the placebo group (p = 0.002). Reversal of dysplasia was observed in 54% (13/24) of the 13-cis retinoic acid group vs. 10% (2/20) in the placebo group (p = 0.01) (Table 1; Figures 1 and 2). Adverse side effects of the retinoid were observed in the skin, eyes, and lips. Hypertriglyceridemia was also detected. All of these were reversed after dose reduction or after treatment was discontinued.

Effects of retinoic acid on the growth and differentiation of established squamous cell carcinoma cell lines in vitro

Although the effects of retinoids on the growth and differentiation of various cultured rodent and human neoplastic cell lines are well documented [33, 34] there are only few reports on the effects of such compounds on human SCC lines. Growth of human skin SCC cultures in the presence of certain retinoids reduced the expression of differentiation markers such as the capability to form cross-linked envelopes (insoluble layer of cross-linked proteins formed under the cell

Table 2. Effect of retinoic acid on the growth of three established human squamous cell carcinomas of the head and neck[a]

RA concentration (μM)	Percent of control cell number		
	UM-SCC 35[b]	UM-SCC 19[c]	UM-SCC 10A[d]
0	100	100	100
0.001	86	91	87
0.01	45	67	48
0.1	10	72	50
1.0	3	68	38

[a] Cells were seeded at 2×10^4 (SCC 19 and 10A) or 1.5×10^5 (35) cells in culture dishes in DMEM medium containing 10% fetal bovine serum, 2μM glutamine, 1x amino acids and antibiotics. After 24 h the medium was replaced with medium containing, in addition to the above constituents, 0.1% dimethylsulfoxide (for controls) or the indicated concentrations of retinoic acid (RA) dissolved in DMSO. The cultures were then incubated at 37°C and refed with fresh medium without or with retinoic acid every 72 h. After 12 days, the cells were detached by a brief exposure to trypsin-2 mM EDTA and counted using an electronic particle counter. The final number of cells in the control cultures was: UM-SCC 35, $2.2. \times 10^6$; UM-SCC 19, 0.9×10^5; and UM-SCC 10A, 7.1×10^5.

[b] Cell line derived from a SCC of the oral-pharynx of a 51-year-old black man.

[c] Cell line derived from a SCC of the tongue of a 67-year-old white man.

[d] Cell line derived from a SCC of the larynx of a 57-year-old white man.

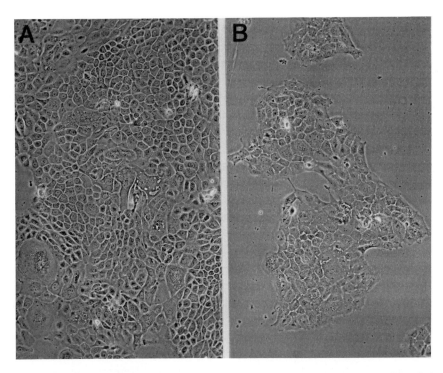

Figure 3. Photomicrographs of UM-SCC 10A head and neck squamous cell carcinoma cell line derived from a tumor in the larynx of a 57-year-old white man. (A) Cells grown for 10 days in control medium; (B) cells grown for 10 days in medium supplemented with 10-μM retinoic acid.

membrane); the level of the protein involucrin, which is one of the cross-linked proteins; and the level of the enzyme epidermal transglutaminase, which is responsible for the cross-linking reactions [98, 99]. The proliferation of the cells was not altered in the presence of 0.3 μM retinyl acetate; however, colony-forming efficiency of cells pretreated with retinyl acetate was lowered by approximately 50%. Similar studies with cells derived from a human squamous carcinoma of the buccal mucosa have shown that treatment with 0.05 μM-all-trans retinoic acid increased cell desquamation and inhibited keratinization by suppressing involucrin expression and decreasing envelope competence [83]. The saturation density of treated cultures was about 50% of that of control cultures; yet, the number of colony-forming cells in cultures pretreated with retinoic acid was almost 10 times higher than in untreated cultures – possibly because the number of terminally differentiated cells was higher in the control cultures. Very recent studies with several other human SCCs, derived from the oropharynx and the esophagus, indicated that retinoic acid inhibits differentiation of various epidermoid carcinoma cells [100].

We have investigated the effects of all-trans retinoic acid on the growth of five cell lines established from human HNSCCs by Dr. Peter Sacks from The University of Texas M.D. Anderson Hospital and Tumor Institute at Houston, and by Dr. Thomas Carey from the University of Michigan, Ann Arbor. The growth rate of four of these cell lines was decreased when the cells were grown in the presence of retinoic acid in a dose-dependent fashion. Fifty percent inhibition of cell growth was observed after a 10-day exposure of the cells to $1 \mu M$ retinoic acid (Table 2). The appearance of control and treated cells is shown in Figure 3. Preliminary results indicate that the ability of some of the cell lines to form colonies in semi-solid medium (0.5% agarose) is suppressed by retinoic acid [101].

Conclusions

The therapeutic application of retinoids to the head and neck cancer patient may have multiple effects. Retinoids will induce cellular differentiation, which may prevent the progression of preneoplastic cells to malignant cells, inhibit the growth of neoplastic cells, and decrease their tendency to metastasize. Retinoids may also exert inhibitory effects on the induction of Epstein-Barr virus by tumor promoters [102], and on the replication of herpes simplex virus type I [103] or of papilloma virus [104], which have been implicated in the causation of some head and neck cancers [20–22].

A potentially unrelated phenomenon to cellular differentiation induced by retinoids may be their effect upon host immunological responsiveness. Retinoids will enhance multiple arms of host defense including lymphokine production, lymphocyte blastogenesis, cell-mediated antitumor cytotoxic response, as well as immunoglobulin production [35, 36].

A consideration of the multiple effects of retinoic acid indicates that retinoids might be useful for the treatment of HNSCC, as well as for the prevention of the progression of premalignant lesions. Since the effect of retinoids on HNSCC is cytostatic, the effectiveness will probably be increased if the retinoids are used in combination with other therapeutic agents.

References

1. Cancer Statistics, 1984.
2. Decker, J. Goldstein, J.C. 1982. Risk factors in head and neck cancers. N. Engl. J. Med. 306: 1151–1155.
3. Rothman, K.J., Cann, C.I., Flanders, D. et al. 1980. Epidemiology of laryngeal cancer. Epidemiol. Rev. 2: 195–209.
4. Wynder, E.L., Hoffman, D. 1976. Tobacco and tobacco smoke. Sem. Oncol. 3: 5–15.
5. Vaughan, C.W., Homburger, F., Shapshay, S.M. et al. 1980. Carcinogenesis in the upper aerodigestive tract. Otolaryngol. Clin. North Am. 13: 403–412.
6. Wyder, E.L., Muchinski, M.H., Spivak, J.C. 1977. Tobacco and alcohol consumption in relation to the development of multiple primary cancers. Cancer 40: 1872–1878.

7. Sellars, S.L. 1979. Epidemiology of oral cancer. Otolaryngol. Clin. North Am. 12: 45–55.
8. Moore, C., Catlin, D. 1967. Anatomic origins and locations of oral cancer. Am. J. Surg. 114: 510–513.
9. Slaughter, D.P., Southwick, H.W., Smejkel, W. 1953. Field cancerization in oral stratified epithelium. Cancer 6: 963–968.
10. Dontenwill, W., Chevalier, H.J., Harke, H.P. 1973. Investigations on the effect of chronic smoke inhalation in Syrian golden hamsters. J.N.C.I. 51: 1781–1832.
11. Auerbach, O., Stout, A.P., Hammond, E.L. *et al.* 1961. Changes in bronchial epithelium in relationship to cigarette smoking in relation to lung cancer. N. Engl. J. Med. 265: 254–267.
12. Vitale, J.J., Gottlieb, L.S. 1975. Alcohol and alcohol-related deficiencies as carcinogens. Cancer Res. 35: 3336–3338.
13. Ketcham, A.S., Wexler, H., Mantel, N. 1963. Effects of alcohol in mouse neoplasia. Cancer Res. 23: 667–671.
14. Wynder, E.L., Covey, L.S., Malbuchi, K. *et al.* 1976. Environmental factors in cancer of the larynx. A second look. Cancer 38: 1591–1601.
15. Rothman, K.J. 1970. The effect of alcohol consumption on risk of cancer of the head and neck. Laryngoscope 88: 51–55.
16. Kisin, B. 1975. Epidemiologic investigations of possible biological interactions of alcohol and cancer of the head and neck. Ann. N.Y. Acad. Sci. 252: 374–377.
17. Klein, G., Giovanella, B., Lindhal, T. *et al.* 1974. Direct evidence for the presence of Epstein-Barr virus DNA and nuclear antigen in malignant epithelial cells from patients with poorly differentiated carcinoma of the nasopharynx. Proc. Natl. Acad. Sci. U.S.A. 71: 4737–4741.
18. Strauss M. 1985. Human papillomavirus in various lesions of the head and neck. Otolaryngol. Head Neck Surg. 93: 342–346.
19. Scully, C. 1983. Viruses and cancer: Herpes viruses and tumors in the head and neck. A review. Oral Surg. 56: 285–292.
20. Scully, C. 1982. The immunology of cancer of the head and neck with particular reference to oral cancer. Oral Surg. 55: 157–169.
21. Hong, W.K., Bromer, R. 1983. Current concepts: Chemotherapy in head and neck cancer. N. Engl. J. Med. 308: 75–79.
22. Goepfert, H. 1984. Are we making any progress? Arch. Otolaryngol. 110: 562–563.
23. Hong, W.K., Popkin, T., Shapshay, S. 1984. Preoperative adjuvant induction chemotherapy in head and neck cancer. In: Head and Neck Oncology. (G. Wolf, ed.). Boston, Martinus Nijhoff, pp. 287–300.
24. Wynder, E.L., Dodo, H., Bloch, D. *et al.* 1969. Epidemiologic investigation of multiple primary cancer of the upper alimentary and respiratory tracts. Cancer 24: 730–739.
25. Schottenfeld, D., Grant, R.C., Wynder, E.L. 1974. The role of alcohol and tobacco in multiple primary cancers of the upper digestive system, larynx and lung. A prospective study. Prev. Med. 3: 277–293.
26. Jesse, R.H., Sugarbaker, E.V. 1976. Squamous cell carcinoma of the oropharynx: Why we fail. Am. J. Surg. 132: 435–458.
27. Shapshay, S., Hong, W.K., Fried, M. *et al.* 1980. Simultaneous carcinomas of the esophagus and upper aerodigestive tract. Otolaryngol. Head Neck Surg. 88: 373–377.
28. Gluckman, J., Crissman, J., Donegan, J.O. 1980. Multicentric squamous-cell carcinoma of the upper aerodigestive tract. Head Neck Surg. 3: 90–96.
29. Vikram, B. 1984. Changing patterns of failure in advanced head and neck cancer. Arch. Otolaryngol. 110: 564–565.
30. Tepperman, B., Fitzpatrick, P. 1981. Second respiratoy and upper digestive tract cancers after oral cancer. Lancet 2: 547–549.
31. Incze, J., Vaughan, C.W., Lui, P. *et al.* 1982. Premalignant changes in normal appearing

188

epithelium in patients with squamous cell carcinoma of the upper aerodigestive tract. Am. J. Surg. 144: 401–405.

32. Lotan, R. 1980. Effects of vitamin A and its analogs (retinoids) on normal and neoplastic cells. Biochim. Biophys. Acta 605: 33–91.

33. Roberts, A.B., Sporn, M.B. 1984. Cellular biology and biochemistry of the retinoids. In: The Retinoids II. (M.B. Sporn, A.B. Roberts, D.S. Goodman, eds.). Academic Press, Orlando, pp. 209–286.

34. Lotan, R. 1986. Immunomodulatory effects of retinoids. J. Nutr. Growth Cancer 3: 29–37.

35. Dennert, G. 1984. Retinoids and the immune system. In: The Retinoids II. (M.B. Sporn, A.B. Roberts, D.S. Goodman, eds.). Academic Press, Orlando, pp. 373–390.

36. Dennert, G. 1985. Immunostimulation by retinoic acid. Ciba Found. Symp. 113: 117–131.

37. Wolbach, S.B., Howe, P.R. 1925. Tissue changes following deprivation of fat soluble vitamin A. J. Exp. Med. 42: 753–777.

38. Lasnitzki, I. 1962. Hypovitaminosis-A in the mouse prostate gland cultured in chemically defined medium. Exp. Cell Res. 28: 40–51.

39. Wong, Y.C., Buck, R.C. 1971. An electron microscopic study of metaplasia of the rat tracheal epithelium in vitamin A deficiency. Lab. Invest. 24: 55–66.

40. Harris, C.C., Silverman, T., Smith, J.M. et al. 1973. Proliferation of tracheal epithelial cells in normal and vitamin A-deficient Syrian golden hamsters. J.N.C.I. 51: 1059–1062.

41. Marchok, A.C., Cone, V., Nettesheim, P. 1975. Induction of squamous metaplasia (vitamin A deficiency) and hypersecretory activity in tracheal organ cultures. Lab. Invest. 33: 451–460.

42. Chopra, D.P. 1982. Squamous metaplasia in organ culture of vitamin A-deficient hamster trachea: Cytokinetic and ultrastructural alterations. J. N.C.I. 69: 895–905.

43. Wolbach, S.B., Howe, P.R. 1933. Epithelial repair and recovery from vitamin A deficiency. J. Exp. Med. 57: 511–525.

44. Sporn, M.B., Clamon, G.H., Dunlop, N.M. 1975. Activity of vitamin A analogues in cell cultures of mouse epidermis and organ cultures of hamster trachea. Nature 253: 47–50.

45. Sporn, M.B., Dunlop, N.M., Newton, D.L. et al. 1976. Relationship between structure and activity of retinoids, Nature 263: 110–113.

46. Chopra, D.P. 1983. Retinoid reversal of squamous metaplasia in organ cultures of tracheas derived from hamsters fed on vitamin A-deficient diet. Eur. J. Cancer Clin. Oncol. 9: 847–857.

47. Lawrence, D.J., Bern, H.A. 1963. Vitamin A and mucous metaplasia. Ann. N.Y. Avad. Sci. 106: 646–653.

48. Hardy, M.H. 1968. Glandular metaplasia of hair follicles and other responses to vitamin A excess in cultures of rodent skin. J. Embryol. Exp. Morphol. 19: 157–180.

49. Barnett, M.L., Szabo, G. 1973. Effect of vitamin A on epithelial morphogenesis in vitro. Fine structural changes in explants of adult mammalian skin. Exp. Cell Res. 76: 118–126.

50. Kubilus, J., Rand, R., Baden, H.P. 1981. Effects of retinoic acid and other retinoids on the growth and differentiation of 3T3 supported human keratinocytes, In Vitro 17: 786–795.

51. Milstone, L.M., McGuire, J., La Vigne, J.F. 1982. Retinoic acid causes premature desquamation of cells from confluent cultures of stratified squamous epithelia. J. Invest. Dermatol. 79: 253–260.

52. Yuspa, S.H., Harris, C.C. 1974. Altered differentiation of mouse epidermal cells treated with retinyl acetate in vitro. Exp. Cell Res. 86: 95–105.

53. Yuspa, S.H., Elgjo, K., Morse, M.A. et al. 1977. Retinyl acetate modulation of cell growth kinetics and carcinogen-cellular interaction in mouse epidermal cell cultures. Chem. Biol. Interact. 16: 251–264.

54. Yaar, M., Stanley, J.R., Katz, S.I. 1981. Retinoic acid delays terminal differentiation of keratinocytes in suspension culture. J. Invest. Dermatol. 76: 363–366.

55. Yuspa, S.H., Ben, T., Steinert, P. 1982. Retinoic acid induces transglutaminase activity but inhibits cornification of cultured epidermal cells. J. Biol. Chem. 257: 9906–9908.

56. Green, H., Watt, F.M. 1982. Regulation by vitamin A of envelope cross-linking in cultured keratinocytes derived from different human epithelia. Mol. Cell. Biol. 2: 1115–1117.

57. Fuchs, E., Green, H. 1981. Regulation of terminal differentiation of cultured human keratinocytes by vitamin A. Cell 25: 617–625.

58. Eckert, R., Green, H. 1984. Cloning of cDNAs specifying vitamin A-responsive human keratins. Proc. Natl. Acad. Sci. U.S.A. 81: 4321–4325.

59. Thivolet, C.H., Hintner, H., Stanley, J. 1984. The effect of retinoic acid on the expression of pemphigus and pemphigoid antigens in cultured human keratinocytes. J. Invest. Dermatol. 82: 329–334.

60. Adamo, S., De Luca, L.M., Silverman-Jones, C.S. et al. 1979. Mode of action of retinol: Involvement in glycosylation reactions in cultured mouse epidermal cells. J. Biol. Chem. 254: 3278–3287.

61. Elias, P.M., Chung, J.C., Topete, R.O. et al. 1983. Membrane glycoconjugate visualization and biosynthesis in normal and retinoid-treated epidermis. J. Invest. Dermatol. 81: 815–855.

62. Robinson, J.K., Freinkel, R.K., Gotschalk, R. 1984. Effect of retinoic acid and low calcium conditions on surface glycoconjugates defined by differential lectin labeling in mouse epidermal cell culture. Br. J. Dermatol. 110: 17–27.

63. Yuspa, S.H., Lichti, U., Ben, T. et al. 1981. Modulation of terminal differentiation and tumor promotion by retinoids in mouse epidermal cell cultures. Ann. N.Y. Acad. Sci. 359: 260–274.

64. Yuspa, S.H., Ben, T., Hennings, H. 1983. The induction of epidermal transglutaminase and terminal differentiation by tumor promoters in cultured epidermal cells. Carcinogenesis 4: 1413–1418.

65. Sporn, M.B., Dunlop, N.M., Yuspa, S.H., 1973. Retinyl acetate: Effect on cellular content of RNA in epidermis in cell culture in chemically defined medium. Science 182: 722–723.

66. Sporn, M.B., Dunlop, N.M., Newton, D.L. et al. 1976. Prevention of chemical carcinogenesis by vitamin A and its synthetic analogs (retinoids). Fed. Proc. 35: 1332–1338.

67. Chopra, D.P., Flaxman, B.A. 1975. The effect of vitamin A on growth and differentiation of human keratinocytes in vitro. J. Invest. Dermatol. 64: 19–22.

68. Taylor, A., Hogan, B.L.M., Watt, F.M. 1985. Biosynthesis of EGF receptor, transferrin receptor and colligin by cultured human keratinocytes and the effect of retinoic acid. Exp. Cell Res. 159: 47–54.

69. Fujimaki, Y. 1926. Formation of carcinoma in albino rats fed on deficient diets, J. Cancer Res. 10: 469–477.

70. Newberne, P.M., Rogers, A.E. 1981. Vitamin A, retinoids, and cancer. In: Nutrition and Cancer: Etiology and Treatment. (G.R. Newell, N.M. Ellison, eds.). Raven Press, New York, pp. 217–232.

71. Lasnitzki, I. 1976. Reversal of methylcholanthrene-induced changes in mouse prostate in vitro by retinoic acid and its analogues. Br. J. Cancer 34: 239–248.

72. Lasnitzki, I., Goodman, D.W. 1974. Inhibition of the effects of methylcholanthrene on mouse prostate in organ culture by vitamin A and its analogs. Cancer Res. 34: 1564–1571.

73. Saffioti, U., Montesano, R., Sellakumar, A.R. et al. 1967. Experimental cancer of the lung. Inhibition by vitamin A of induction of tracheobronchial squamous metaplasia and squamous cell tumors. Cancer 20: 857–864.

74. Stich, H.F., Stich, W. 1982. Chromosome-damaging activity of saliva of betel nut and tobacco chewers. Cancer Lett. 15: 193–202.

75. Genta, V.M., Kaufman, D.g., Harris, C.C. et al. 1974. Vitamin A deficiency enhances the binding of benzo [a]pyrene to tracheal epithelial DNA. Nature 247: 48–49.

76. McCormick, D.L., Sowell, Z.L., Thompson, C.A. et al. 1983. Inhibition by retinoid and ovariectomy of additional primary malignancies in rats following surgical removal of the first mammary cancer. Cancer 51: 593–599.

77. Lotan, R., Nicolson, G.L. 1977. Inhibitory effects of retinoic acid or retinyl acetate on the growth of untransformed, transformed and tumor cells in vitro. J.N.C.I. 59: 1717–1722.

78. Lotan, R. 1979. Different susceptibilities of human melanoma and breast carcinoma cell lines to retinoic acid-induced growth inhibition. Cancer Res. 39: 1014–1019.

79. Lacroix, A., Lippman, M.E. 1980. Binding of retinoids to human breast cancer cell lines and their effect on cell growth. J. Clin. Invest. 65: 586–591.

80. Lotan, R., Kramer, R.H., Neuman, G. et al. 1980. Retinoic acid-induced modifications in the growth and cell surface components of a human carcinoma (HeLa) cell line. Exp. Cell Res. 130: 401–414.

81. Marchok, A.C., Clark, J.N., Klein—Szanto, A. 1981. Modulation of growth, differentiation and mucous glycoprotein synthesis by retinyl acetate in cloned carcinoma cell lines. J.N.C.I. 66: 1165–1174.

82. Rudland, P.S., Paterson, F.C., Twiston-Davies, A.C. et al. 1983. Retinoid-specific induction of differentiation and reduction of the DNA synthesis rate and tumor-forming ability of a stem cell line from a rat mammary tumor. J.N.C.I. 70: 949–958.

83. Reiss, M., Pitman, S.W., Sartorelli, A.C. 1985. Modulation of the terminal differentiation of human squamous carcinoma cells in vitro by all-trans retinoic acid. J.N.C.I. 74: 1015–1023.

84. Kim, K.H., Schwartz, F., Fuchs, E. 1984. Differences in keratin synthesis between normal epithelial cells and squamous cell carcinomas are mediated by vitamin A. Proc. Natl. Acad. Sci. U.S.A. 81: 4280–4284.

85. Clamon, G.H. 1980. Retinoids for the prevention of epithelial cancers: Current status and future potential. Med. Pediatr. Oncol. 8: 177–185.

86. Moon, R.C., Itri, L.M. 1984. Retinoids and cancer. In: The Retinoids II, (M.B. Sporn, A.B. Roberts, D.S. Goodman, eds.). Academic Press, Orlando, pp. 327–371.

87. Moriarty, M., Dunn, J., Darragh, A. et al. 1982. Lancet 1: 364–365.

88. Bollag, W. 1979. Retinoids and cancer. Cancer Chemother. Pharmacol. 3: 207–215.

89. Peck, G.L. 1981. Chemoprevention of cancer with retinoids. Gynecol. Oncol. 12: 5331–5340.

90. Meyskens, F.L., Alberts, D.S., Salmon, S.E. 1982. Effect of 13-cis retinoic acid and 4-hydroxy-phenyl-all-trans retinamide on human tumor colony formation in soft agar. Int. J. Cancer 32: 295–299.

91. Meyskens, F.L., Gilmartin, G., Alberts, D.S. et al. 1982. Activity of 13-cis-retinoic acid against squamous epithelial premalignancies and malignancies. Cancer Treat, Rep. 66: 1315–1319.

92. Koch, H. 1978. Biochemical treatment of precancerous oral lesions: the effectiveness of various analogues of retinoic acid. J. Maxillofac. Surg. 6: 59–63.

93. Shah, J.P., Strong, E., Decosse, J.J. et al. 1903. Effect of retinoids on oral leukoplakia. Am. J. Surg. 146: 466–470.

94. Gold, E.J., Mertelsman, R.H., Itri, L. et al. 1983. Phase I clinical trial of 13-cis-retinoic acid in myelodysplastic syndrome. Cancer Treat. Rep. 67: 981–986.

95. Surwit, E.A., Graham, V., Droegemuller, W. et al. 1982. Evaluation of topically applied trans-retinoic acid in the treatment of cervical intraepithelial lesions. Am. J. Obstet. Gynecol. 143: 821–823.

96. Gouveia, J., Mathe, G., Hercent, T. 1982. Degree of bronchial metaplasia in heavy smokers and its regression after treatment with a retinoid. Lancet 1: 710–712.

97. Hong, W.K., Itri, L., Endicott, J. et al. 1986. The effectiveness of 13-cis retinoic acid (13-CRA) in the treatment of premalignant lesions in oral cavity. N. Eng. J. Med. 315: 1501–1505.

98. Cline, P.R., Rice, R.H. 1983. Modulation of involucrin and envelope competence in human keratinocytes by hydrocortisone, retinyl acetate, and growth arrest. Cancer Res. 43: 3203–3207.

99. Thacher, S.M., Coe, E.L., Rice, R.H. 1985. Retinoid suppression of transglutaminase activity and envelope competence in cultured human epidermal carcinoma cells. Differentiation 29: 82–87.

100. Reiss, M., Sartorelli, A.C., 1985. Effects of epidermal growth factor (EGF) and all-trans retinoic acid (RA) on growth and differentiation of human squamous carcinoma (SqCC) cell lines in vitro (Abstr.). Proc. Am. Assoc. Cancer Res. 26:40.

101. Lotan, D., Sacks, P., Lotan, R., Hong, K.W. 1986. Differential effects of retinoic acid on the growth of two human head and neck squamous cell carcinoma (HNSCC) lines (Abstr.). Proc. Am. Assoc. Cancer Res. 27: 1627.

102. Yamamoto, N., Bister, L., Zur Hausen, H. 1979. Retinoic acid inhibition of Epstein-Barr virus induction, Nature 278: 553–554.

103. Taylor, J.L., O'Brien, W.J. 1984. The effects of retinoids on the replication of herpes simplex type 1. Curr. Eye Res. 3: 481–488.

104. Gross, G., Pfister, H., Hagedorn, M. *et al.* 1983. Effect of oral aromatic retinoid (Ro 10–9359) on human papilloma virus 2-induced common warts. Dermatologica 166: 48–53.

13. Avoiding biostatistical pitfalls in the design and analysis of head and neck cancer clinical trials

ROBERT MAKUCH and MARY JOHNSON

Introduction

The ultimate objective of any clinical trial is to obtain the correct answer to an important medical question. The science of biostatistics plays an important role in helping to meet this fundamental objective. By properly applying sound statistical principles to clinical research in oncology, one can insure that results of completed studies are valid and convincing to others in the scientific community. To this end, the biomedical literature contains several excellent and thorough discussions regarding the design, execution, and analysis of cancer clinical trials and methods of data acquisition [1–3]. These references draw attention to certain basic components of a successful clinical trial, including: (1) a clear, unambiguous protocol which addresses a significant medical question, (2) well-defined conditions for entry of patients on-study, (3) sample sizes sufficiently large and duration of follow-up adequate to detect treatment effects if they are present, (4) a clear description of treatment regimens and experimental design, (5) explicit definition of endpoints used for efficacy and safety evaluation, (6) patient record forms and data management procedures which enhance data quality, (7) appropriate methodology for data monitoring and statistical analysis to account for incomplete data, and (8) appropriate consideration of ethical issues. While there may be a variety of equally plausible ways to satisfy each of these criteria, their precise specification will depend on the goals of the particular trial, its administrative structure, and the nature of the treatment and disease under study.

This chapter will focus on biostatistical issues that arise in planning and interpreting phase III comparative clinical trials for new treatments of head and neck cancer. Due to the numbers of patients, cost, and length of time typically required to complete these studies, the best and most pertinent statistical methodology must be employed. It is our intent to highlight specific approaches to study design, sample size, patient allocation, statistical analysis, and determination of treatment-of-choice. Rather than provide an exhaustive overview of methodology in each area, we will present a number of currently popular methods and

C. Jacobs (ed) Cancers of the head and neck.
© 1987, Martinus Nijhoff Publishers, Boston. ISBN 0–89838–825–2. Printed in the Netherlands.

emphasize biostatistical pitfalls which can be avoided through their proper use in the design and analysis of clinical trials in head and neck cancer.

Study design

A crucial stage in evaluating new therapies for head and neck cancer involves the planning of phase III comparative clinical trials. Proper planning will minimize bias in the study design and thus lead to more persuasive study conclusions. Fundamental to attaining this goal is the use of a 'control' group to serve as a standard to which results of a new, experimental treatment will be compared. While 'historical' controls (i.e., patients who received the standard therapy under previous protocols) may be the quickest and simplest control group to assemble, control patients arising from a concurrently randomized clinical trial are generally favored as a comparison group because the randomization helps guard against both selection bias in the assignment of treatments and accidental bias. In spite of the controversy surrounding the use of historical controls, advocates of the design cite the following advantages [4]: (1) without a concurrent control group, all patients receive the new treatment, thereby shortening the overall completion time and accrual objectives relative to those required for a randomized study, (2) the control and experimental groups can be guaranteed to be comparable in regard to those characteristics used as a basis for selecting the control patients, and (3) such studies are more ethical since all new patients are given the experimental (and often thought to be the better) treatment.

Nevertheless, serious disadvantages of historical controls which may ultimately compromise the results of such studies include [5]: (1) the inability to account for imbalances in important but currently unrecognized prognostic factors, (2) the need to adjust for differences in the prognostic profile between the control and experimental treatment groups using complex statistical techniques which entail strict and possibly untenable statistical assumptions about the data, (3) the presence of many errors and missing values in factors required for adjustment in historical data, and (4) the lack of protection from potential biases introduced into treatment comparisons by changes over time in diagnostic methods, staging criteria, supportive care, referral patterns, and effects of unmeasured or unknown prognostic factors. Clearly, the inability to control for biases due to unmeasured or unknown prognostic factors is a major drawback of historical controls. This point was illustrated by Farewell and D'Angio [6] using data from two consecutive randomized studies conducted by the same research group, each employing the same control treatment arm. They found that conclusions of the second study differed materially if the control group from the first study had been used for comparison rather than the concurrent randomized controls. A review of the cancer clinical trial literature by Pocock [7] further illustrates the lack of reproducible results with the same treatment in consecutive trials. Thus, one must question the notion of Gehan and Freireich [4] that historical controls are acceptable, even if they arise from the most recent in a sequence of previous studies in which similar kinds of patients were admitted and similar evaluation criteria were used.

While we prefer the concurrently randomized control group, there are some fairly specialized situations where historical control groups serve a useful purpose. For instance, historical controls can be valuable in the study of diseases so rare that sufficient patient accrual over a reasonable period of time is impossible in a prospective, randomized clinical trial. Another valid reason for using historical controls as a comparison group is if one can identify a subset of patients for which death (or any other well-defined outcome event) is inevitable within a relatively short and predictable period of time. Then any new treatment that prolongs survival beyond that point can be recognized quickly as a therapeutic advance. This holds since any dramatic change in the endpoint can reasonably be attributed to the new therapy by virtue of the fact that the outcome is inevitable and not subject to much variability, selection bias or other unknown patient features. However, this situation is generally inapplicable for patients with head and neck cancer, given that the disease course is highly variable and influenced by many treatment-related and non-treatment-related factors.

Since the advantages of randomization are well-recognized [8], the concurrently randomized, parallel-group controlled trial is generally the preferred choice for the experimental design of a phase III study. But, to circumvent certain practical as well as ethical problems with the traditional approach, many variations on this design have been proposed, each with its own set of desirable properties and potential drawbacks. For example, the randomized consent design of Zelen [9] was created to enhance the physician's role as a competent decision-maker and the patient's right to make an informed choice. Yet, there is a price to be paid in terms of possible bias in treatment assignments and the dilution of real treatment differences. The institutional choice design [10] was developed so that institutions participating in a multi-center study would be allowed to randomize patients to a subset of the treatments under study, but this approach suffers from some of the same limitations as historical controls when treatments not common to all centers are compared [11]. The design chosen for emphasis here is the factorial design, since it is often overlooked by many investigators, and it has many positive features which make it a viable candidate for more frequent use in clinical trials for head and neck cancer.

The simplest and most commonly used form of factorial design is the 2×2 factorial, in which there are two controllable treatment options, each having two levels. This experimental design is especially attractive in that it allows the simultaneous evaluation of several treatment strategies in the same clinical trial. To illustrate this feature, assume that interest centers on the relative merits of two distinct treatment options for patients with head and neck cancer. The first question may involve whether or not immunotherapy (e.g., thymosin fraction V) should be given in addition to standard therapy of surgery and radiation therapy, while the second may involve whether or not induction chemotherapy should be given in addition to the standard therapy. This particular realization of a 2×2 factorial design is given in Table 1. Patients are assigned to one of the four treatment groups based on every combination of the two treatment options. Each treatment group appears in the Table, and the groups are: (1) standard therapy alone, (2) standard therapy plus immunotherapy, (3) standard therapy plus induction chemotherapy, and (4) standard therapy plus induction chemotherapy and immunotherapy.

For evaluating treatment efficacy, assume that $\bar{x}_i$ is the mean value for some normally distributed response among patients in group i ($i = 1,2,3,4$ as above). From the Table, one estimates the comparative effect of immunotherapy as $\bar{x}_2 - \bar{x}_1$, while another independent estimate is obtained by calculating $\bar{x}_4 - \bar{x}_3$. Assuming that the same number of patients is in each group, and averaging these two independent estimates of treatment efficacy, one calculates the overall average effect of immunotherapy to be

$$\frac{(\bar{x}_2 - \bar{x}_1) + (\bar{x}_4 - \bar{x}_3)}{2}.$$

Thus patients in groups 1 and 3 combined are compared to patients in groups 2 and 4 combined. Similarly the overall average effect of chemotherapy is obtained by calculating

$$\frac{(\bar{x}_3 - \bar{x}_1) + (\bar{x}_4 - \bar{x}_2)}{2}.$$

Thus two independent treatment questions are answered for the price of one. Of course, this would hold true only if the various treatments under study can be delivered to the patients without any reduction in dose. Otherwise, one should plan on carrying out two single-treatment studies.

Another positive feature of the factorial design is that the effects of two important treatment interventions can be examined separately as well as in

Table 1. A 2×2 factorial design: treatment groups consist of all combinations of the two factors

Immunotherapy	Induction chemotherapy	
	no	yes
no	$\bar{x}_1$ [a]	$\bar{x}_3$
yes	$\bar{x}_2$	$\bar{x}_4$

[a] $\bar{x}_1$ defines the average value for some normally distributed response to treatment.

combination. For example, with this design one can evaluate the effect of immunotherapy in the presence or absence of induction chemotherapy, or equivalently, the effect of induction chemotherapy can be examined in the presence or absence of immunotherapy. If immunotherapy provides a similar benefit to patients, regardless of whether or not they receive chemotherapy, then the two treatments are said to be independent. If the effect depends on whether or not chemotherapy is given, then a treatment interaction exists. In this situation, Peto claims that '2 × 2 designs will point unbiasedly to the complicated truth while misleading conclusions could well emerge from other designs' [12]. That is, without use of a factorial design or some variation of it, one would not discover that the effects of a particular treatment modality vary according to its use in conjunction with a particular level of another treatment modality.

The concept of interaction will be discussed more fully later in the chapter. For now, the important point to emphasize is that the overall treatment comparisons given above are useful summaries of overall treatment efficacy if no marked interactions are present. If interactions are present, then the overall treatment comparisons usually are of secondary importance since they may not be representative of any patient studied. To demonstrate this point, assume immunotherapy has no effect in patients not receiving chemotherapy (i.e., $\bar{x}_2 - \bar{x}_1 = 0$), and the effect in those receiving induction chemotherapy is to raise by two units the average value of the endpoint under consideration (i.e., $\bar{x}_4 - \bar{x}_3 = 2$). Then the overall average treatment effect for immunotherapy is calculated to be

$$\frac{(\bar{x}_2 - \bar{x}_1) + (\bar{x}_4 - \bar{x}_3)}{2} = 1,$$

indicating that immunotherapy raises the endpoint value by one unit on average. However, this overall average treatment effect is representative of neither patient subgroup!

In practice, the major statistical problem with the 2 × 2 factorial design is the difficulty of determining whether or not an interaction actually exists. The interaction of two treatments is estimated by the quantity $(\bar{x}_2 - \bar{x}_1) - (\bar{x}_4 - \bar{x}_3)$, implying that the variance is four times as great as for the overall main treatment effects. As a result, the ability, or power, to detect a significant interaction, if it exists, is markedly less than the power to detect main effects. Byar and Piantadosi provide an example where a treatment interaction is present, and the power for testing the main effects is 92%, while it is only 18% for testing the interaction [13]. To overcome this problem, one might consider expanding the sample sizes in each group to increase the power for detecting interaction. We recommend this particular maneuver, especially if *a priori* evidence suggests that such an interaction is likely to arise. Although the total sample size required may be larger than that required for two single-factor studies, one can obtain a broader knowledge of treatment interrelationships using this design by examining whether two combined therapies are simply additive or synergistic in their effects on patient outcome. If no interaction is anticipated, then the total sample size required in a 2×2 factorial study will be less than that required for two single-factor studies.

Sample size requirements

During the planning stages of a controlled trial, it is imperative that a statistical rationale be utilized in the determination of the proposed sample size. Even though practical or financial restrictions may limit the number of patients that can be enrolled and treated, every effort should be made to achieve the sample size required on statistical grounds to meet the intended objectives of the trial. Such steps might include modifying patient eligibility criteria, lengthening the accrual period, or enlisting more investigators to recruit patients. The lack of adequate statistical input into the determination of sample size requirements can be a major pitfall in trial design since it frequently leads to entirely inconclusive results in studies that would otherwise be sound and defensible. Freiman *et al.* highlight this problem in a review of 71 'negative' trials in major journals, pointing out that 66 of these trials carried a substantial ($>20\%$) risk of missing a 25% true therapeutic improvement [14].

The usual approach for sample size estimation in comparing two treatments requires specifying a true treatment difference, D, which is considered important to detect, as well as the type-I and type-II error rates associated with the statistical tests to be used. The type-I error represents the event of falsely rejecting the null hypothesis that the treatments are equivalent. The probability of making this error is denoted by α. The other type of decision-making error occurs when the null hypothesis is not rejected even though the alternative hypothesis that a difference exists between the treatments is, in fact, true. This is called the type-II error, and the probability of making this error is specified as β. The power of the test, i.e., the probability of detecting a true treatment difference, is $(1 - \beta)$. Underlying this hypothesis-testing framework is the notion that a statistical test is performed at the end of the trial on a major endpoint of interest, and one wishes to test the null hypothesis of no difference in treatment efficacy. This is done by calculating the p-value corresponding to the value of the test statistic for the observed data. The conventionally accepted p-value to reject the null hypothesis is 0.05. This implies that, assuming that there is no true difference in treatment efficacy, the probability of obtaining a difference in the data as extreme as that observed is 0.05. Thus the p-value does not describe the probability that the null hypothesis is true, but rather the probability of obtaining a difference as large as that observed when the null hypothesis is true.

In principle, one can determine the sample size from the quantities α, β and D along with knowledge of the probability distribution of the test statistic used to test the null hypothesis. An excellent general review of these areas is provided by Lachin [15] and the references therein. Commonly used endpoints for sample size planning in clinical trials for head and neck cancer are either dichotomous (e.g., success versus failure, where 'success' may be defined as tumor response or survival to a fixed time T) or the time to some critical event (e.g., tumor recurrence or death). In the absence of any complicating factors such as patients being lost to follow-up or dropping out of the study, tables for the required number of patients are readily available. Some of the most widely used tables are presented below.

For comparing two treatment groups with a dichotomous endpoint, assume that p_T is the proportion of 'success' patients in the experimental treatment group and p_C is the corresponding proportion in the control treatment group. One wishes to have a total of N patients in each group so that, with high probability, we can detect a true difference of absolute magnitude $D = |p_T - p_C|$. This probability is the power of the test, $1 - \beta$, and is usually specified for planning purposes between 0.80 and 0.95. One must also specify the significance level α of the test; it is usually chosen to be 0.05 or 0.01. Table 2 indicates the number of patients required per group in order to achieve a specified power and significance level as a function of the true success rates. These values were obtained using the approximation formula of Casagrande, Pike, and Smith [16], and the table is used in the following way.

Suppose we wish to detect an increase in the complete response rate from 40% to 70% between a standard and new induction chemotherapy regimen for patients with stage III or stage IV head and neck squamous carcinoma. Although one expects the new regimen to provide a higher response rate, unexpected morbidity or mortality could arise in this group, and the response rate could be lower than that for the standard group. A two-sided significance level is therefore selected. Two-sided significance levels should be used for planning purposes unless a strong justification exists for expecting a difference in only one direction between the two treatments. With these specifications, Table 2 shows that 62 patients are needed in each group to detect a difference, $D = 0.30$ ($= 0.70 - 0.40$) with power of 0.90 for $\alpha = 0.05$. Forty-eight patients are required per group if one is willing to have probability 0.80 (rather than 0.90) of detecting a difference in the response rates, keeping all other parameters unchanged. When the success rate exceeds 0.50, the table is used by considering the failure rate and entering the table with $1 - (\text{success rate})$.

Note that the number of patients decreases as the magnitude of the true treatment difference increases between the two treatment groups. Thus, one must avoid specifying a larger treatment difference for planning purposes than may be realistic in order to justify that study accrual can be completed within a reasonable period of time (e.g., 3 years). Such optimistic projections during the planning stages of a clinical trial can be very damaging, since the power of the study will be low for detecting differences of a more reasonable magnitude. With such experimental design characteristics, it is quite likely that a truly superior new experimental treatment will not be found to differ significantly from the standard therapy. As a consequence it may be wrongfully excluded from any further clinical evaluation.

In contrast to the above setting for demonstrating the superiority of an experimental treatment over a control treatment, a fairly recent phenomenon in cancer clinical trial research is the search for new therapeutic strategies that are less toxic but otherwise equivalent to a standard therapy. A different perspective for sample size calculation is required in this evaluation of 'conservative' or less intensive treatments. For instance, in the treatment of stage II head and neck cancer patients with oral cavity sites of primary disease, the hypothesis that radiotherapy produces as good a survival result as surgery may be of interest. For this setting, Makuch and Simon [17] propose that enough patients be entered so that the confidence interval on the difference in success rates is nearly certain to

Table 2. Number of patients in each of two treatment groups (two-sided test)

Smaller success rate	Larger minus smaller success rate									
	0.05	0.10	0.15	0.20	0.25	0.30	0.35	0.40	0.45	0.50
0.05	620[a]	206	113	74	54	42	33	27	23	19
	473[b]	159	88	58	43	33	27	22	18	16
0.10	956	285	146	92	64	48	38	30	25	21
	724	218	112	71	50	38	30	24	20	17
0.15	1250	354	174	106	73	53	41	33	26	22
	944	269	133	82	57	42	32	26	21	18
0.20	1502	411	197	118	79	57	44	34	27	22
	1132	313	151	91	62	45	34	27	22	18
0.25	1712	459	216	127	84	60	45	35	28	23
	1289	348	165	98	65	47	36	28	22	18
0.30	1880	495	230	134	88	62	46	36	28	22
	1414	375	175	103	68	48	36	28	22	18
0.35	2006	522	239	138	89	63	46	35	27	22
	1509	395	182	106	69	49	36	28	22	18
0.40	2089	537	244	139	89	62	45	34	26	21
	1571	407	186	107	69	48	36	27	21	17
0.45	2132	543	244	138	88	60	44	33	25	19
	1603	411	186	106	68	47	34	26	20	16
0.50	2132	537	239	134	84	57	41	30	23	17
	1603	407	182	103	65	45	32	24	18	14

[a] Upper figure: significance level 0.05, power 0.90.
[b] Lower figure: significance level 0.05, power 0.80.

be less than some specified length. This approach is appropriate if 'equivalence' of the two treatments is taken to mean simply that the success rate on the new treatment is very close (not necessarily identical) to that of the standard treatment. The anticipated overall proportion of successes P (e.g., proportion alive at three years) is specified, along with a value d such that if the two treatments are truly equally effective the upper $100 \cdot (1 - \alpha)$ percentage confidence level for the true difference in proportion of successes on the two treatments does not exceed d with probability $(1 - \beta)$. Then the required number of patients, N, per treatment group

Table 3. Number of patients in each of two treatment groups required to demonstrate treatment equivalence for various values of P[a], d[b], α[c], and β

Proportion of successes (P)	d = 0.10	d = 0.05
0.95	75[d]	298
	100[e]	400
0.90	142	565
	190	757
0.85	200	800
	269	1073
0.80	251	1004
	337	1346
0.75	294	1176
	395	1577
0.70	330	1318
	442	1766
0.65	357	1427
	479	1913
0.60	377	1506
	505	2019
0.55	389	1553
	521	2082

[a] P = the overall proportion of successes that one anticipates will occur.
[b] d = a prespecified value such that if 2 treatments are truly equally effective, the upper $100 \cdot (1 - \alpha)$ percentage confidence limit for the true difference in proportion of successes on the 2 treatments does not exceed d with probability $(1 - \beta)$.
[c] $\alpha = 0.05$.
[d] $(1 - \beta) = 0.80$
[e] $(1 - \beta) = 0.90$.

202

is $2 \cdot P \cdot (1.0 - P) \cdot (z_{\alpha/2} + z_\beta)^2/d^2$, where z_α is the upper α tail point of the standard normal distribution (e.g., for $\alpha = 0.05$ and $\beta = 0.20$, $z_{\alpha/2} = 1.96$ and $z_\beta = 0.84$). Sample sizes based on this confidence interval approach are presented in Table 3 for various choices of P, d, α and β.

To demonstrate the required calculations, assume that the proportion of stage II patients who receive either radiotherapy or surgery alone and are alive at 3 years is $P = 0.75$. We wish the sample to be large enough so that with a high degree of confidence $(1 - \beta = 0.80)$, one can conclude that the treatments differ in regard to 3-year survival by no more than $d = 0.10$. For $\alpha = 0.05$, we calculate the number of patients required in each group to be $2 \cdot (.75) \cdot (.25) \cdot (1.96 + .84)^2/.1^2 = 294$. All of the per group sample sizes in Table 3 are calculated similarly. As many trial planners fail to appreciate, this example demonstrates that large sample sizes are often needed in 'conservative' clinical trials to demonstrate the similarly of two treatments with a high level of confidence. An important corollary is that a lack of statistical significance should not be taken as evidence of equivalence unless sufficient numbers of patients have been studied. Without large enough sample sizes, the width of the confidence interval around the observed difference between treatments will tend to be broad. In order to conclude that treatments have equivalent effects, the confidence interval, which indicates the range of true treatment differences consistent with the observed data, should not only include zero but should also be of narrow width. This point is frequently overlooked in clinical trial design as well as the interpretation of results. Articles by Detsky and Sackett [18] and Makuch and Johnson [19] contain further discussions concerning the design and interpretation of 'equivalence' trials.

Although many clinical studies in head and neck cancer are planned using a dichotomous response, published studies almost always include analyses with survival or other types of time-to-failure as the endpoints of primary importance. To incorporate this type of endpoint in the sample size consideration of a study, several different approaches are available. George and Desu [20] developed sample size requirements for the two-treatment situation where the failure distribution is assumed to be exponential, and all patients are followed until failure. The assumption of exponential survival in each treatment group implies that the risk of death is identically constant in each interval of time. Without any loss in generality, we will assume failure to imply death. For determining the number of deaths required in each treatment group, one specifies the type I error rate (α) and the ratio of median survival times (Δ) for the two groups that one wishes to detect with power $(1 - \beta)$. Any Δ greater than 2.0, implying that the true median for one group will be twice as large as that for the comparison group, is unrealistic for most planning situations. Table 4 provides the required numbers of deaths in each of two treatment groups for various choices of α, β and Δ. For example, suppose one wants 90% power ($\beta = 0.10$) to detect a 40% increase in survival attributable to a new therapy as compared to a standard ($\Delta = 1.4$). For a two-sided

$\alpha = 0.05$, one would need to have 187 patients per treatment group, all followed until death. When two or more treatment groups are under study, Makuch and Simon [21] generalized the results of George and Desu [20] to account for the multiple comparisons possible among k treatment groups.

Of course, it is rare that survival comparisons are deferred until all patients have died. Since patients enter a study serially, complete survival times for all patients frequently are not known at the time of analysis. This practical consequence of clinical trial execution bears on sample size estimation since the ability to detect treatment differences is a function only of the number of deaths, not of the number of patients, under the assumption that survival curves follow the exponential distribution.

To account for this in one's sample size considerations, a simple alteration to Table 4 provides a good approximation to the actual patient numbers required using more complicated formulae. Quite simply, one divides the appropriate number in Table 4 by the overall proportion of deaths expected at the time of analysis. If the study is to be analyzed after all patients have died, then the overall expected proportion is 1, and so the sample sizes are precisely those given in Table 4. If one anticipates that roughly 50% of the patients will have died at the time of analysis, then the sample sizes in Table 4 must be doubled, in order to have approximately the same power and α-level of detecting the ratio Δ of median survival times. This result follows from the work of Schoenfeld [22], who derived a sample size formula for the more general situation where no specific distributional form for the survival times was required.

In addition to the fact that not all patients may have died by the final analysis time, another factor to be considered when estimating sample sizes is the continuation period, which is defined to be the length of time after accrual has stopped and prior to the time of analysis. Though often ignored in planning a study, varying the length of the continuation period can have a sizeable impact on the required size and duration of the study. To illustrate, assume the median time for patients receiving standard therapy is 1 year, and we wish to detect with power

Table 4. Number of patients required on each of two treatment groups to compare survival distributions, all followed to failure

Δ = ratio of median survival times

1.1	1.2	1.3	1.4	1.5	1.6	1.8	2.0	3.0
1731[a]	473	230	140	96	72	46	34	14
2361[b]	633	306	187	129	96	62	45	18
2574[c]	704	340	207	143	107	69	50	20

[a] Upper figure: 2-sided $\alpha = 0.05$, $\beta = 0.20$.
[b] Middle figure: 2-sided $\alpha = 0.05$, $\beta = 0.10$.
[c] Lower figure: 2-sided $\alpha = 0.01$, $\beta = 0.20$.

0.80 an increase in median survival to 2 years ($\Delta = 2$) for patients receiving an experimental therapy, with $\alpha = 0.05$. Assume the loss to follow-up rate is 0, the yearly accrual rate is 60 patients, and there is no continuation period. Once can then demonstrate that the estimated total required trial length is 2.3 years. If one were to specify a 1-year continuation period, while leaving all other design parameters unchanged, the total trial time becomes 2.6 years. However, because of the one year continuation period, the accrual period would be only $2.6 - 1.0 = 1.6$ years instead of 2.3 years. It follows that fewer patients would be entered on-study in this situation, since accrual is shortened by roughly three-fourths of a year. Thus, the continuation period is an important parameter to consider when designing a study, since it can reduce the total number of patients required for the study, while extending the total trial length only slightly. Rubinstein, Gail and Santner [23] give a thorough review of these issues and provide an extensive set of tables to illustrate the various trade-offs that occur as one varies loss to follow-up, the accrual period, and the continuation period.

The importance of sample size planning and its impact on practical and scientific aspects of a clinical trial cannot be over-stated. This section provided a brief outline of the general principles involved, and helpful references dealing with the subject in greater depth. Factors that complicate the determination of appropriate study size and length include the effects of drop-outs due to non-adherence, the need for stratification by important risk-groups, the effects of slow or uneven accrual rates, and the use of sequential procedures for monitoring an on-going study. While beyond the scope of this chapter, excellent references are available on these topics [24, 25]. Given the complexity of sample size considerations in long-term follow-up studies, it is usually advisable to seek advice from a statistician who is acquainted with the literature in this area and is experienced in planning such trials.

Allocation

When designing a comparative clinical trial, one must decide on a particular method of allocating the treatments to the patients. Since a major objective of such trials is to provide a precise and valid treatment comparison, an allocation method should contribute to this objective by preventing bias and insuring an efficient treatment comparison. Any allocation method based on a systematic approach (e.g., alternating treatment assignments or assigning one treatment on even-numbered days and the other on odd-numbered days) can introduce selection bias. Such bias can easily occur when an investigator's *a priori* knowledge of the next treatment assignment affects his decision to enter the next eligible patient on-study. For example, if it is known that the next treatment assignment will be to a more aggressive treatment, a good prognosis patient might be accepted on-study, consciously or unconsciously, more readily than might a poor prognosis patient unable to receive the full treatment course. Thus, initial allocation to treatment groups using a formal randomization process is recommended to avoid such a potential for selection bias. Also, randomization provides a statistical foundation for assessing error, so that one can evaluate the extent to which an observed difference is larger than random allocation would produce ordinarily.

The most straightforward method for randomly allocating patients involves assigning each patient to one of T treatment groups with probability 1/T. The distinguishing feature of this method, referred to as 'pure' randomization, is that the allocation depends neither on patient characteristics nor on previous treatment assignments. Peto *et al.* support the use of this approach, since they contend that any imbalance in prognostic factors can be adjusted for in the analysis and that the method possesses sufficient simplicity to encourage participation in the study and minimize errors in assigning treatment [26].

Implicit in this recommendation is the notion that only large trials which tend to insure balance of important prognostic factors between treatment groups are worthwhile, and that the interim analysis for detecting unexpected toxicities and early treatment differences is of little interest. Such is usually not the case in the head and neck cancer research area. For clinical trials with a relatively small number of patients, Grizzle showed that accounting for stratification at the time of randomization is significantly more efficient than using pure randomization and stratifying at the time of analysis [27]. The medical audience to whom the study is addressed also may find the study results less convincing when an imbalance is present in the prognostic profile of the two treatment groups, an event which becomes more likely as the number of patients becomes smaller. Brown states '... there is much to be gained in persuasiveness or credibility by presentation of data that show the number of patients assigned to the several treatments to be closely balanced with regard to the variable commonly felt to be related to the course of the disease and the response to treatment. No amount of post-stratification and covariance analysis... will be as convincing as the demonstration that the groups were balanced in the beginning...' [28].

In addition, pure randomization has the rare but unfortunate potential for producing a severe imbalance in the number of patients in each treatment group. For example, with a total of 50 patients, there is greater than a 5% chance that an 18:32 split will occur; for 100 patients, the split could be 40:60. This outcome could prove troublesome to the medical investigator, especially if the smaller number of patients received the experimental treatment for which crucial information about efficacy and tolerance is most desired. Further, with a significant imbalance in prognostic factors or the number of patients in each group, the comparison between groups would be less efficient, and the statistical power of a test to detect differences in the performance of two therapies would be diminished. Thus, randomized treatment assignment usually is restricted in some way to insure prognostic comparability among the treatment groups, as well as fairly equal numbers of patients in each group.

206

Perhaps the most commonly used method to achieve comparability is the random permuted blocks design. It ensures exactly equal numbers of treatment assignments at certain equally spaced points in the sequence of patient entries. This process helps protect against 'accidental bias' caused by unknown time trends that may occur in the characteristics of arriving patients over time. By randomly assigning patients to all T groups within small lengths of time relative to the entire accrual period, one need not worry as in pure randomization that the treatment assignments are confounded with changes in patient characteristics. Severe confounding is highly detrimental to a clinical trial because it then becomes quite difficult to ascribe differences in patient outcome to the effects of treatment as opposed to non-treatment-related effects caused by imbalances in prognostic factors.

The first step in implementing a random permuted blocks design involves defining strata, where each stratum comprises a different combination of levels of each factor on which balance is desired. Then treatment assignments are independently and randomly generated within each stratum using random permuted blocks. Each random permuted block is composed of $b \cdot T$ random treatment assignments subject to the constraint that each of the T treatment groups has been assigned to b patients. Selecting a particular value of b is related to the conflicting needs between balance and minimizing bias. A large value of b will reduce bias since it will be harder to guess what the next treatment will be, but it also increases the chances of producing a significant imbalance in the distribution of prognostic factors the treatment groups. On the other hand, if b is too small, an investigator might be able to keep track of the assignments and guess the next treatment. Good balance will be achieved in this situation at the expense of introducing an unacceptably high degree of bias. Depending on the size of the study and the number of strata, the values of b usually selected lie between 2 and 4 inclusive.

To demonstrate this method of patient allocation, assume that two treatment groups (C = control and E = new experimental treatment) are to be compared for patients with advanced (stages III and IV) resectable head and neck cancer in the larynx or oropharynx. Two important prognostic factors for this disease are stage and site. Thus the total number of strata defined by all combinations of levels of these two factors is $2 \times 2 = 4$. If $b = 2$ then after every four treatment assignments in each stratum, two patients will be assigned C and two patients will be assigned E. Every possible ordered treatment assignment per block must be one of the following: CCEE, CECE, CEEC, ECEC, EECC, and ECCE. The overall list of treatment assignments for each stratum is formed by repeatedly and randomly selecting among these six possible ordered treatment assignments. For example, the first 12 treatment assignments for stage III patients with a primary of the oral cavity might be CEEC EECC CECE. This same process is used to independently produce a randomization list for every stratum. To minimize the potential for bias, an impartial individual should be given the responsibility of generating the treatment assignment list. Also, the investigator should be kept unaware of the next treatment assignment on the list until the patient is deemed eligible and willing to enter the study, and an informed consent has been obtained.

Note that the total number of strata is the product of the number of levels in each factor, and consequently the total number of strata increases dramatically with every additional factor. One must appreciate that as the total number of strata increases, a stratified randomization becomes more and more similar to pure randomization where substantial imbalances in important factors may occur. Secondly, sizable differences can appear in the overall number of patients in each treatment group, leading to a statistically inefficient design. Either of these situations can result when a large number of randomized blocks have many unassigned treatments; this is known as overstratification.

To see how overstratification can defeat the the intent of stratified randomization, we consider the following example. A sequence of treatment assignments was generated using the permuted block method for $b = 3$ and $T = 2$, where four factors (primary site, nodal status, stage, and performance status) believed to be predictive for survival were selected as stratification factors. Primary site was divided into larynx and oropharynx, nodal status was divided into N0 and N1 versus N2 and N3, stage was categorized into stage III and stage IV, and performance status was split into < 90 vs. 90 or more. Since each factor has two levels, there are $2 \times 2 \times 2 \times 2 = 16$ strata. Table 5 gives one realization of a permuted block randomization list for 16 strata, and the check marks show the treatment assignments made thus far. The number of patients assigned to either C or E is given in the bottom of the table, and it shows a marked treatment imbalance in the proportion of patients with a particular characteristic. Thus, the prognostic profile of patients is quite dissimilar between the treatment groups when site and stage are considered.

Although few would consider stopping a study after only 31 patients were entered on-study, it is not unusual for some investigators participating in a multi-institutional study to enter only a few patients. Since stratified randomization is almost always performed separately within each institution, such imbalances in many institutions could lead to serious overall imbalances in prognostic profiles for the entire study. Solutions to this dilemma include: (1) reducing the number of strata, (2) generating for each patient an overall score (based on a statistical model of prognostic factors from previous trials) which summarizes several patient characteristics into a single stratification factor, and (3) using alternative randomization methods. Other more complex procedures have been described by, among others, Pocock and Simon [29] and Wei [30]. All have the property that randomization can be dynamically weighted to insure greater likelihood of balance of prognostic factorsbetween groups. These methods are useful when there are many stratification factors or many levels of a particular factor which result in a large number of strata. However, they will not be discussed further since their technical aspects extend beyond the scope of this chapter.

A final topic for brief discussion is unequal randomization, where patients are randomized to one of two treatments with unequal probability. Roughly equal-sized treatment groups using a 1:1 treatment allocation ratio provide the most efficient means for comparing treatments under most standard conditions. Nevertheless, other factors may influence the choice of allocation ratio in favor of more patients receiving the new therapy, such as the need to motivate investigators to enter patients on-study, gather relatively more information quickly about the new treatment, and gain greater experience regarding its use. To this end, a commonly proposed alternative to equal allocation is a 2:1 randomization weighting, where on average two patients are placed on the new treatment for every patient assigned to the control treatment. Statistically speaking, the loss in power to detect differences of some prespecified magnitude is quite modest when the treatment

Table 5. Imbalance of prognostic profile between two treatment groups in an overstratified design

	Stage III				Stage IV			
	PS 80 or below		PS 90 or above		PS 80 or below		PS 90 or above	
	N 0+1	N 2+3	N 0+1	N 2+3	N 0+1	N 2+3	N 0+1	N 2+3
Oropharynx	C√	C√	E√	C√	E√	C√	E√	E√
	C√	C√	C√	C√	E	E	C√	C√
	C√	E	C√	E	C	E	E	C
	E	C	C	E	C	C	C	E
	E	E	E	E	E	C	E	E
	E	E	E	C	C	E	C	C
Larynx	C√	C√	E√	E√	E√	E√	E√	E√
	E	C√	E√	C√	E√	C	E√	E√
	C	E	C	E	C	E	C	E√
	E	C	E	C	C	C	E	C
	E	E	C	E	E	C	C	C
	C	E	C	C	C	E	C	C

		C	E
Site:	oropharynx	12	4
	larynx	4	11
Stage:	III	13	4
	IV	3	11
PS:	80 or below	9	4
	90 or above	7	11
N status:	0 or 1	7	9
	2 or 3	9	6
Total, within each treatment		16	15

allocation ratio is 2:1 or less. For ratios greater than 2:1, the loss in power increases more dramatically, and few statisticians would recommend exceeding it.

Though several statisticians claim that unequal randomization should be used more widely provided that statistical efficiency is not seriously impaired, important non-statistical issues should also be considered. For example, during a recent study in which, on average, two patients were randomized to the experimental therapy for every one control patient, there was a period of time early in the trial when practically all the patients were randomized to receive the experimental therapy. Unfortunately, unexpected life-threatening toxicities (pneumocystis carinii pneumonia) occurred overwhelmingly in the experimental treatment group, and it was impossible to ascertain whether these toxicities were a sufficient drug-related cause for alarm to necessitate terminating the study prematuraly, or whether they simply appeared to predominate in the experimental group because so few had been randomized to the control treatment. Thus, due to power considerations as well as potential problems with imbalances in the number of patients exposed to the therapies under study, we recommend that equal allocation be used under most circumstances.

Statistical analysis

There are a variety of statistical methods used to analyze and interpret clinical trial data, but we will focus on some aspects of statistical analysis involving time-to-failure data since this type of data is frequently encountered in head and neck cancer trials. Failure is a general term which encompasses a variety of endpoint events including death or tumor relapse. We will use failure to imply death unless explicitly mentioned otherwise, since most of the comments apply equally to disease-free survival curves, freedom-from-relapse curves, or any other type of endpoint data involving time. Because the methods to be described are broadly applicable and relatively straightforward to put into practice, they are frequently misused with potentially dramatic adverse consequences. Some computational mechanics associated with these analytical tools will be described, followed by general comments on the conditions under which these methods can be applied properly.

Survival data may be distinguished from most other types of data on the basis of two characteristics. First, the data assume non-negative values only and they can be highly skewed in the positive direction. This suggests the need to use nonparametric statistical techniques, which reduce the influence of an infrequent, uncommonly large survival period. The second distinction involves the definition of a 'failure', since whether or not a patient is observed to fail affects the way the calculations proceed. For calculating survival curves, a patient failure is usually, though not always, defined to be a patient who dies from any cause. This is called an uncensored observation, and one usually calculates the interval of time from entry on-study (or some other relevant start point) to the death date as the length of observation. Patients who are known to be alive at the most recent date prior to analysis represent 'incomplete censored observations', implying that a *possible* change in status could occur during subsequent follow-up. The length of the censored observation is calculated from some relevant start date to the date the patient was last known alive. Thus, censoring occurs whenever the investigator is unable to observe the endpoint of interest. For example, for patients who survive 12 months from the start of treatment, the analysis must distinguish between those patients who die at the end of those 12 months and those patients who were last known to be alive at that time. Any analysis which does not discriminate between these two situations (and almost *all* standard statistical analytic techniques and summary statistics assume no such distinction) would be clearly misleading.

The most common technique for estimating and graphically displaying the survival experience of a group of patients is the 'product-limit' method developed by Kaplan and Meier [31]. Although there are other methods for estimating survival curves, the product-limit estimate is recommended for most situations since it is an empirical approach which avoids parametric model assumptions that may be difficult to justify for relatively small datasets. To estimate the survival curve for N patients, a time t for each patient is first calculated from the start of therapy to either the date of death or the last date of follow-up if death was not known to have occurred. Then the N times are ordered in increasing magnitude, and the number of patients (N_i) alive just prior to time t_i and the number of deaths (d_i) occurring at time t_i are recorded. The conditional probability of surviving at least to time t_i, given survival up to time t_{i-1}, is estimated by $(N_i - d_i)/N_i = P_i$. The probability of surviving beyond time t_i, $S(t_i)$, is estimated by the product of all the conditional probabilities of surviving intervals of time up to and including time t_i, that is, $\hat{S}(t_i) = P_1 \cdot P_2 \cdot ... \cdot P_i$. Note that $P_i = 1$ for all times t_i when a death does not occur, so $\hat{S}(t_i)$ changes value only at observed death times, not at censoring times. The values of $\hat{S}(t_i)$ lie between 0 and 1 inclusive, and the estimated survival curve is plotted with $\hat{S}(t_i)$ on the vertical axis and t_i on the horizontal axis. The coordinates $[t_i, \hat{S}(t_i)]$ are joined by a step function in which the value of $\hat{S}(t_{i-1})$ is drawn horizontally from t_{i-1} to t_i when it drops to $\hat{S}(t_i)$.

Some calculations are provided in Table 6 to illustrate the method using survival data for advanced stage, non-metastatic cancer patients who received surgery and radiation therapy in a multi-institutional randomized trial. The corresponding survival curve is presented in its entirety in Figure 1. One important feature of the product-limit survival estimate is that each portion of the curve depends on the preceding segments. If most patients have been on-study for only a short period of time and have not had an adequate opportunity to fail, then the estimated curve is subject to more variability than if the majority of patients were followed for a longer period. Glatstein and Makuch point out that this variability due to insufficient patient follow-up can lead to overly optimistic results in estimating the probability of surviving beyond time t_i, particularly in study reports that are published too soon due to early findings that appear strikingly positive [32]. A minimum period of follow-up (e.g., at least as long as the anticipated median survival time for the disease under study) should be specified to guard against over-interpretation of premature results.

One way to measure the extent of variability associated with points on the curve is to calculate confidence intervals. The usefulness of a confidence interval is that it indicates the range of true values that is reasonably consistent with the observed data. Because the median survival, defined as the value of t for which $S(t) = 0.50$, is a frequently chosen point to summarize survival experience, we have selected the method developed by Brookmeyer and Crowley [33] to calculate a 95% two-sided confidence interval for the median survival estimate in Figure 1. The method is straightforward to use and merely requires that each point estimate $(\hat{S}(t_i))$ and its standard error (s.e.) be known. For each t_i, one first calculates $(\hat{S}(t_i) - 1/2)^2$. If this quantity is less than $(3.84) \cdot [(\text{s.e. } \hat{S}(t_i))^2]$, then that value of t_i lies within the 95% confidence interval of the median. One can see in Figure 1

Table 6. Survival data for patients with head and neck cancer: calculations to produce Kaplan-Meier survival estimates

$t_i{}^a$	$d_i{}^b$	$c_i{}^c$	$N_i{}^d$	$\hat{P}_i \dfrac{(= N_i - d_i)^e}{N_i}$	$\hat{S}(t_i)^f$
12	1	0	152	0.9934	$0.993 (= 151/152)$
19	1	0	151	0.9934	$0.987 (= 151/152 \cdot 150/151)$
23	1	0	150	0.9933	$0.980 (= 151/152 \cdot 150/151 \cdot 149/150)$
56	1	0	149	0.9933	0.974
137	1	0	148	0.9932	0.967
.	.	.	.	.	.
.	.	.	.	.	.
.	.	.	.	.	.
225	1	0	133	0.9925	0.868
237	1	0	132	0.9924	0.862
291	3	1	131	0.9769	0.842
305	1	0	127	0.9921	0.835

[a] t_i = ordered, distinct death time.
[b] d_i = number of deaths at t_i.
[c] c_i = number of observations censored at t_i.
[d] N_i = number of patients alive and followed just before t_i.
[e] $\hat{P}_i$ = estimated probability of surviving the internal (t_{i-1}, t_i), given that the patient was alive at t_{i-1}.
[f] $\hat{S}(t_i)$ = product-limit survival estimate of the probability of exceeding time t_i.

212

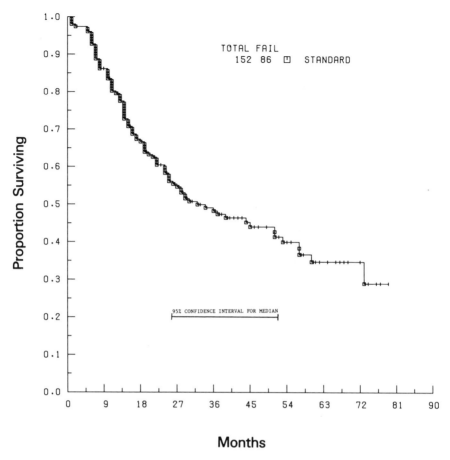

Figure 1. Kaplan-Meier survival curve.

that the estimated median survival is 32 months and the 95% confidence interval ranges from 25 months inclusive to 51 months. Even with a relatively large number of patients at risk, these calculations demonstrate that the range of true median values consistent with the observed median is fairly broad. As the number of patients at risk becomes smaller, the confidence interval becomes even broader. Thus, knowledge of the median survival time alone, with no indication of its variability, is of limited utility in gauging the success of a new treatment.

The comparison of medians may be misleading and usually is statistically inefficient. More generally, it is usually inappropriate to conduct statistical tests of significance comparing treatments at any individual point along the curves. This approach to comparative analysis can introduce subjectivity, especially if comparisons are chosen at specific time points where the treatment differences are largest, or smallest, to confirm one's *a priori* opinion regarding relative treatment efficacy. P-values obtained from such comparisons cannot be interpreted in a standard fashion due to the data-dependent nature of the comparison. The analysis should be based on methods which compare the entire curve to another. Two commonly applied techniques for comparative analysis are Gehan's generalized Wilcoxon test [34] and the logrank test described by Mantel [35]. Since the latter test is frequently used and relatively easy to describe, it will now be summarized.

To calculate the logrank statistic comparing two treatment groups, a 2×2 table is formed at each death time as depicted in Table 7. The quantity a_i is the observed number of deaths at time t_i and b_i is the number of patients alive at time t_i in the experimental treatment group; c_i and d_i are the corresponding quantities in the control group. For each table, one calculates the expected number $E(a_i)$ of deaths in the experimental treatment group as $(a_i + c_i) \cdot (a_i + b_i)/N_i$, where $N_i = a_i + b_i + c_i + d_i$. This is the expected number of deaths assuming that no survival difference exists between the two groups. The variance of a_i is

$$V(a_i) = (a_i + c_i) \cdot (b_i + d_i) \cdot (a_i + b_i) \cdot (c_i + d_i)/N_i^2 \cdot (N_i - 1).$$

The logrank statistic is calculated as

$$(\sum_i a_i - \sum_i E(a_i))^2 / \sum_i V(a_i).$$

The application of the logrank test to the analysis of clinical trial data is summarized in Peto et al. [26].

As we have seen, the calculations involved in graphically displaying and analyzing time-to-failure data are relatively straightforward. But their proper application requires knowledge about the assumptions underlying these methods. The proper use and interpretation of these statistical methods for evaluating time-to-failure data depends on a number of factors, including (1) the appropriate choice of patients for inclusion in the analysis, and (2) attention to the manner in which censored observations arise, that is, consideration of other risks operating which might alter the results for the particular endpoint analyzed. These two issues will be introduced by way of an example.

In a large randomized study for patients with advanced, operable head and neck cancer, patients were randomized to receive surgery and radiation therapy (stan-

Table 7. Distribution of patients at death time t_i, according to treatment and survival status

Treatment group	No. of deaths at time t_i	No. of survivors at time t_i	No. of patients at risk just prior to time t_i
Experimental	a_i	b_i	$a_i + b_i$
Control	c_i	d_i	$c_i + d_i$

dard therapy) or induction chemotherapy plus standard therapy plus maintenance chemotherapy. Upon completion of surgery, the patient was either rendered disease-free or not, based upon examination of the tumor specimen. Among those not disease-free, there were eight patients of 152 (5.3%) in the standard therapy arm (S) and 19 of 151 (12.6%) in the experimental treatment arm (M). A standard approach to disease-free analysis would exclude these 27 patients. For the remaining patients, the disease-free interval was calculated from the time of surgery (removal of all gross tumor) to the date of relapse or most recent follow-up. The logrank test gave some indication that the experimental therapy was superior to the standard in prolonging disease-free survival time ($p = 0.16$), although further follow-up and more patients might ultimately lead to a more definitive statement. See the top panel in Figure 2. However, when all the patients randomized to each of these two treatments were analyzed with respect to disease-free survival, and the 27 patients never rendered disease-free were assigned a disease-free period of zero, then there was no treatment difference whatsoever ($p = 0.92$). See the bottom panel in Figure 2. The interpretation of these data is now considered in light of the issues mentioned above.

Although randomization was used to help insure comparability of the treatment groups, a greater proportion of patients receiving experimental therapy was never rendered disease-free following surgery than in the standard treatment group. If those patients with persistent disease also tended to have a poorer prognosis, there would be a relatively more favorable prognostic group of patients in the remainder of the experimental group, inducing a bias in any comparison other than one based on all randomized patients. It is possible that such a bias was operating in our example since the two analyses yield strikingly different evidence regarding relative treatment efficacy. What makes this example quite dramatic is that such a distinction arose between the two analyses, although the number of patients responsible for the difference in results is quite small.

This example also demonstrates that randomization will not provide any guarantee of comparability among subsets of the overall randomized groups. A standard technique to see if comparability is not violated is to compare statistically the distribution of known risk factors in the two subsets, where the patients not rendered disease-free are excluded. If there are no apparent imbalances, many analysts will routinely evaluate these subsets and interpret the data as if they arose from a direct randomized comparison. In our example there were no marked prognostic imbalances in any important features including performance status, stage, site of primary disease, T or N class, between the two treatment subsets at $p = 0.60$ or greater. Thus the standard analytic approach would have provided a misleading overall finding with a trend favoring the experimental treatment. The major emphasis should always be on the randomized comparison of all patients, with the observation that, for a subset of patients who were rendered disease-free, an interesting finding suggests that a new study should be designed to examine this issue directly.

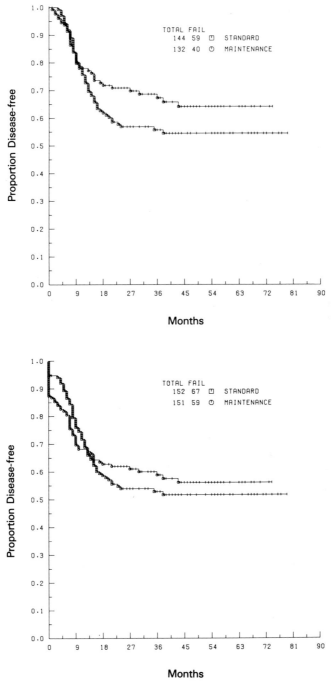

Figure 2. Disease-free period, by treatment group. Upper panel excludes patients never rendered disease-free. Lower panel includes patients never rendered disease-free. For these patients, a time of 0 is assigned for their disease-free interval.

Related to issues regarding the propriety of excluding patients from analysis is the distinction made by Schwartz and Lellouch between pragmatic and explanatory trials [36]. The former type of trial assumes that human experimentation is imperfect and that some patients wil deviate in some way from the study protocol. The purpose of such trials is to compare the *policy* of giving one treatment versus another treatment. This approach in therefore directed towards the comparison of treatments under presumably realistic conditions that a clinician faces in practice, and it is argued that a realistic measure of treatment efficacy is obtained as a result. The explanatory viewpoint is biologically purer, in the sense that one wishes to know the effect of treatment for all patients who followed the protocol exactly. Although both approaches are useful in understanding treatment efficacy and in providing new directions for future research, it is by no means clear that explanatory answers can be obtained in the inherently imperfect clinical trial setting. Thus the pragmatic approach involving the analysis of all randomized patients should be the dominant basis for interpreting data.

A second issue in the analysis of failure data involves understanding the nature of censored observations. The need for thorough patient follow-up is particularly important if losses to follow-up are related to patient outcome. Returning to the example, assume that disease-free patients do not return for their scheduled visit when they become ill and that the illness is a precursor of tumor recurrence. Then, only the censored observation (i.e., non-failure) obtains, and tumor recurrence is by definition a nonobservable event. The analysis of these data would therefore show an overly optimistic effect of treatment in preventing tumor recurrence because a crucial condition for proper survival analysis has been violated. Namely, an individual who is censored at some time, t say, should be representative of all patients who have not yet recurred and are available for follow-up at time t. This condition does not hold in our hypothetical consideration since the censoring time carries prognostic information about the individual's tumor status. To minimize this problem, every effort should be made to obtain the necessary endpoint information for each patient.

Treatment-covariate interaction

A treatment-covariate interaction is said to occur when the treatment effect depends on particular characteristics of the patient. Peto has classified treatment-covariate interactions into two general classes: quantitative and qualitative [37]. A quantitative interaction arises when the magnitude of the treatment effect varies according to the patient's characteristics, but the direction of the effect does not. For example, the addition of induction chemotherapy to surgery and radiation therapy may benefit all patients with advanced head and neck cancer, but the treatment efficacy is more pronounced in N0 and N1 patients than in N2 and N3 patients. A qualitative interaction, on the other hand, describes a change in the direction of the treatment effect based on the particular characteristics of the patient. An illustration of a qualitative interaction is to assume the addition of maintenance adjuvant chemotherapy following surgery and radiotherapy is beneficial for good performance status patients while it is actually harmful to poor performance status patients.

The identification of a qualitative interaction, if it exists, is crucial from a clinical viewpoint since it implies that the optimal treatment for any given patient will depend on his particular set of characteristics. However, leaving aside differences in costs of treatment, toxicity, and other relevant factors that may play an important role in the decision to select one treatment over another, awareness of a quantitative interaction may cause less concern since one treatment is always superior to the other, regardless of patient characteristics, and it is only the magnitude of its superiority which is likely to vary. Another reason for less concern is that quantitative interactions are model dependent; that is, the interaction could disappear with a change in the scale of measurement or the selection of an alternative statistical model. However, this is not true for qualitative interactions unless improper statistical methods are employed.

An example of a qualitative·treatment-covariate interaction is given in Table 8. Assume that the proportion alive at 2 years among good performance status patients is 0.75 for patients receiving maintenance chemotherapy following surgery and radiation therapy (MSR) and 0.60 for patients receiving surgery and radiation therapy alone (SR). Conversely, the same two-year proportions for the poor prognosis patients are 0.25 and 0.40, respectively. The overall level of statistical significance comparing the two treatments is given in the table, as well as the corresponding p-values for the comparison of treatments within each of the two covariate strata separately. Although the overall test of significance does not reveal a dramatic difference in favor of one treatment or the other, a formal test of interaction is highly significant, as are the treatment differences in each of the two subsets. Thus an important result would have been overlooked if the subsets were not analyzed separately, since the data strongly suggest that a patient's prognostic category is crucial to selecting appropriate treatment.

This type of example is used frequently to justify an investigator's request that statisticians thoroughly explore treatment effects within a variety of patient subsets. Although it is an entirely reasonable wish on the part of the clinician that

Table 8. Example of qualitative interaction: proportion alive at 2 years

Subset	Maintenance	No maintenance	p-value[a]
Good performance status	0.75 (100[b])	0.60 (100)	0.024
Poor performance status	0.25 (200)	0.40 (200)	0.002
All patients	0.42 (300)	0.47 (300)	0.23

[a] Chi-squared test unadjusted for continuity; [b] number of patients.

a medical trial should provide reliable and precise predictions of clinical outcome for various combinations of treatment and patient characteristics, the extent to which a statistician can help in this regard is limited by a number of statistical facts. As Tukey stated [38], 'It is right for each physician to want to know about the behavior to be expected from the intervention or therapy when applied to his particular individual patient ... It is not right, however, for a physician to *expect* to know this – except, possibly, for the most dramatically effective and time-tested interventions or therapies'. Some of the non-trivial statistical issues associated with these comments are touched upon below.

One often unappreciated fact is that treatment-covariate interactions, both quantitative and qualitative, can arise much more frequently by chance alone than one might expect. Assume that MSR is compared to SR in regard to the proportion alive at 2 years. Denote the observed treatment difference in favor of MSR as $D = (p_1 - p_2)$, and let the standard error of D be D/2. The overall significance test is obtained by dividing D by its standard error, giving a standardized z-value of 2 which corresponds to a two-sided p-value of 0.045. Now, let us randomly divide the data into two subsets of equal size and consider separately the two quantities D_1 and D_2 corresponding to the observed treatment difference in proportion alive at 2 years in each of the two subsets. In one realization of this hypothetical split, let us assume that the observed difference in subset 1 is 1.5 times the observed overall treatment difference, and in subset 2 the observed difference is half the observed overall treatment difference (i.e., $D_1 = 3/2 \cdot D$ and $D_2 = 1/2 \cdot D$). The one can readily calculate the two-sided p-value for subset 1 to be 0.034 while for subset 2 the two-sided p-value is 0.48. Such quantitative differences in each of the two subsets might lead one to recommend that most of the treatment benefit of maintenance chemotherapy is in subset 1 while there is not treatment benefit in subset 2 attributable to maintenance chemotherapy. But statistical significance is a function of the sample size as well as the observed difference obtained in a study. Merely examining p-values within subsets can be misleading unless one forms a statistical link to combine results or investigate variation across the subsets using formal techniques of statistical inference.

A test of interaction serves as a useful guide in evaluating whether the variability in comparative treatment efficacy across subgroups is real or represents random fluctuation. Its strength lies in the fact that it uses all the data, and thus it quantitates formally the extent to which chance alone might account for the degree of heterogeneous treatment response observed among subgroups. A formal test for interaction in the foregoing example of quantitative interaction gives a p-value of 0.32, indicating that variability in relative treatment efficacy as extreme as that observed between subsets could occur by chance alone approximately one-third of the time! Thus, in the absence of additional information, an appropriate interpretation of these data would indicate that the benefit of maintenance chemotherapy is not restricted to any particular subset of patients, but rather that it may be generalized to the overall population of patients represented in the study. One must always keep in mind, however, that quantitative interactions depend on the particular scale of measurement used in the analysis, and that an apparent interaction could disappear if a different scale of measurement for relative treatment efficacy (e.g., the ratio of p_1 and p_2) were used instead.

Whether apparent reversals of treatment benefit in various subsets of patients are a product of chance fluctuations or represent a true qualitative interaction is a complex issue which recently has begun to receive wider statistical attention [39–41]. The issue arises naturally in the context of clinical trial research when, for example, interest focuses on defining groupings of patient characteristics for which treatment superiority switches. Ingelfinger *et al.* framed the treatment-covariate qualitative interaction problem in the following manner [42]. They assumed that an overall treatment difference exists, and that the treatment effect is the same across all strata. They calculated the probability that a significant treatment reversal obtains by chance alone in the least favorable stratum, where 'least favorable' is defined as that stratum in which the treatment reversal is largest. Their method requires that the data be divided into k strata of equal size, and that the overall treatment effect and its standard error be specified as well. For this situation they show that, if the overall treatment difference is significant at $p = 0.045$ and one has eight strata, there is an 89% chance that the least favorable stratum will have the overall treatment benefit reversed due to random fluctuation. Even if the overall treatment difference was significant at the $p < 0.001$ level, there would be a 48% probability that a treatment reversal in the least favorable stratum would occur by chance alone.

The assessment of treatment-by-covariate interaction effects is a complex issue, usually requiring input from a qualified biostatistician. In general, before one can conclude that the treatment-of-choice policy holds in a particular setting, two general concepts should be adhered to. First, one must demonstrate that the relative treatment efficacy varies significantly among the subgroups, that is, a significant treatment-covariate interaction exists. Second, unless a plausible biological explanation is present or a treatment-covariate interaction was anticipated prior to the start of the study, a significant interaction should be considered in the spirit of exploratory data analysis. This implies that its medical plausibility should be considered and future studies should be designed to confirm or refute these initial observations. Finally, since interactions often are detected only after a very thorough analysis of the data has been carried out, statistical issues involving multiplicities add an additional layer of complexity to the proper interpretation of p-values.

The researcher should be alert to the hazards of basing conclusions on 'significant' results discovered after applying multiple tests of hypotheses across various subgroups and outcome variables. This multiplicity problem, often facetiously referred to as 'data-dredging' or 'ransacking the data', has serious implications. The more significance tests that are conducted, the greater the possibility of drawing erroneous conclusions unless certain precautions are taken. For example, if two treatment groups are compared within only ten subgroups defined by age, sex, and disease stage, there is a 40% chance that at least one of the ten subgroups would turn up a significant treatment difference at the 5% level, even though the treatments had equivalent therapeutic value. This problem may be overcome by the choice of a more stringent nominal significance level for each test, so that the overall significance level is maintained at some desired level such as 0.05. For example, if there are k patient subgroups that would have been looked at for treatment differences seriously if results for them appeared interesting, Tukey requires significance at the 0.05/k level before claiming significance at the 0.05 level in any one of the k subgroups [38]. Note that this is an especially stringent criterion if there are several outcome variables, since k would be inflated as the product of the number of plausible end-points multiplied by the number of plausible patient subsets. An alternative approach to this multiplicity problem is to properly focus trial objectives on a well-defined class of patients and clearly identify at most two or three primary end-points in the study protocol to assess treatment efficacy. Prespecification of study hypotheses is a crucial aspect of study planning in that it offsets multiplicity problems that would otherwise arise in the analysis.

Acknowledgement

This work was supported bu grant CA-16359 from the National Cancer Institute.

References

1. Buyse, M.E., Staquet, M.J., Sylvester, R.J. 1984. Cancer Clinical Trials: Methods and Practice. Oxford University Press, Oxford.
2. Mike, V., Stanley, K.E. 1982. Statistics in Medical Research: Methods and Issues, with Applications in Cancer Research. John Wiley and Sons, Inc., New York.
3. Symposium on Methodology and Quality Assurance in Cancer Clinical Trials. 1985. Cancer Treat. Rep. 69: 1039–1233.
4. Gehan, E.A., Freireich, E.J. 1974. Non-randomized controls in cancer clinical trials. N. Engl. J. Med. 290: 198–203.
5. Byar, D.P., Simon, R.M., Friedewald, W.T. et al. 1976. Randomized clinical trials. N. Engl. J. Med. 295: 74–80.
6. Farewell, V.T., D'Angio, G.J. 1981. A simulated study of historical controls using real data. Biometrics 37: 169–176.
7. Pocock, S.J. 1977. Randomized clinical trials (letter). Br. Med. J. 1 (6077): 1661.
8. Byar, D.P. 1979. Necessity and justification of randomized clinical studies. In: Controversies in Cancer Treatment (H.J. Tagnon, M.J. Staquet, eds.). Mason Publishing, New York, pp. 75–82.
9. Zelen, M. 1979. A new design for randomized clinical trials. N. Engl. J. Med. 300: 1273–1275.
10. Schoenfeld, D., Gelber, R. 1979. Designing and analyzing clinical trials which allow institutions to randomize patients to a subset of the treatments under study. Biometrics 35: 825–829.

11. Makuch, R.W., Simon, R.M. 1978. A note on the design of multi-institution three-treatment studies. Cancer Clin. Trials 1: 301–303.
12. Peto, R. 1978. Clinical trial methodology. Biomedicine 28: 24–36.
13. Byar, D.P., Piantadosi, S. 1985. Factorial designs for randomized clinical trials. Cancer Treat. Rep. 69: 1055–1062.
14. Freiman, J.A., Chalmers, T.C., Smith, H., Jr., et al. 1978. The importance of beta, the type II error and sample size in the design and interpretation of the randomized control trial: Survey of 71 'negative' trials. N. Engl. J. Med. 299: 690–694.
15. Lachin, J.M. 1981. Introduction to sample size determination and power analysis for clinical trials. Controlled Clin. Trials 2: 93–113.
16. Casagrande, J.T., Pike, M.C., Smith, P.G. 1978. An improved formula for calculating sample size for comparing two binomial distributions. Biometrics 34: 483–486.
17. Makuch, R.W., Simon, R.M. 1978. Sample size requirements for evaluating a conservative therapy. Cancer Treat. Rep. 62: 1037–1040.
18. Detsky, A.S., Sackett, D.L. 1985. When was a 'negative' clinical trial big enough? How many patients you needed depends on what you found. Arch. Intern. Med. 145: 709–712.
19. Makuch, R.W., Johnson, M.F. 1986. Some issues in the design and interpretation of 'negative' clinical studies. Arch. Intern. Med. 146: 986–989.
20. George, S.L., Desu, M.M. 1974. Planning the size and duration of a clinical trial studying the time to some critical event. J. Chronic. Dis. 27: 15–24.
21. Makuch, R.W., Simon, R.M. 1982. Sample size requirements for comparing time-to-failure among k treatment groups. J. Chron. Dis. 35: 861–867.
22. Schoenfeld, D. 1981. The asymptotic properties of nonparametric tests for comparing survival distributions. Biometrika 68: 316–319.
23. Rubinstein, L.V., Gail, M.H., Santner, T.J. 1981. Planning the duration of a comparative clinical trial with loss to follow-up and a period of continued observation. J. Chronic. Dis. 34: 469–479.
24. Palta, M., McHugh, R. 1980. Planning the size of a cohort study in the presence of both losses to follow-up and non-compliance. J. Chron. Dis. 33: 501–512.
25. Bernstein, D., Lagakos, S.W. 1978. Sample size and power determination for stratified clinical trials. J. Stat. Comput. Simu. 8: 65–73.
26. Peto, R., Pike, M.C., Armitage, P. et al. 1976. Design and analysis of randomized clinical trials, requiring prolonged observation of each treatment. I. Introduction and design. B. J. Cancer 34: 585–612.
27. Grizzle, J.E. 1982. A note on stratifying versus complete random assignment in clinical trials. Controlled Clin. Trials 3: 365–368.
28. Brown, B.W., Jr. 1980. Statistical controversies in the design of clinical trials – some personal views. Controlled Clin. Trials 1: 13–27.
29. Pocock, S.J., Simon, R. 1975. Sequential treatment assignment with balancing for prognostic factors in the controlled clinical trial. Biometrics 31: 103–115.
30. Wei, L.J. 1978. An application of an urn model to the design of sequential controlled clinical trials. J. Am. Stat. Assn. 73: 559–563.
31. Kaplan, E.L., Meier, P. 1958. Nonparametric estimation from incomplete observations. J. Am. Stat. Assn. 53: 458–481.
32. Glatstein, E., Makuch, R.W. 1984. Illusion and reality: Practical pitfalls in interpreting clinical trials. J. Clin. Oncol. 5: 488–497.
33. Brookmeyer, R., Crowley, J. 1982. A confidence interval for the median survival time. Biometrics 38: 29–41.
34. Gehan, E.A. 1965. A generalized Wilcoxon test for comparing arbitrarily singly censored samples. Biometrika 52: 203–224.
35. Mantel, N. 1966. Evaluation of survival data and two new rank order statistics arising in its consideration. Cancer Chemother. Rep. 50: 163–170.

222

36. Schwartz, D., Lellouch, J. 1967. Explanatory and pragmatic attitudes in therapeutic trials. J. Chronic. Dis. 20: 637–648.
37. Peto, R. 1982. Statistical aspects of cancer trials. In: Treatments of Cancer (K.E. Halnan, ed.). Chapman and Hall, London, pp. 867–871.
38. Tukey, J.W. 1977. Some thoughts on clinical trials, especially problems of multiplicity. Science 198: 679–684.
39. Gail, M., Simon, R. 1985. Testing for qualitative interactions between treatment effects and patient subsets. Biometrics 41: 361–371.
40. Shuster, J., van Eys, J. 1983. Interaction between prognostic factors and treatment. Controlled Clin. Trials 4: 209–214.
41. Byar, D.P. 1985. Assessing apparent treatment-covariate interactions in randomized clinical trials. Stat. Med. 4: 255–263.
42. Ingelfinger, J.A., Mosteller, F., Thibodeau, L.A., Ware, J.H. 1983. Biostatistics in Clinical Medicine. MacMillan, New York, pp. 253–260.

14. Management of orbital rhabdomyosarcoma

MOODY D. WHARAM JR. and HAROLD M. MAURER

Introduction

Rhabdomyosarcoma (RMS) is a soft tissue sarcoma that arises from the same mesodermal tissues that form striated skeletal muscle. It typically arises in the pediatric age group and can originate in virtually any anatomic location. The management of the child with orbital or eyelid RMS has changed substantially in the past two decades. Formerly dismal, the prognosis is now excellent. Advances have resulted from the application of two modern concepts in cancer management: first, multidisciplinary management including surgery, radiation oncology, and pediatric oncology; second, application of the methodology of the clinical research cooperative group. Principles of diagnostic evaluation, local tumor control, and treatment of disseminated but occult metastases have been developed and refined. Important information regarding etiology, histologic subtypes, treatment, and late effects continues to accrue.

History

Calhoun and Reese reported five cases of orbital RMS in 1942 [1]. In their literature review, they found only 14 previously reported patients. In 1958, Blaxter and Smith reported two additional cases and noted only 33 reported to that time [2]. A year later, 12 more were reported by Frayer and Enterline [3]. The first large series of cases was reported from the Armed Forces Institute of Pathology in 1962 [4]. The report of 55 cases does not indicate the time period over which the patients were accrued. Thirteen patients were apparently cured by orbital exenteration. No patient initially receiving radiotherapy was cured. The largest report from a single institution was by Jones *et al.* from the Institute of Ophthalmology at Columbia-Presbyterian Medical Center, New York City [5]. Again, the time period during which their 62 cases were accrued is not given. Thirty of their patients were apparently cured. Exenteration was the standard operative proce-

C. Jacobs (ed) Cancers of the head and neck.
© *1987, Martinus Nijhoff Publishers, Boston. ISBN 0–89838–825–2. Printed in the Netherlands.*

dure, and radiation treatment was of no apparent benefit. Also in 1965, 34 patients were reported from the Institute of Ophthalmology, University of London [6]. Only eight patients were apparently cured. The authors advocated the approach of Lederman [7] that initial treatment consist of simple excision and radiation therapy, with exenteration reserved for local treatment failures. They also advocated investigation of the potential role of chemotherapy.

The first report of the disciplined application of modern megavoltage radiation therapy to orbital RMS was published by Cassady et al. from Columbia-Presbyterian Medical Center in 1968 [8]. They documented a 50% local tumor control rate after postoperative local recurrence. More importantly, they demonstrated that definitive radiation therapy (5000 rad in 5 weeks) preceded only by tumor biopsy rendered five of five patients disease-free with follow-up from 1.3 to 4.5 years. Subsequent publications from the same institution in 1972 and 1979 confirmed the favorable outcome of the initial series in a larger number of newly diagnosed patients [9, 10]. By 1979 they had achieved a local control rate of 91% in 58 patients [10].

The concept of adjuvant chemotherapy for pediatric RMS was advanced by Pinkel and Pickren in 1961 [11]. The concept was tested prospectively by Children's Cancer Study Group A in a randomized trial which accrued patients for 4 years beginning in 1967 [12]. All patients under age 21 with RMS were eligible. Patients receiving 1 year of vincristine and actinomycin-D courses after complete tumor excision plus postoperative radiation had a 2-year disease-free survival rate of 82%, compared to 53% for patients not receiving chemotherapy. When the same two drugs plus cyclophosphamide were administered to patients with orbital RMS after definitive radiotherapy (mean dose 5500 rad in 5 to 6 weeks), the 3-year survival rate for patients with localized tumor (normal tomography) improved from 66% (4 of 6) (radiation only) to 91% (10 of 11) [10].

To accelerate patient accrual and to facilitate randomized, prospective clinical trials, three clinical cooperative groups (Children's Cancer Study Group A, Southwest Oncology Group, and The Cancer and Leukemia Group B) created the Intergroup Rhabdomyosarcoma Study Committee (IRS) in 1972. The first study (IRS I) concluded in 1978, having enrolled 690 eligible patients. IRS-II concluded in 1984 and enrolled 912 eligible patients. Much of the information in this chapter is from publications and reports of the IRS.

Incidence

The incidence of RMS in white American children under age 15 is 4.5% of all malignancies [13]. RMS of the eyelid and orbit comprises 8% of all children with RMS. The annual incidence of orbital RMS is estimated to be one in 4.4 million [14]. It is the most common malignant orbital tumor in children and the most common site of RMS among all head and neck sites.

Etiology

The etiology of orbital RMS is unknown. Environmental factors associated with the risks of having RMS at any site were described by Grufferman *et. al.* [15]. They noted the association of cigarette smoking by fathers (not mothers) and a variety of factors indicative of low socioeconomic status in North Carolina. The associated factors included fewer immunizations than controls, more preventable infections, chemicals exposure, dietary organ meats, maternal age greater than 30 and antibiotic usage before birth.

Normal and tumor anatomy

The walls of the bony orbit approximate a four-sided pyramid with the eyelids at its base and the apex corresponding to the optic canal. The roof of the orbit is composed of the frontal bone. Above it is the anterior cranial fossa. The floor of the orbit lies just above the maxillary sinus. The lateral wall is composed of the frontal bone and the zygoma. Just lateral to these bones is the temporal fossa. Posteriorly the lateral wall borders the middle cranial fossa. The medial wall is thin and affords little resistance to invasive tumors. Anteriorly it borders the nasal cavity. Posteriorly it borders the ethmoid air cells and more posteriorly the sphenoid sinus. The contents of the orbit consist of the eyeball and optic nerve, the six extra-ocular muscles and associated nerves, arteries, and veins. The majority of orbital RMS arise within the orbital cavity. In a summary of seven series totaling 191 cases, 21% appeared to arise from the lids and 8% from the conjunctiva [16]. When the primary originates in the orbital cavity, it does not usually arise from the extraocular muscles. Rather, it seems to originate in orbital connective tissue [4, 6]. The early literature suggested a predominant presentation in the upper and medial portions of the orbit [4]. Two series refute this observation [5, 6]. In the 62 cases reported by Jones *et al.,* one-half of the tumors were central, one-quarter superior, and the rest inferior or other [5].

Lymphatics have not been described within the orbital cavity. The association of nodal metastases at presentation from orbital RMS is rare and is generally associated with primary lid tumors. Lymphatics of the lid follow two routes. The medial group follows the facial vein to the submaxillary nodes. A lateral group drains to the deep parotid lymph nodes.

Pathology

The conventional classification of RMS includes four histologic subtypes: embryonal, alveolar, botryoid, and pleomorphic. *Embryonal:* this type is characterized by long, spindle-shaped cells with acidophilic cytoplasm. The cell may assume

226

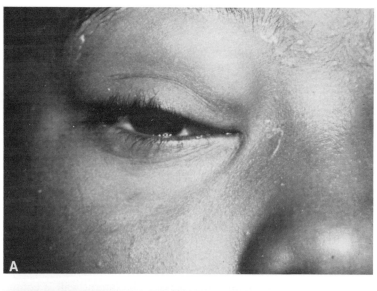

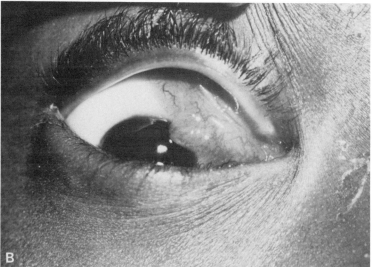

Figure 1. (A) A 10-year-old black female with RMS of the orbit presenting in the lid and causing ptosis. (B) The lesion involves the conjunctiva.

a racquet shape or may be small and round; neither cross-striations nor mitoses are frequent. *Alveolar:* the cellular distribution in this type is determined by connective tissue trabeculae which result in septal divisions of tumor resembling lung alveoli. The rhabdomyoblasts are usually small and round, but may be multinucleated with both cross and longitudinal striations. *Botryoid:* this type is typically seen in genitourinary sites but does occur in the head and neck. Grossly, it has a characteristic polypoid ('grape cluster') appearance. Centrally, the tissue

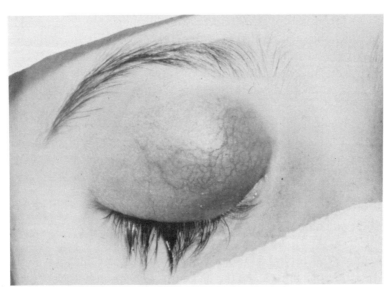

Figure 2. Rhabdomyosarcoma arising in the right upper lid of a 9-year-old white female and causing marked edema and erythema.

is myxomatous with few cells. Peripherally and just beneath the mucosal surface is a layer of rhabdomyoblasts with a typical small, round cell character and relatively frequent mitotic figures. The absence of the loose, myxomatous stroma in metastases suggests that the botryoid subtype is a morphological variant of embryonal RMS. *Pleomorphic:* typically found in adults, this subtype features large rhabdomyoblasts that can have a strap shape with multiple nuclei in tandem, a simple round shape with an eccentric nucleus, or a racquet shape with a tapering cytoplasmic body [4, 5, 17].

In the second Intergroup RMS Study (IRS II), 51% of all patients were embryonal in histology and 19% were alveolar. The remaining patients were other types (24%) or unknown (6%). For patients with orbital RMS, only 6% were alveolar. Although historically this subtype has carried a worse prognosis, this has not been true in the IRS I and II trials for orbit RMS patients.

A new cytologic classification of RMS which defines a subset of patients with unfavorable prognosis histology (UH) has been proposed by the IRS pathology subcommittee [18]. However, the few IRS I and II orbit patients (8%) with one of these subtypes were without relapse.

Clinical manifestations

The differential diagnosis of proptosis in a child is extensive. It includes developmental, inflammatory, metabolic, neoplastic, osseous, and vascular disorders, and orbital hemorrhage of various causes, including trauma. Iliff and Green summarized four series of 358 children with histologically documented orbital lesions to which they contributed 174 cases [19]. The most frequent diagnosis was dermoid cyst (37%) followed by hemangioma (12%) and RMS (9%).

Rapid progression of unilateral proptosis in a child is the initial and major presenting symptom of orbital RMS (Figure 1). Jones *et al.* describe ptosis in 33% and a palpable nodular subconjunctival or lid mass in 25% [5] (Figure 2). Lid and conjunctival edema and redness of the eye are less often seen [4, 20]. Tearing is uncommon (10%), but may occur early [5]. Vision loss and papilledema are similarly uncommon [3]. The average duration of symptoms before diagnosis is 6 weeks [3].

Diagnostic evaluation

The infrequency of orbital RMS must not dissuade the clinician from having a high index of suspicion to make the diagnosis. Nicholson and Green emphasize the obligation of the examining ophthalmologist:

'The history or observation of rapid increase in observable tumor size or degree of proptosis advances rhabdomyosarcoma to the top of any list of differential diagnoses and demands immediate histologic confirmation or exclusion of this possibility' [21].

Histologic diagnosis requires only a biopsy and not tumor excision or debulking. Excision does not contribute to improved prognosis nor does it permit reduction of radiation portal size. The surgical approach for tumor biopsy is determined by the position of the mass and the direction of eye displacement. The several biopsy approaches are described by Harley [22].

The physical examination must include height and weight. Computed tomography is the preferred imaging technique [23] and may be superior to magnetic resonance imaging [24]. Plain X-rays may disclose bone destruction but seldom demonstrate a mass. Tomographically, orbital tumors are described as within or outside the cone formed by the six extraocular muscles (*intraconal* or *extraconal*), or anterior to the fibrous septum of the orbit rim (*preseptal*). In one series, RMS was extraconal in four patients and also involved the preseptal space in two [23] (Figure 3). Extension to adjacent structures such as the medial air sinuses and the cavernous sinus is uncommon but should be carefully sought. Other radiographic studies include chest X-ray and bone scan. Necessary laboratory studies are complete blood count, urinalysis, creatinine, hepatic enzymes, bilirubin, uric acid, calcium, phosphorus, and alkaline phosphatase. Baseline bone marrow aspiration or biopsy is needed. Cerebrospinal fluid chemistry and cytology is essential if the primary tumor has extended to or near to the meninges. The toxicity associated with particular chemotherapeutic agents requires appropriate baseline studies: for adriamycin, radionuclide angiography or echocardiography; for cisplatin, serum magnesium and audiologic exam.

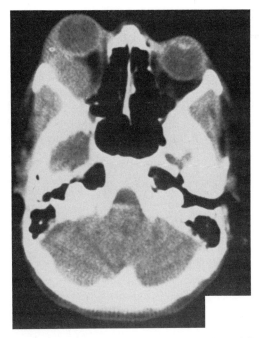

Figure 3. A right orbital RMS imaged by computerized tomography and demonstrating significant proptosis.

The most widely accepted staging system for RMS is the IRS surgical-pathological clinical grouping classification. The group is used to determine therapy and to report and compare treatment outcome.

The IRS clinical groups are:

– *Group I:* Localized disease, completely resected (regional nodes not involved). (a) Confined to muscle or organ of origin. (b) Contiguous involvement – infiltration outside the muscle or organ of origin, as through fascial planes. This includes both gross inspection and microscopic confirmation of complete resection. Any nodes that may be inadvertently taken with the specimen must be negative. If the latter should be involved microscopically, then the patient is placed in group IIb or c (see below).

– *Group II:* (a) Grossly resected tumor with microscopic residual disease (surgeon believes that he has removed all of the tumor, but the pathologist finds tumor at the margin of resection). No evidence of gross residual tumor. No evidence of regional node involvement. Once radiotherapy and/or chemotherapy have been started, reexploration and removal of the area of microscopic residual does not change the patient's group. (b) Regional disease, completely resected. Regional nodes involved and/or extension of tumor into an adjacent organ. All tumor completely resected with no microscopic residual. Complete resection with microscopic confirmation of no residual disease makes this different from groups IIa and IIc. Additionally, in contrast to group IIa, regional nodes (which are completely resected, however) may be involved. (c) Regional disease with involved nodes, grossly resected, but with evidence of microscopic residual. The presence of microscopic residual disease makes this group different from group IIb, and nodal involvement makes this group different from group IIa.

- *Group III:* Incomplete resection or biopsy with gross residual disease.
- *Group IV:* Distant metastatic disease present at onset (e.g., lung, liver, bones, bone marrow, brain, distant muscle, and nodes). This excludes *regional* nodes and adjacent organ infiltration which places the patient in a more favorable grouping (as noted above under group II).

With modern management of orbital RMS, extensive surgery that would render a patient group I or group II is not needed. Distant metastatic tumor at presentation is rare. In the IRS series of 132 patients, only three patients (2.3%) were in group IV. Thus, virtually all patients would be in group III.

Population characteristics

The first IRS protocol began accruing patients in November 1972, and the second in November 1978. Through June 1983, 132 patients with orbital RMS were entered and had confirmation of histologic diagnosis by a pathology review panel. The upper age limit for registration was 20 years. The treatment results (described on pages 15–18) are restricted to those patients without distant metastases (three eliminated) and to those not lost to follow-up in the first month (two eliminated) leaving a population of 127 patients treated primarily at medical institutions throughout the United States but including some from the United Kingdom and Canada. The mean age of the group is 7 years (median 6 years). In the review of 161 patients by Knowles, the mean age was 7.8 years, but five patients over age 20 were included. The same review gave a ratio of male to female patients of 1.7: 1 [17]. In contrast, the IRS series was males, 60, to females, 67 (0.9: 1).

The rarity of orbital RMS occurring in non-Caucasians was attributed to socioeconomic factors by Knowles [17]. In the IRS, 16% were non-Caucasian children.

Treatment methods

Surgery

The essential role of the surgeon in obtaining tissue to establish histologic diagnosis is noted in the section on Diagnostic evaluation. A potentially curative procedure, orbital exenteration, is frequently followed by local recurrence and therefore has not been practiced since the 1960s [25]. It remains, however, the only method to treat the occasional patient with locally persistent or recurrent disease. It involves removal of all the orbital contents including periosteum and, if required, portions of the bony walls and sinuses [22].

Radiation therapy

The 1968 report by Cassady *et al.*, that biopsy followed by high dose megavoltage radiation controlled orbital RMS in five of five patients established that radiation was the primary modality for local control and that a tumor dose of approximately 5000 rad in 5 weeks was required [8]. Their technique consisted of a direct anterior portal employing either 22.5 MeV photons or ^{60}Co teletherapy equipment. When required, supplemental treatment was given laterally to augment dose to the posterior orbit to ensure homogeneity. A subsequent publication from the same institution described a similar technique and a tumor dose of 5800 rad in 29 fractions (200 rad/day, 5 days/week) [9].

In the first IRS protocol, the recommended radiation dose to the primary tumor site was 5000 to 6000 rad using conventional fractionation. It was restricted to 4000 rad for children less than age 5. Patients in clinical group I were randomized to receive or not receive radiotherapy. Analysis of the study indicated that radiotherapy was not needed for group I patients. For patients in groups II and III, tumor doses less than 4000 rad were retrospectively compared to doses of 4001 to 5000 rad and greater than 5000 rad. Although the local recurrence rate was highest with the lowest dose range, the differences were not of statistical significance. At the lowest dose category, the local recurrence rate increased for children age 6 and older (again not statistically significant) [26]. These findings and, in addition, the observation of an adverse impact on survival due to tumors greater than 5 cm diameter in group III patients, led to revised radiotherapy doses in IRS II. Radiotherapy was omitted for group I patients. The dose for group II was 4000 to 4500 rad. For group III (and primary site treatment of group IV patients), the dose depended on age at diagnosis and post-surgery (pre-chemotherapy) tumor size (Table 1).

Table 1. Primary site total tumor dose for clinical groups III and IV patients treated in accordance with the IRS II protocol

Age	Tumor size	
	< 5 cm	⩾ 5 cm
< 6 years	4000–4500 rad	4500–5000 rad
⩾ 6 years	4500–5000 rad	5000–5500 rad

The daily dose was 180–200 rad/day, five fractions/week.

Local and local plus regional recurrence rates were tabulated for the first 640 IRS II patients evaluated in groups II, III and IV. The overall local and local plus regional recurrence rates were 12% and 18%, respectively. Though the local recurrence rate was higher (15%) in patients receiving less than 4000 rad, there was no statistical evidence that it differed according to radiotherapy dosage (p > 0.3). It also did not differ within clinical groups, or by tumor size (greater or less than 5 cm). There was moderately strong evidence that local recurrence rates differed significantly by age group (p < 0.02), the highest local recurrence rate being 28% in patients under age 1 year. Within each age group, however, there was no significant variation by radiation dose. For the category of patients under age one year, those that got less than 4000 rad (median 2000 rad) had a local recurrence rate of 50%. It was 20% in the remainder of the under 1 year olds who got more than 4000 rad [27]. However, all these infants also received lower doses of chemotherapy than children over a year of age.

Among the IRS group I and II patients with orbital RMS, the local plus regional recurrence rate did not differ significantly whether the tumor dose was less than or greater than 4500 rad. In fact, the only relapses in the lower dose group were in patients getting 3000 rad or less. The lowest doses at which control was achieved were 3600 to 3900 rad.

Additional analysis of all IRS I and II group I patients not getting radiotherapy revealed that local plus regional recurrence was significantly higher in unfavorable histology patients compared to favorable histology patients (p < 0.001) [28].

These various observations have led the IRS committee to establish specific tumor doses in the study (IRS III) which began entering patients November 1984. All radiation treatments to primary tumors are to be administered at 180 rad/day, 5 days/week. For group I (unfavorable histology patients only) and group II patients, the tumor dose is 4140 rad. The total doses for clinical groups III and IV (primary site) are listed in Table 2. Doses vary according to age and pre-chemotherapy size but not histology. Orbital RMS will rarely exceed 5 cm diameter so that the tumor dose will be 4140 rad for about one-half of patients and will be 4500 rad for most of the remainder.

Table 2. Primary site total tumor dose for clinical groups III and IV patients treated in accordance with the IRS III protocol

Age	Tumor size	
	< 5 cm	≥ 5 cm
< 6 years	4140 rad	4500 rad
≥ 6 years	4500 rad	5040 rad

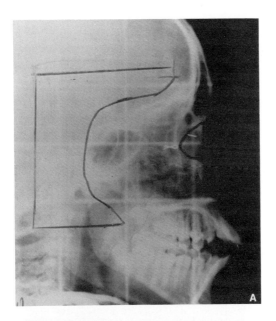

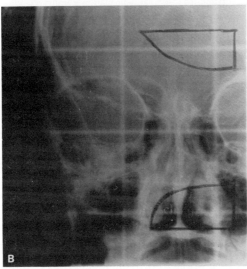

Figure 4. (A) A right lateral radiation therapy simulator X-ray indicating the generous margins employed in encompassing the orbit as part of a wedged-field, two-port plan. The dark, crayoned lines posteriorly indicate the position of a shield to protect portions of the frontal lobe, brain stem and temporal lobe. Anteriorly, the shield lines denote protection of the lens. (B) The companion anterior simulator film shows that the medial border extends to the opposite bony canthus.

Proper radiation technique requires that the child be immobilized with a method that is reproducible on a daily basis. A custom prepared plaster-of-Paris cast is ideal [29]. The child must be supine with the neck slightly extended so that

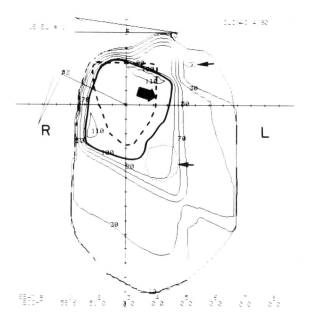

Figure 5. A computerized radiation isodose treatment plan in a transverse plane through the orbits. The limits of the right orbit are denoted by the dotted line (large arrow) and the contralateral lens and sella turcica by small arrows. The 100% isodose line (dark, solid line) encompasses the orbit. 'R' and 'L' indicate 'right' and 'left'.

the eye at rest looks vertically. If under age 3 years, sedation will probably be required [29, 30]. An occasional 2-year-old child may require Ketamine anesthesia [31].

Treatment planning should be done with the patient in the immobilization cast to be used during actual treatment. The six borders of the treatment volume are defined at the time of simulation [32] (Figure 4). They will generally be 2 cm beyond the bony borders of the orbit but this will vary with the size of the tumor, extent of invasion, patient age, and machine characteristics. Superiorly, the port must be above the orbital roof which is slightly above the superior orbital rim. Inferiorly, it is below the orbital floor and includes the infraorbital foramen. Laterally, it includes the ascending zygomatic bone. Medially, it extends to the opposite medial canthus in order to provide a generous margin beyond the thin bones of the ethmoid sinuses. Posteriorly, the portal must be behind the orbital fissure. The anterior border will be anterior to the tumor mass. When a lateral treatment portal is used, it must be angled posteriorly to avoid radiation to the contralateral lens. The use of megavoltage treatment equipment (^{60}Co to 6 MeV) is mandatory. This will minimize photoelectric absorption of radiation dose in bone and afford a skin-sparing effect which will reduce corneal and conjunctival dose from an anterior port. The lids of the treated eye should be held open to eliminate the bolus effect they would have so as to preserve maximal dosage sparing of the cornea.

Computerized treatment planning should be performed to determine the best method to achieve homogeneous coverage of the treatment volume. In small children, a single, direct anterior port may suffice, but in general a wedged-pair technique employing a lateral port in addition to an anterior port will ensure full tumor dose posteriorly (Figure 5). At the time of first treatment, and at least weekly thereafter, portal verification X-rays should be taken by the treating technologist and compared to the simulation films by the radiation oncologist. The physician must also personally assess the patient in the treatment position and the technical set-up periodically. He should also re-examine the patient once a week. The tumor may regress rapidly during radiotherapy necessitating revision of the technical set-up parameters.

Chemotherapy

The landmark study of Heyn *et al.* demonstrated that chemotherapy eradicated occult, metastatic RMS [12]. Orbital RMS probably has a lower rate of occult disseminated tumor than most other sites based on the finding of Abramson *et al.* that, with radiation alone, 70% of children receiving radiotherapy were 5-year survivors [10]. Since all tumor deaths occurred within 3 years, the survivors are presumed to have been disease-free. This finding would imply that as many as 30% of similar patients would harbor occult metastases at diagnosis. When these patients received adjuvant chemotherapy, they had a better 3-year survival rate if their primary disease was limited to the orbit (without sinus invasion). Although the trial was not randomized, and the relapse sites by treatment group were not specified, one may safely assume that the chemotherapy played a role in reducing local or distant treatment failure or both.

Abramson *et al.* began vincristine and cyclophosphamide on the day of diagnosis and radiotherapy within 24 h. Actinomycin D was begun after radiation (week 18) and continued for 9 months. Vincristine was stopped after 12 weeks and cyclophosphamide after 2 years [10].

In both IRS I and IRS II, patients were randomized by clinical group and not by primary site. For that reason, children with RMS of the orbit could have received one of five regimens in the first study or one of six regimens in the second study. The specific drugs, doses, and schedules are described for IRS I in reference 33 and IRS II in reference 34.

The majority of the orbital RMS patients were in group III. In IRS I, radiotherapy began 6 weeks after the first day of chemotherapy. The group III chemotherapy was either 'pulse' VAC:
- vincristine, $2\,mg/m^2$ i.v. weekly × 12 (top dose 2 mg);
- actinomycin D, $0.015\,mg/kg/day$ i.v. × 5 (top dose 0.5 mg); course repeated
  × 4 in 54 weeks;

- cyclophosphamide, 10 mg/kg/day i.v. days 1–5; course repeated orally days 84–90, then 2.5 mg/kg/day p.o. from day 140 to 24 months;

or, 'pulse' VAC as above plus:

- adriamycin, 60 mg/m^2 i.v. (single dose) at weeks 5, 18, 27, 39, and 51.

In IRS II, group III patients received either repetitive 'pulse' VAC courses:

- vincristine, 2 mg/m^2 i.v. weekly × 12 (top dose 2 mg);
- actinomycin D, 0.015 mg/kg/day i.v. × 5 (top dose 0.5 mg);
- cyclophosphamide, 10 mg/kg/day i.v. × 3;
- cyclophosphamide, 20 mg/kg i.v. days 21, 42 and 63.

Beginning week 12 and every 4 weeks to 24 months:

- vincristine, 2 mg/m^2 i.v. days 0 and 4 (top dose 2 mg);
- actinomycin D, 0.015 mg/kg/day i.v. × 5 (top dose 0.5 mg);
- cyclophosphamide, 10 mg/kg/day i.v. × 3;

or they received repetitive 'pulse' VADRC courses substituting adriamycin for actinomycin D (above) in alternate courses for the first year of treatment. The adriamycin dose is 30 mg/m^2 i.v. on days 0 and 1, then 21 and 22 initially, and then on days 0 and 1 of each VADRC course.

In both IRS I and II, and subsequently in IRS III (*vide infra*), drug dosages are reduced by 50% in children under a year of age to reduce toxicity. If tolerated, dosages are increased to 75% and then 100% of recommended amounts.

In each schedule, radiotherapy would begin at week 6.

Even more intensive chemotherapeutic regimens were devised for IRS III, group III patients; however, recognizing the success attained for patients with orbital primary (see 'Treatment results') and selected other head and neck sites [35], these patients were exempted from the randomization for other group III patients if the tumor was favorable histologically. Instead, they receive:

- actinomycin D, 0.015 mg/kg/day i.v. × 5 (top dose 0.5 mg), initially, then every 9 weeks × 5 courses;
- vincristine, 2 mg/m^2 i.v. (top dose 2 mg) weekly × 6 beginning each 6-week course on days 21, 84, 147, 210, 273 and 336.

Radiotherapy begins on day 14. In the initial 14 days of treatment, determination of histology (favorable or unfavorable) is made. Orbit RMS patients with unfavorable histology would be randomized to one of three regimens each featuring a 'backbone' of vincristine, actinomycin D, and cyclophosphamide to which is added (in the second regimen) cisplatin, and (in the third) cisplatin and VP-16.

All the drug regimens described and, in particular, the ones for patients with unfavorable histology, carry a risk of lethal toxicity and must therefore be administered only by pediatric oncologists. The treatment concepts of IRS III are investigational and should not be employed for non-study patients until the results are known to be better than those achieved in IRS I and II.

Treatment results

The patients entered on IRS I and II with orbital RMS each met three eligibility requirements: age less than 21; no prior chemotherapy or radiotherapy; and submission of their histologic material to an expert panel of referee pathologists who confirmed the diagnosis. The resulting group of 132 children and adolescents constitute the largest series of patients with orbital RMS reported.

Study population

As noted above (Population characteristics), five patients were excluded from the analysis of results. Three had distant metastases at diagnosis, and two were withdrawn from the study in the first month and were lost to follow-up. The remaining 127 patients had been randomized to particular treatment regimens based on their clinico-pathologic group. Actual treatment administered, however, may have differed substantially in some cases from the written requirements due to either patient or physician non-compliance. For purposes of this analysis, however, no additional patients were excluded even though their treatment may have been inadequate by protocol requirements.

Of the 127 patients, 87% were Caucasian, 47% were male, and 53% were female. The mean age was 7 years, the median age was 6 years, and 90% were age 12 or less. Seven patients had unfavorable histology (alveolar) by conventional classification, and ten different patients had unfavorable histology by the proposed cytologic classification [18]. Clinical group distribution was: I, 6%; II, 24%; and III, 70%. Median follow-up was 5 years (range 1 week to 11 years).

Only seven patients had exenteration at diagnosis. One hundred twenty-two patients received radiotherapy, with a dose range from 3000 to 6400 rad. About one-half of patients received a dose from 4500 to 5500 rad. All patients received at least one chemotherapy course.

Results

Of the seven children who had orbital exenteration at diagnosis, two were rendered clinical group I (no gross or microscopic residual tumor), and both were randomized to receive local radiotherapy on IRS I [33]. Neither relapsed. The remaining five patients were clinical group II and therefore received radiation. One relapsed locally. Thus no child avoided radiotherapy because of exenteration.

Five patients were group I as a result of surgery that spared the eye. Three who were randomized to receive radiation are disease-free. Of the two not given radiation, one relapsed locally. Another local relapse occurred among the 26 group II patients who had an eye-sparing operation.

LOCALIZED ORBITAL RHABDOMYOSARCOMA
DISEASE-FREE SURVIVAL

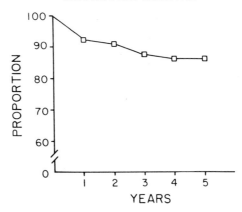

Figure 6. Actuarial plot of disease-free survival of 127 children with orbital RMS. At 5 years, the proportion alive and continuously disease-free is 88%.

Eighty-nine patients were in group III. Of the total of only ten relapses (8%) in the entire study, seven were in this group. The relapse risk was not influenced by clinical group. The actuarial (Kaplan-Meier estimate) 5-year relapse-free survival rate is 88% (Figure 6). The 13 patients who comprise the 'not disease-free' group include three who died without evidence of disease (sepsis, two; second malignancy, one). Another four who relapsed in the orbit had successful salvage therapy (exenteration in three; radiotherapy in one) and remained disease-free an additional 4 to 32 months. The remaining six patients died of disease. Their site of initial relapse was orbit in three and regional nodes in three. One of the three orbital relapses and two of the three nodal relapses occurred in children less than age 12 months. Not one child had an initial relapse in the form of distant metastasis.

Local-regional control was achieved initially or by salvage therapy in 121 patients (95%). The efficacy of radiotherapy and chemotherapy in achieving local control is best assessed in group III patients (biopsy only). Of 87 such patients, five had relapse in the orbit, for a local control rate of 94% which increased to 98% after salvage surgery.

All relapses occurred by 4 years. None were in the 17 patients who had unfavorable histology by either classification system. Nine of the ten relapses were seen in girls (p <0.001). There is no explanation for this observation, although a similar disparity in relapse risk by gender was found for RMS patients with primary tumors in other head and neck sites except for those in the high risk parameningeal sites [35]. Three of ten relapses were among the five children 12 months or younger at diagnosis (p <0.01).

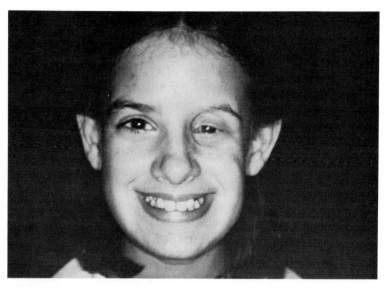

Figure 7. Five years after radiotherapy (5600 rad) and chemotherapy in accordance with IRS protocol I, this 14-year-old white female exhibits the sequelae of enophthalmos, ptosis, and partial eyebrow and eyelash epilation.

Treatment morbidity and complications

Treatment morbidity may be classified according to location (local, systemic); etiology (surgery, radiation, chemotherapy); and time (acute, chronic). Systemic toxicity related primarily to chemotherapy is beyond the scope of this chapter. The reader is referred to standard texts [29, 36]. Of the 127 IRS patients with orbital RMS, two died of sepsis while on therapy. Two others subsequently developed acute myelogenous leukemia of whom one died.

In the absence of radiation, systemic chemotherapy can produce ocular morbidity [37]. Changes including blurred vision, conjunctivitis, photophobia, eye pain, and diplopia have been described [38]. These are unlikely to be distinguished in the child also receiving orbital radiotherapy; however, chemotherapy of the types used for RMS may enhance the ocular side effects of radiation [39, 40].

Acute toxicities of orbital radiation include keratitis, conjunctivitis, tearing, and photophobia [17]. Erythema and dermatitis occur and are potentiated by actinomycin D. Chronic changes may include conjunctival neovascularization, corneal ulceration, xerophthalmia, and vaso-obliterative retinopathy [17, 25]. All patients develop cataracts 1 to 3 years post treatment which are amenable to surgery if required. In younger children, impaired growth of facial and orbital bones occurs with a resulting cosmetic deformity. This varies with age at treatment and radiation dose.

At worst, corneal, retinal, and lacrimal gland changes may leave a painful eye without useful vision. Enucleation may be necessary, as it was for one-third of the 58 patients in the series reported by Abramson *et al.* [10].

Heyn *et al.* have tabulated the late effects of therapy in 50 IRS I orbital RMS patients. Patients experienced infections, structural, and functional problems. Chronic infections were most frequent following exenteration, but in a patient who had less extensive surgery, cellulitis developed and necessitated enucleation. Numerous structural defects occurred, the most common being cataracts in 90%. Bony hypoplasia was seen in half the patients with most having consequent facial asymmetry. Less frequent changes were seen in the cornea, and ten children had enophthalmos (Figure 7). Seven had lacrimal duct stenosis. Vision loss (complete or partial) occurred in 90% of the patients evaluated and correlated closely with the presence of cataracts. Eight children had cataract surgery and improvement was observed in those patients in whom postoperative vision testing was reported. Secondary enucleation was performed in four of 44 children. Twenty-seven of the 44 children (61%) had reduction in growth velocity sufficient to reduce their expected height by more than 20 percentile levels. In 12 of the patients, the decrement exceeded 40 percentile levels [41]. This complication follows the impairment of growth hormone production that is a known consequence of incidental pituitary radiation [42]. Its recognition is imperative, since it is reversible with the administration of growth hormone [42].

Summary

Prior to the 1960s, the child with orbital RMS would inevitably face surgery entailing sacrifice of the eye with only a modest prospect for local tumor control or survival. The fundamental concept of radiation dose response was tested and affirmed by Drs. Cassady, Sagerman, Tretter, and Ellsworth [8]. They established that orbital RMS had a high rate of local control with carefully planned megavoltage radiotherapy and that the affected eye could continue to function. Heyn and her colleagues in the Children's Cancer Study Group employed the concept of combination chemotherapy and demonstrated in an early, prospectively randomized trial that adjuvant chemotherapy was an essential component to the multimodality treatment of RMS [12]. With the advent of the single disease clinical cooperative group (IRS) in 1972, it became immediately possible to extend the modern management of RMS nationwide and to begin refining, and eventually reducing, the treatment for RMS of the orbit. The improvement in survival achieved by the first and second IRS protocols for orbital RMS is virtually without precedent in modern oncology. The management outlined in 'Treatment methods' constitutes the current standard of care. Reduction of morbidity and late effects, and improvement in vision remain crucial, but attainable goals.

Acknowledgements

This work was supported in part by U.S. Public Health Service Grants CA-24507, CA-30138, CA-30969, CA-29139, and CA-13539.

The membership of the Intergroup Rhabdomyosarcoma Study Committee is gratefully acknowledged: Mohan Beltangady, William Crist, Edmund Gehan, Denman Hammond, Daniel Hays, Ruth Heyn, Walter Lawrence, Jr., Pat Morris-Jones, William Newton, Nigel Palmer, Abdel Ragab, Beverly Raney, Jr., Fred Ruymann, Melvin Tefft, and Bruce Webber.

The secretarial assistance of Yvonne Greene and Bert Fields is gratefully acknowledged.

References

1. Calhoun, F.P., Reese, A.B. 1942. Rhabdomyosarcoma of the orbit. Arch. Ophthalmol. (Chicago) 27: 558–578.
2. Blaxter, P.L., Smith, J.L. 1958. Rhabdomyosarcoma of the orbit. Report of two cases. Trans. Ophthalmol. Soc. U.K. 78: 83–97.
3. Frayer, W.C., Enterline, H.T. 1959. Embryonal rhabdomyosarcoma of the orbit in children and young adults. Arch. Ophthalmol. (Chicago) 62: 203–210.
4. Porterfield, J.F., Zimmerman, L.E. 1962. Rhabdomyosarcoma of the orbit. Virchows Arch. Path. Anat. 335: 329–344.
5. Jones, I.S., Reese, A.B., Krout, J. 1965. Orbital Rhabdomy osarcoma: an analysis of sixty-two cases. Trans. Am. Ophthalmol. Soc. 63: 223–255.
6. Ashton, N., Morgan, G. 1965. Embryonal sarcoma and embryonal rhabdomyosarcoma of the orbit. J. Clin. Pathol. 18: 699–714.
7. Lederman, M. 1956. Radiotherapy in the treatment of orbital tumours. Br. J. Ophthalmol. 40: 592–610.
8. Cassady, J.R., Sagerman, R.H., Tretter, P., Ellsworth, R.M. 1968. Radiation therapy for rhabdomyosarcoma. Radiology 91: 116–120.
9. Sagerman, R.H., Tretter, P., Ellsworth, R.M. 1972. The treatment of orbital rhabdomyosarcoma of children with primary radiation therapy. Am. J. Roent, Nucl. Med. Radiat. Ther. 114: 31–34.
10. Abramson, D.H., Ellsworth, R.M., Tretter, P. et al. 1979. The treatment of orbital rhabdomyo-sarcoma with irradiation and chemotherapy. Ophthalmology 86: 1330–1335.
11. Pinkel, D., Pickren, J. 1961. Rhabdomyosarcoma in children. J.A.M.A. 175(4): 293–298.
12. Heyn, R.M., Holland, R., Newton, W.A. et al. 1974. The role of combined chemotherapy in the treatment of rhabdomyosarcoma in children. Cancer 34: 2128–2142.
13. Young, J.L., Miller, R.W. 1975. Incidence of malignant tumors in U.S. children. J. Pediatr. 86(2): 254–258.
14. Ghafoor, S.Y.A., Dudgeon, J. 1985. Orbital rhabdomyosarcoma: improved survival with combined pulsed chemotherapy and irradiation. Br. J. Ophthalmol. 69: 557–561.
15. Grufferman, S., Wang, H.H., DeLong, E.R. et al. 1982. Environmental factors in the etiology of rhabdomyosarcoma in childhood. J.N.C.I. 68: 107–113.
16. Schuster, S.A.D., Ferguson, E.D., Marshall, R.B. 1972. Alveolar rhabdomyosarcoma of the eyelid. Diagnosis by electron microscopy. Arch. Ophthalmol. 87: 646–651.
17. Knowles, D.M., Jakobiec, F.A., Potter, G.D., Jones, I.S. 1978. The diagnosis and treatment of rhabdomyosarcoma of the orbit. In: Ocular and Adnexal Tumors (F.A. Jakobiec, ed.). Aesculapius Publishing Company, Birmingham, pp. 708–734.

18. Palmer, N.F., Foulkes, M.A., Sachs, N., Newton, W.A. 1986. Rhabdomyosarcoma: a cytologic classification of prognostic significance. A report of the Intergroup Rhabdomyosarcoma Studies I and II (1972–1983). Cancer (in press).

19. Iliff, W.J., Green, W.R. 1978. Orbital tumors in children, In: Ocular and Adnexal Tumors. (F.A. Jakobiec, ed.). Aesculapius Publishing Company, Birmingham, pp. 669–684.

20. Adhikary, H.P., Fitzmaurice, D.J. 1982. Presentation of orbital rhabdomyosarcoma. Clin. Oncol. 8: 21–23.

21. Nicholson, D.H., Green, W.R. 1983. Tumors of the eye, lids, and orbit in children, In: Pediatric Ophthalmology (second edition) (R.D. Harley, ed.). W.B. Saunders Company, Philadelphia, pp. 1223–1271.

22. Harley, R.D. 1983. Diseases of the orbit. In: Pediatric Ophthalmology (second edition) (R.D. Harley, ed.). W.B. Saunders Company, Philadelphia, pp. 349–388.

23. Lallemand, D.P., Brasch, R.C., Char, D.H., Norman, D. 1984. Orbital tumors in children. Characterization by computed tomography. Radiology 151: 85–88.

24. Sobel, D.F., Kelly, W., Kjos, B.O. et al. 1985. MR imaging of orbital and ocular disease. A.J.N.R. 6: 259–264.

25. Tretter, P. 1976. Radiotherapy of ocular and orbital tumors. In: Tumors of the Eye (third edition) (A.B. Reese, ed.). Harper and Row, Hagerstown, pp. 373–386.

26. Tefft, M., Lindberg, R.D., Gehan, E.A. 1981. Radiation therapy combined with systemic chemotherapy of rhabdomyosarcoma in children: local control in patients enrolled in the Intergroup Rhabdomyosarcoma Study. Natl. Cancer Inst. Monogr. 56: 75–81.

27. Tefft, M., Wharam, M., Gehan, E. 1986. Radiation therapy in embryonal rhabdomyosarcoma: local control in children less than one year of age and in children with tumors of the orbit. (Abstr.) Proc. Am. Soc. Clin. Oncol. 5: 205.

28. Tefft, M., Wharam, M., Ruymann, F., Foulkes, M., Gehan, E. 1984. Radiotherapy for rhabdomyosarcoma in children: a report from the Intergroup Rhabdomyosarcoma Study #2 (Abstr.). Int. J. Radiat. Oncol. Biol. Phys. 10 (Suppl. 2): 86.

29. Wharam, M.D. 1983. Radiation therapy. In: Malignant Diseases of Infancy, Childhood and Adolescence (second edition) (A.J. Altman, A.D. Schwartz, ed.). W.B. Saunders Company, Philadelphia, pp. 96–110.

30. Bilenki, M.E., Ziegfeld, C. 1986. Managing sedation in the pediatric radiation patient (Abstr.). Oncology Nursing Forum Supplement 13 (2): 99.

31. Cronin, M.M., Bousfield, J.D., Hewett, E.B. et al. 1972. Ketamine anaesthesia for radiotherapy in small children, Anaesthesia 27(2): 135–142.

32. Wharam, M.D., Order, S.E. 1980. Treatment planning in radiation therapy: maximization by CT. Appl. Radiol. May-June: 50–56.

33. Maurer, H.M., Moon, T., Donaldson, M. et al. 1977. The Intergroup Rhabdomyosarcoma Study. A preliminary report. Cancer 40: 2015–2026.

34. Maurer, H.M. 1980. The Intergroup Rhabdomyosarcoma Study II: objectives and study design. J. Pediatr. Surg. 15: 371–372.

35. Wharam, M.D., Foulkes, M.A., Lawrence, W. et al. 1984. Soft tissue sarcoma of the head and neck in childhood: nonorbital and nonparameningeal sites. A report of the Intergroup Rhabdomyosarcoma Study (IRS)-1. Cancer 53: 1016–1019.

36. Jaffe, N. 1984. Late sequelae of cancer therapy. In: Clinical Pediatric Oncology (third edition) (W.W. Sutow, D.J. Fernbach, T.J. Vietti, ed.). The C.V. Mosby Company, St. Louis, pp. 810–832.

37. Griffin, J.D., Garnick, M.B. 1981. Eye toxicity of cancer chemotherapy: a review of the literature. Cancer 48: 1539–1549.

38. Vizel, M., Oster, M.W. 1982. Ocular side effects of cancer chemotherapy. Cancer 49: 1999–2002.

39. Chan, R.C. and Shukovsky, L.J. 1976. Effects of irradiation on the eye. Radiology 120: 673–675.

40. Parsons, J.T., Fitzgerald, C.R., Hood, C.I. *et al.* 1983. The effects of irradiation on the eye and optic nerve. Int. J. Radiat. Oncol. Biol. Phys. 9: 609–622.
41. Heyn, R., Ragab, A., Raney, R.B. *et al.* 1986. Late effects of therapy in orbital rhabdomyosarcoma in children: a report from the Intergroup Rhabdomyosarcoma Study (IRS). Cancer 57: 1738–1743.
42. Wara, W.M., Richards, G.E., Grumbach, M.M. *et al.* 1977. Hypopituitarism after irradiation in children. Int. J. Radiat. Oncol. Biol. Phys. 2: 549–552.

15. Current management of cutaneous melanomas of the head and neck

SAMUEL R. FISHER, CAMERON A. GILLESPIE, HILLIARD F. SEIGLER and IAN R. CROCKER

Epidemiology and etiology of cutaneous melanomas of the head and neck

Cutaneous melanoma is a malignant neoplasm arising from melanocytes, which are the melanosome-containing cells that synthesize and transport melanin pigment. Whereas Carswell [1] is credited with the first modern clinical description of a malignant melanocyte neoplasm and suggested the term melanoma in 1834, Pemberton [2] in 1855 wrote one of the first reports of such a lesion originating in the head and neck region.

Each year four of every 100,000 people will develop a malignant melanoma, accounting for approximately 1% of all the cancers recorded in the United States, with approximately the same percentage of cancer deaths. Representing only 3% of all cutaneous neoplasms, its malignant potential can readily be appreciated when one considers that it is responsible for 65% of all skin cancer deaths [3, 4].

The global incidence of melanoma appears to be doubling every 10 to 17 years, evidenced by a rapid increase in the incidence of melanoma in Caucasians in Southern Arizona, quadrupling between 1969 and 1978 [5]. Increased awareness, more complete reporting, and alterations in diagnostic criteria do not appear to have caused an artifactual increase in the reported incidence, which is confirmed by the concomitant, commensurate increase in melanoma mortality [6].

Melanoma affects men and women with equal frequency; however, there are striking differences in distribution of the primary lesion by skin sites. There are a larger number of lower extremity lesions in women and a proponderance of truncal lesions in men [7]. Melanomas occurring on the head and neck account for 15–30% of all melanomas, and in the Duke University Medical Center review of 399 cases of head and neck melanomas, the ratio of males to females for this anatomic site was 1.8 to 1 [8]. The greatest percentage of cases occurred during the sixth and seventh decades of life for both males and females. The average age of the males was 52.4 years at the time of diagnosis, and the average age of the females was 54.6 years.

In this series only 0.75% of cases were in non-Causasians, demonstrating the

C. Jacobs (ed) Cancers of the head and neck.
© 1987, Martinus Nijhoff Publishers, Boston. ISBN 0–89838–825–2. Printed in the Netherlands.

protective role of skin pigmentation [8–10]. When non-Caucasians develop melanoma, they do so in less deeply pigmented parts of the body, and in the head and neck region, specifically in the oral mucosa [10]. The etiology of the disease in non-Caucasians is presumably different from that in Caucasians. Although conclusive proof is lacking, by epidemiologic observation, solar exposure is strongly implicated as the most significant etiologic factor. Lancaster first described the significant effect on the incidence and mortality of melanoma by the latitude of residence [11]. Within each region studied, both mortality and incidence increased significantly as the equator was approached. This observation has been corroborated by many investigators. The significance of the duration of exposure to sunlight is underscored by the observation that in Israel the incidence of melanoma is highest among Israeli natives of European extraction, intermediate for those European-born but long-term residents in Israel, and lowest for the newly arrived European-born immigrants [12].

Despite these data, the role of cumulative sun exposure in melanoma pathogenesis has been questioned because of the high incidence in urban dwellers and in professional and administrative workers who would not be expected to have protracted solar exposure [13–15]. It has been observed that melanoma patients have had a greater number of sunburns than controls, and it appears that the pattern of solar exposure may be as important as the total duration of exposure [16]. Hormonal factors have been implicated in the etiology of melanoma, since the prognosis is better for women than men, even when corrected for stage and age [17, 8]. Interestingly, the survival advantage noted for women disappears in the post-menopausal subgroup [17].

Clinical differential diagnosis

There are many pigmented cutaneous skin lesions that must be distinguished from melanoma, and if doubt exists as to the true nature of a lesion, consultation with a dermatologist should be obtained and a biopsy performed. Common acquired nevi, pigmented seborrheic keratoses, and pigmented basal cell carcinomas often resemble superficial spreading melanomas; likewise, dermatofibromas, Spitz nevi, and hemangiomas may resemble nodular melanomas.

Common acquired nevi, which are proliferative aggregates of normal-appearing melanocytes, are of three types – junctional, compound, and dermal. These distinctions are made primarily by the histological appearances, which correlate with the clinical appearance [18]. Histologically, junctional nevi consist of aggregates of morphologically normal melanoctyes in the basal layer of the epidermis with foci of extension into the upper dermis. Clinically, these lesions are flat, circular, small (usually less than 5 mm in diameter), and a homogeneous tan or brown in color. A superficial spreading melanoma, on the other hand, is mottled and variegated in coloration, with a notched irregular margin.

Compound nevi have melanocytes in both the epidermis and dermis, and in the deeper dermis, the cells may lose pigment and have a clear cytoplasm. These lesions are distinguished from superficial spreading melanomas in vertical growth phase by the slowness of nodule development and by the orderly pattern of coloration and regular margin.

Dermal nevi, as the name suggests, have only a dermal component that in histologic appearance is similar to the dermal component of a compound nevus. Usually these lesions are devoid of pigment, and, since an entirely amelanotic primary melanoma is such a rare lesion, it may be differentiated on this basis.

Pigmented seborrheic keratoses have a dull, waxy surface that is studded with keratin plugs. The lesions are tan to dark brown in color and appear to be only stuck to the skin surface. Indeed, the lesions can be scraped from the skin surface, in contradistinction to melanomas which are firmly anchored to the skin and cannot be scraped off.

Pigmented basal cell carcinomas, because the melanin pigment is confined to the dermis, are not true brown or black, but bluish, red-brown, or gray-white. Careful examination with side-lighting and a hand lens may reveal the peripheral ring of tumor ('pearling' of the border) and telangiectasis that are characteristic only of basal cell carinoma [19].

Dermatofibromas are firm nodules, usually less than 1 cm in diameter, with a uniform moderate or dark pigmentation. Commonly they occur on the extremities of middle-aged women, and the application of lateral pressure will produce dimpling, in contrast to melanomas, which protrude above the skin [20].

The Spitz nevus, first described in 1948 and known by a variety of names, including juvenile melanoma, presents a major problem in clinical and histologic diagnosis [21]. A rapidly growing, small (6–7 mm), dome-shaped, pink to red lesion suggests the diagnosis. Histologically, the cells are often fat, elongated, and devoid of pigment; multinucleated giant melanocytes are frequently present [22]. The treatment of choice is excision.

Hemangiomas can be differentiated from nodular melanomas by their globoid, dark blue-red or purple color and by significant blanching of the lesion when pressure is applied with a glass slide.

Classification of head and neck melanoma

On histological and clinical grounds, the most common head and neck cutaneous melanomas are superficial spreading melanomas (SSM), nodular melanomas (NM), and lentigo maligna melanomas (LMM). At Duke, 49% (196 of 399) were superficial spreading melanomas, 35% (140 of 399) were nodular melanomas, and only 16% (63 of 399) were diagnosed as lentigo maligna melanoma [8]. The correct recognition of the three dominant types of head and neck melanoma will allow for clinical diagnosis at a stage of development when the disease is curable. SSM and LMM are characterized by the gradual and indolent peripheral enlargement of flat, irregularly pigmented, primary lesions. This period of centrifugal growth lasts for years and is known as the radial growth phase. During this time, it acquires little or no competence to metastasize and may be treated by local excision. Focal, deep penetration begins the vertical growth phase, and it is the extent of this growth phase that forms the basis for the Clark's level of invasion and the Breslow tumor thickness measurements that presently are used for prognosis and contribute to staging of the disease. Since NM is composed exclusively of a vertical growth phase, it is the most malignant of the three varieties; in our series, both SSM and LMM had a better prognosis than NM (p = 0.03). There was no significant difference in survival between SSM and LMM [8].

SSM accounts for approximately 70% of all cutaneous melanomas in Caucasians, and in many series is intermediate in survival prognostication. Early lesions appear as irregular combinations of tan, brown, blue, and black, with shades of rose and pink usually being present. Marked variation in color, marginal notching, and loss of skin creases distinguish this lesion from the more common intraepidermal or junctional nevus.

NM, constituting 12% of all cutaneous melanomas is the second most common head and neck melanoma, and has the worst prognosis. NM is composed exclusively of a vertical phase, with melanoma cells generally producing little host cellular response as deep dermal invasion proceeds. The lesions progress rapidly over several months to a year, with even the earliest lesions being raised. Earlier lesions are gray and pink, while later lesions give way to a blueberry-like, blue-black color. Early diagnosis and therapy are thwarted by the lack of an indolent radial growth phase.

The best prognostic type of head and neck melanomas is LMM. Constituting approximately 15% of all melanomas, it occurs most commonly on areas heavily exposed to the sun, such as the head, neck, and dorsum of the hands. The median age of patients with LMM, approximately 70 years, tends to be older than that of patients with SSM or NM. The radial growth phase of LMM precedes the development of vertical growth by decades, thereby facilitating early diagnosis and treatment. The vertical growth phase, however, is associated with metastases in 25% of cases [23]. The early lesions are large, flat, and tan or brown in color. Later, focal elevation occurs as the vertical growth phase is entered, while the original tan-brown pattern of the radial growth phase persists. The minimal elevation of the radial growth phase and the lack of rose or pink colors distinguishes LMM from SSM.

Definitive diagnosis and staging

Careful clinical examination is still the foundation of accurate staging. The site, size, color, and topography of the lesion should be carefully noted. Head and neck melanomas are often conspicuous on examination and account for approximately 25% of all cutaneous melanomas. The majority of head and neck melanomas occur on the face [24]. Of head and neck sites, the cheek is the most common site, with the neck (7%), external ear (7%), and scalp (3%) being much less frequent [25, 26]. Posterior scalp, neck, and ear lesions carry a significantly poorer prognosis than other head and neck sites [8, 27]. The surrounding skin and subcutaneous tissues should be visually examined and palpated to locate any satellite lesions or regional metastases, and the entire body surface should be examined for additional precursor lesions or primary melanomas.

The nodal groups should be examined, since as many as 36% of patients will demonstrate clinical evidence of nodal metastatic disease at the time of the initial presentation. The primary lesion is occult in up to 15% of patients [28, 29]. In such cases, a careful history with regard to complete regression or previous excision of a pigmented lesion should be obtained, and careful examination of the anatomic sites which drain to the affected lymph nodes should be performed. If metastatic disease is suspected, laboratory studies should include a chest film, a complete blood count, and a blood chemistry profile. Liver function tests, particularly the lactic dehydrogenase (LDH) and gamma glytamyl transpeptidase (GGTP) are of use in detecting liver metastases, although any elevation in LFT's should be followed up by radionuclide scan or CT [30, 31]. Routine liver, bone, and brain scans are not helpful in detecting metatases [32, 33]. Tomographic gallium-67 citrate scanning, however, may help to locate visceral metastases other than brain [34]. Computed lung tomography has been shown to be of diagnostic value in detecting occult metastasis in patients without suggestive routine chest roentgenograms [35].

The use of lymphangiography in the pre treatment evaluation of melanoma patients remains problematic, although it has been reported to be of benefit in directing the subsequent therapy in cervical melanomas [36]. Little data is available on head and neck lymphangiography, and even in anatomic sites where it is frequently used (such as the lower extremities), false positive and false negative diagnoses are common. While metastases could not be dependably identified, useful information for the design and execution of lymphadenectomy operations can be derived from lymphangiography in sites where primary drainage routes could be quite variable [37].

Lymphoscintigraphy, using technetium-99 antimony sulfur colloid, is frequently utilized at the Duke University Comprehensive Center to identify patterns of regional lymphatic drainage [38]. For lesions of the posterior scalp, or areas of indeterminate primary drainage, lymphoscintigraphy is helpful in determining the primary afferent lymphatic channels. With this information therapeutic decisions can be made about which areas (posterior neck dissections, standard neck dissections, and superficial parotidectomies) should be included in the lymphadenectomy. Lymphoscintigraphy is thus an excellent *in vivo* test for demonstrating the functional anatomy of the reticuloendothelial system and the nodal groups at risk for developing metastatic disease. While it does not prove that a nodal group is harboring metastases, lymphoscintigraphy can direct the surgical effort and often results in a decrease in the extent of the indicated surgical procedure.

Any lesion suspected of being a malignant melanoma should be biopsied, and, when feasible, an excisional biopsy with adequate uninvolved margins should be performed [39–41]. If a lesion is too large or located in a functionally or cosmetically critical area, an initial incisional or punch biopsy may be performed. In either event, wide local excision for definitive management of malignant melanoma should not be performed without a biopsy-proven diagnosis. Patient prognosis, it should be recognized, is not adversely affected by either prior excisional or incisional biopsy [41].

Both adequate surgical sampling and proper histologic sectioning are required to give accurate microstaging: The surgical specimen must be cut at frequent intervals, perpendicular to the skin surface, at right angles to the long axis throughout its entire length.

Clark *et al.* proposed five anatomic levels of tumor invasion in malignant melanoma, and noted that the level of invasion correlated with the prognosis [42]. With increasing level of invasion, survival decreases, although not necessarily in a linear manner [42]. The levels are defined as follows:
- *Level I:* malignant cells extend to the dermoepidermal junction but are limited to the epidermis;
- *Level II:* malignant cells extend into the papillary dermis;
- *Level III:* malignant cells fill the papillary dermis and impinge upon the reticular dermis without actually invading it;
- *Level IV:* malignant cells extend into collagen bundles of the reticular dermis;
- *Level V:* malignant cells extend into the subcutaneous tissue.

Breslow noted that the prognosis correlates well with tumor thickness as measured by an ocular micrometer and concluded that prognostic information provided by thickness was easier for histopathologists to determine, less subjective, and more reproducible than determination of Clark level [43–46]. In fact, within individual Clark levels of invasion, there can be primary melanomas of widely varying tumor thicknesses [43]. The non-linear, stepwise rise in mortality rate with increasing tumor thickness for a large group of patients with stage I melanoma has been analyzed by Day *et al.* to develop four divisions [47]. The respective 8-year survival rates (%) are as follows: less than 0.85 mm (99 ± 1%); 0.85 – 1.69 mm (93 ± 2%), 1.70 – 3.64 mm (69 ± 5%), and greater than 3.64 mm (38 ± 6%). Site, cell type, nodal findings, number of mitoses, inflammatory reaction, and ulceration also correlate significantly with the prognosis of head and neck melanomas [47–49].

Most centers evaluate melanomas on both Clark's level and Breslow thickness which makes comparison easier. Much useful information is also provided by the following commonly used clinical staging system:

1. local disease
    A. solitary primary lesion only,
    B. primary with satellites within a 5 cm radius of the primary,
    C. local recurrence within a radius of 5 cm from the resected primary,
    D. metastases within the regional lymphatic drainage area of the primary but not more than 5 cm from the primary site;
2. regional nodal disease;
3. disseminated disease.

The clinical and surgical TNM staging system proposed by Beahrs and Myers (1983) uses both the level of invasion and maximum measured thickness to determine the T classification [50]. Primary tumors with satellite lesions or nodules within 2 cm of the primary tumor are considered as T_4. Satellite lesions or nodules within the regional nodal distribution, beyond two centimeters from the primary, are considered to be in-transit metastases and are included under the N categories. Stage grouping is designed to reflect the differing prognoses for patients with specific amounts of localized disease, as quantified by histologic microstaging. The delineation of prognostic groups by this staging system is more accurate than by any previous staging system [50].

The TNM classification (AJC, 1983) is as follows [50]:

Primary tumor (T)

T_x No evidence of primary tumor (unknown primary or primary tumor removed and not histologically examined)

T_0 A typical melanocytic hyperplasia (Clarck level I); nota malignant lesion

T_1 Invasion of papillary dermis (Clark level II) or 0.75 mm thickness or less

T_2 Invasion of papillary-reticular-dermal interface (level III) or 0.76–1.5 mm thickness

T_3 Invasion of the reticular dermis (level IV) or 1.51 to 4.0 mm thickness

T_4 Invasion of subcutaneous tissue (level V) or 4.1 mm or more in thickness and satellite(s) within 2 cm of any primary melanoma

Nodal involvement (N)

N_x Nodes cannot be assessed

N_0 No regional lymph node involvement

N_1 Involvement of only one regional lymph node station; node(s) movable and not over 5 cm in diameter or negative regional lymph nodes and the presence of less than five in-transit metastases beyond 2 cm from primary site

N_2 Any one of the following: (1) involvement of more than one regional lymph node station, (2) regional node(s) over 5 cm in diameter or fixed, (3) five or more in-transit metastases or any in-transit metastases beyond 2 cm from primary site with regional lymph node involvement

Distant metastasis (M)

M_x Not assessed

M_0 No known distant metastasis

M_1 Involvement of skin or subcutaneous tissue beyond the site or primary lymph node drainage

M_2 Visceral metastasis (spread to any distant site other than skin or subcutaneous tissues)

Stage grouping

IA	$T_1N_0M_0$
IB	$T_2N_0M_0$
IIA	$T_3N_0M_0$
IIB	$T_4N_0M_0$
III	Any TN_1M_0
IV	Any T, N_2M_0 or any T, any N_0M_1 or M_2

Treatment

Currently, head and neck melanomas are treated by four modalities: surgery, immunotherapy, chemotherapy, and radiotherapy. In our series, all modalities were used as indicated with a five-year actuarial survival for the entire population of head and neck cases of 55%, and with a median survival of 67.1 months [8]. Median survival was 63.5 months for males, and 81.4 months for females – statistically not significant because of the population size, but with a clear trend to greater longevity for females. Five-year actuarial survivals of 65.4%, 80% and 33.5% have been reported by Ames [51], Das Gupta [52] and Knutson [53].

Surgery for head and neck melanomas

Margins of resection
Historically, Handley, in 1907, in his treatise on the pathologic evaluation of the centrifugal dermal lymphatic permeation of malignant melanoma, recommended wide local excision [54]. His treatise, however, was based on a single autopsy study of the distribution of tumor in the lymphatics surrounding cutaneous metastases, not primary tumors. More convincing than the theoretical reasons for wide excision of a primary melanoma are the empirical justification for it: limited excision has a high likelihood of recurrence associated with it, and local recurrence has exceedingly bad prognostic implications. Wilson reported a 57% local recurrence rate in 49 patients whose primary melanoma was treated by excisional biopsy alone, as compared to only 3% in 73 patients treated by wide excision of the primary [55]. Local recurrence, after excision of the primary, may be within 5 cm of the site and be termed arbitrarily 'satellitosis'. Also by convention, recurrence more than 5 cm from the primary is termed 'in-transit' metastatic disease. Either pattern of local recurrence is associated with a very poor prognosis, with reported 5-year survival rates for patients with local recurrence ranging from

14–45% [56–61]. Nevertheless, it is becoming clear that local recurrence of a thin (1 mm) melanoma is rare, regardless of the extent of resection [62, 63]. In the head and neck, to preserve functionally and cosmetically significant structures, not excising large areas (the traditional 5 cm margins) of surrounding tissue unnecessarily is to be greatly encouraged. Minimal safe margins have not been established for thin lesions (< 0.76 mm), since local recurrence is so rare, but it is generally recommended that for lesions less than 0.76 mm and for lentigo maligna melanoma, 1–2 cm margins are acceptable. The limited surgical defects created by narrower margins around a melanoma may be closed primarily or by local flaps, and split thickness skin grafting is not required. Neither the method of closure not the removal of fascia alters the prognosis [64, 65].

Treatment of regional lymph nodes
Correct management of the regional lymphatics in the treatment of head and neck melanoma is controversial. Although the regional lymph nodes are the most common sites of initial metastases, it is controversial as to whether lymphadenectomy for occult lymph node metastases is of benefit [66]. Guidelines for performing a therapeutic neck dissection are the following: (1) the primary lesion and/or the regional lymph nodes are surgically resectable; (2) survival time is expected to be greater than 6 months in duration; (3) distant metastases are limited; (4) the general medical condition of the patient permits surgery. Local control of the disease can prevent skin breakdown and disfigurement. It should be emphasized that approximately 20–30% of these patients will survive for 5 years, and all tumor burden should therefore be eliminated.

Factors such as type of melanoma, presence or absence of ulceration, level and depth of invasion, size and location of the primary, age, sex and condition of patient, are all important prognostic indicators. There is confusion in the literature regarding the value of immediate or delayed cervical lymphadenectomy because of the lack of controlled studies taking into account the numerous prognostic indicators. Also many series evaluating the effectiveness of elective neck dissection include the head and neck area with other body sites. Data from this institution indicate that melanomas of the head and neck are biologically different from trunk and extremity primaries and should be analysed independently [8].

Patel reported that the cervical lymph nodes are the primary site of metastases from head and neck primaries [66]. The theoretical basis for elective neck dissection (END) is based on the assumption that the natural history of melanoma develops in an orderly course of metastasis first to regional lymph nodes and then to distant sites. Thus, by removing micrometastases and occult disease within regional lymph nodes, survival should increase and metastatic disease lessen. This is suggested by the poor survival statistics for delayed lymphadenectomy and the decreasing survival rates as the number of pathologically involved lymph nodes increases [67, 68].

The incidence of occult disease increases in proportion to increasing thickness of the primary lesion. It has been reported for all head and neck sites that the risk of regional metastases varies with thickness: 0% for lesions less than 0.75 mm; 24% for lesions 0.76 mm to 1.49 mm; 57% for lesions 1.5 mm to 3.99 mm; 62% for lesions greater than 4 mm [69, 70, 72]. Since the incidence of metastatic spread is so low for lesions less than 0.76 mm, elective neck dissection would not be of significant benefit. Likewise END for lentigo maligna is not necessary.

For superficial spreading and nodular melanomas of the head and neck, lesions 0.76 mm to 4.0 mm have reported rates of occult nodal metastasis at surgery ranging from 14–44% [67, 72]. The precise metastatic rate may be higher since 50–60% of patients who did not undergo END for intermediate thickness melanomas developed clinical evidence of nodal involvement [69, 73]. Thus for localized intermediate thickness melanomas (0.75 mm to 4.0 mm) elective neck dissection appears to be indicated on the basis of the likelihood of occult nodal involvement.

For deeply invasive head and neck melanomas (thickness greater than 4.0 mm), improved survival with elective lymph node dissection has been suggested by a number of authors [67, 74, 75]. Ames' study points out that it has been consistently reported that the survival of patients who have only microscopically positive nodes is better than the 5-year salvage in patients who have evolved positive nodes [73]. This comparison has been a traditional part of the rationale for elective neck dissections, and this seems to be sound logic. Unfortunately, since only 20–30% of patients actually have regional subclinical disease, 70–80% of patients would undergo neck dissection without the presence of any nodal disease. Even if subclinical disease is discovered, elective neck dissection is not a guarantee of survival. The key is that if the findings of subclinically positive nodes could direct effective subsequent adjuvant therapy for those who actually have regional disease, elective neck dissection will have a certain and beneficial role. It is for this reason that at Duke University Medical Center chemotherapy is recommended for those cases with five or more positive nodes on elective neck dissection, and data is being collected by protocol.

Some authors assert that there is no benefit from elective neck dissection (END) as compared to therapeutic neck dissection, since in their series 5-year survival rates are similar for patients with either END or therapeutic neck dissection (TND) [76]. Data from this institution does not support this contention, since patients with stage I disease who received an END had significantly better prognosis than patients who underwent TND for clinical stage II disease. The tendency toward better 5-year survival has been reported for patients who underwent an END with lesions less than 3.5 mm deep and who had fewer than two nodes pathologically involved [67, 73, 77]. Since prognosis is so poor for patients with metachronous regional metastases, END has been supported by several authors at the time of wide excision of the primary [78, 79].

Historically, Clark level, Breslow thickness and stage have been dependable prognostic indicators of survival. Other factors which have been demonstrated to affect the prognosis adversely are: (1) presence of ulceration, (2) nodular melanoma, (3) advanced age, (4) male sex, (5) location on the posterior scalp and ear. Ulceration of even a thin melanoma (less than 0.75 mm) may indicate need for elective node dissection. This is supported by Balch, who reported ten year survival rates of 60–70% for non-ulcerated axial (head and neck and trunk) melanoma patients compared to 25% for ulcerated lesions [73].

In view of these accumulated data, elective node dissection can be recommended for situations in which the risk of occult regional metastases is known to be high. Thus, those patients with lesions 1.5 mm to 4.0 mm in thickness arising from any head and neck site should be considered for END. Patients with lesions 0.75 mm to 1.5 mm thick need to have individualized treatment plans, with elective node dissection advised particularly for lesions approaching 1.5 mm in thickness, having ulceration, of the nodular type, or located on the posterior scalp or ear. In patients with thick (greater than 4.0 mm) melanomas, occult regional and distant metastases is likely (80%) and prognosis is poor [73]. Elective neck dissection in these cases is unlikely to improve prognosis, but does offer improved local control, staging information, and preparation for specific active immunotherapy or adjuvant chemotherapy.

Modifications of the standard classic radical neck dissection (RND) have been shown to reduce the deformity inherent with RND, and to decrease the associated morbitity by preserving the spinal accessory nerve. Recent evidence is accumulating to show that modified neck dissection is efficacious in controlling both squamous cell carcinoma and selected melanomas [80–82]. Unfortunately, the term 'modified neck dissection' may denote preservation of structures such as the spinal accessory nerve, the sternocleidomastoid muscle, and the internal jugular vein or any combination of these structures. Whereas the modified neck dissection may provide a functionally and cosmetically preferable alternative, statistical analysis of the effectiveness of these procedures in regard to survival, disease-free interval and local control is difficult due to small patient numbers and variations in the definition of a modified neck dissection at different centers.

Immunotherapy

Historically, the most effective immunotherapy has been active immunization against a specific disease. Melanoma is a highly antigenic tumor. For over two decades it has been realized that melanoma tumor associated antigens exist. This has stimulated an intense research effort investigating the recognition of human melanoma antigens by a patient's immune system and it is the basis of immunotherapy of malignant melanoma. Seigler reported the results for specific active immunization in 719 patients with invasive malanoma [83]. In this series, the patients were sequentially immunized with 2.5×-10^7 X-irradiated neuraminidase treated melanoma cells, and BCG was used for its adjuvant effect.

Head and neck sites constituted 15% of the cases. Although the results are encouraging, further controlled studies using this approach are presently underway. Currently, at Duke University Medical Center, those patients with stage I (greater than 0.75 mm thickness) and stage II with less than four lymph nodes positive are treated with a total of four innoculations at monthly intervals. Those with secondary lesions are treated with seven innoculations at the rate of one each month. If these patients develop recurrent disease during treatment, they receive three additional treatments.

Pre-operatively many investigators have performed intra-lesional adjuvant therapy using adjuvants such as vaccinia, dinitrochlorobenzene (DNCB), and Bacillus Calmette-Guerin (BCG). Everall and co-workers performed a prospective study of the efficacy of pre-operative injection of vaccinia virus into the primary melanomas with definitive surgery performed 2 weeks post-innoculation [84]. Forty-eight patients were studied, and the disease-free intervals were compared. At 4 years, a significant benefit was noted for the vaccinia-treated group with relapses of 20% as compared to 50% for surgery alone. Allocation, however, in the two treatment groups was not random, and, although the two treatment groups were comparable in age, the vaccinia virus-treated group contained significantly more tumors of the superficial spreading type.

DNCB has been used in the pre-operative period by Castermans-Elias to treat 37 patients with clinical stage I melanoma. Of these, 23 were clinically diagnosed and treated with DNCB before excisional biopsy. In this group of patients, 2 mg of DNCB was applied to the primary lesions for 48 h and repeated twice at weekly intervals. After 8 to 19 days, definitive surgery was performed. This was compared to the 14 patients who were surgically diagnosed and who received DNCB after surgery. A significant benefit was noted after 3 years of observation, with none of the 23 pre-operatively treated patients relapsing and four of 14 post-operatively treated patients relapsing [85].

Intralesional BCG has been evaluated by Rosenberg and associates, with 26 patients randomized to receive intralesional BCG or no treatment prior to definitive surgical excision [86]. The number of patients is small; however, the therapeutic benefit appears to be significant, with only five of 13 of the BCG group relapsing and ten of 13 of the control group relapsing

Based on the above observations, presurgical intralesional therapy and postsurgical specific active immunotherapy warrant further investigation in the treatment of high-risk melanoma patients.

Systemic chemotherapy

Since prognosis for disseminated melanoma is dismal (generally 6–8 months), initiation of systemic chemotherapy should be guided by drug toxicity and morbitity versus objective benefit. The single most active agent for the treatment of metastatic malignant melanoma is dimethyl triazene imidazole carboxamide (DTIC) with a reported response rate of 20–30% [87]. The median duration of response in favorable sites is 5.7 months [88, 89]. The apparent effectiveness of DTIC prompted several investigators to combine DTIC with other chemotherapeutic agents with response rates ranging from 19 to 48% in patients with disseminated melanoma [90–93].

Complications of DTIC include GI and hematologie toxicities. Liver dysfunction can be caused by DTIC, and rarely it may cause acute liver failure secondary to liver necrosis and veno-occlusive disease [94–97].

Other single agents with well-documented activity against malignant melanoma are the nitrosoureas, of which BCNU, CCNU, methyl CCNU, and chlorozoticin are the best known [98–101]. The response rates for these single agent therapies range from 10% to 18%, with a median response duration of 2–6 months. The oral nitrosoureas are much more convenient to administer than intravenous DTIC, but, unfortunately, are not quite as effective and have greater hematologic toxicity.

Most other single agents have demonstrated little if any antitumor action against melanoma. Several regimens combining these agents have been used in phase II and controlled clinical trials to determine which agents potentiate the activity of DTIC with the least synergistic toxicity [104–115]. Bleomycin, vincristine, and CCNU all have activity against melanoma, although as single agents, they are not as effective as DTIC [116, 117]. Wasch and associates reported response rates of 48.5% in stage III melanoma when bleomycin, vincristine, and CCNU were combined with DTIC [118].

Currently at Duke University Medical Center, a chemotherapeutic protocol is underway to determine the response rate of patients with disseminated metastatic melanoma to a combination of bleomycin, vincristine, CCNU, and DTIC (BOLD) [119]. DTIC is given at $200\,mg/m^2$/day IV push for days 1–5, with a maximum single dose of 400 mg; CCNU is given at $80\,mg/m^2$ p.o. on day 1, with a maximal single dose of 150 mg; bleomycin, in the first course, is given at a dose of 7.5 units subcutaneously on days 1 and 4, and on the second course at 15 units subcutaneously on days 1 and 4 with a maximum cumulative dose of 400 units; and vincristine is given at $1\,mg/m^2$ IV on days 1 and 5, with a maximum single dose of 2.5 mg. These drugs are given in cycles which are repeated every 6 weeks.

There is a real need for the development of more effedtive chemotherapeutic agents in melanoma therapy. Further research may find a way to exploit the tyrosinase-catalyzed pigment biosynthesis mechanism that is unique to both normal and malignant melanocytes [120].

Hormonal therapy

There appears to be a relationship between the biologic behavior of melanoma and sex hormones. Several factors imply this relationship. First, the female patient generally has a better prognosis than the male petient with increased survival noted for premenopausal females compared with postmenopausal females [121]. Second, melanoma is rare before puberty [122]. Third, clinical exacerbations during pregnancy have been often reported. This relationship is, however, not clear, since pregnancy and exogenous estrogen use have been shown to have varying effects on melanoma [123–125]. Recent studies have demonstrated estrogen receptor binding in melanoma tumor cytosols; yet this finding is weakened in significance by the finding that the enzyme tyrosinase binds estradiol in a specific, saturable, and inhibitable manner [126]. Zava and Goldhirsch have presented a model system to explain how tyrosinase, an enzyme unique to pigmented cells, such as normal and malignant melanocytes, can oxidize (3H)-estradiol to radiolabeled products which closely resemble the tight binding of (3H)-estradiol to estrogen receptor [127]. McCarty *et al.* noted that purified tyrosinase, which mimicks estrogen-binding in estrogen cytolsols, was inhibited by DOPA, while the binding of estradiol to estrogen receptor preparations was not [126]. Thus, gradient analysis and DOPA inhibition studies should be included in evaluating the estrogen-binding phenomenon in human melanoma.

The data to support hormonal therapy is fragmentary. The responses are infrequent, but when measured, seem to occur with no correlation to the hormone receptor status. The objective response rates in clinical trials using hormonal therapies (Tamoxifen, Medroxy progesterone acetate, Diethylstilbestrol, Estramustine, and Pregnanetrione) averages 10% [128–134]. Additional research will be required to clarify this area.

Radiotherapy

Malignant melanoma has classically been felt to be a radioresistant tumor. This may be explained by the disappointing clinical response to conventionally fractionated radiation (180 to 200 rad per fraction), 'historial opinion', and possibly a case selection bias [135]. Although not a universally held opinion, most radiation biologists have noticed an enhanced shoulder on *in vitro* survival curves of melanoma cells [136, 137]. This results from a melanoma cell's ability to efficiently repair sublethal radiation damage [136, 141]. These data would lead one to predict that large doses per fraction would be necessary to observe any significant response to fractionated radiation therapy. A number of clinical studies looking at the dose per fraction effect in irradiation of skin and nodal metastases have been performed. These are summarized in Table 1.

Although most of the data suggest the benefit of large dose per fraction treatment [138–140], Lobo found quite satisfactory responses with normal fraction size. Trott in reviewing his material found a positive association with increasing N.S.D. and most strikingly with reduced treatment times as opposed to large fraction size. It should be emphasized that none of the above studies were prospective or randomized.

Radiation therapy has been used in the treatment of melanoma as follows: (1) primary treatment; (2) adjuvant treatment; and (3) palliative treatment in melanoma of the head and neck.

1. Primary treatment

Lentigo maligna (LM) and lentigo maligna melanoma (LMM)
Harwood and his colleagues at the Princess Margaret Hospital in Toronto have written extensively on the treatment of these disorders with conventional X-ray treatment in the recent years [135, 143, 144]. In their most recent report [151], only two recurrences were encountered in 21 cases of lentigo maligna. Similarly, of 28 cases of lentigo maligna melanoma, local control was achieved in 26 cases with the median follow-up in both series of approximately 30 months. Similar results have been achieved in Europe using the Miescher (contact kilovoltage therapy) technique [145]. These lesions tend to regress very slowly with the median time to regression of 7 to 8 months. These data suggest the possible role of radiotherapy for LM or LMM in lesions which are difficult to approach surgically or in patients who are medically inoperable.

Superficial spreading and nodular melanoma
The accumulated experience in radiation therapy of primary lesions of this type is limited and in some cases of dubious value [135]. In one series biopsy confirmation is lacking in approximately 30% of cases and the doses advocated would appear to exceed conventional skin tolerance Table 2 [146].

Table 1.

Author	Size of daily fraction	Response rate
Habermals and	600	28/31
Fisher [138]	500	4/19
Overgaarde [139]	500	17/34
	500	15/15
Hornsey [140]	300	15/28
	300–400	22/29
	400	30/37
Lobo [141]	200–300	14/21
Trott [142]	300	10/28
	300–400	6/6
	400	4/10

In light of the above noted deficiencies and preliminary nature of these reports, there appears to be little basis for treating these lesions primarily with irradiation on a routine basis.

2. Adjuvant radiotherapy

Gordon Richards from the Toronto General Hospital pioneered the use of limited local excision followed by postoperative irradiation, particularly in the head and neck area, to preserve structure and function. Dickson reported on their results in 1958, concluding that 5-year survivals with this treatment (41%) were better than with local excision alone (19.7%) and comparable to radical surgery (26.2%) [148]. Achievement of local control by local excision and pre- or postoperative irradiation has been reported by Nitter, Hellriegel and Jorgsholm [146, 147, 149]. They felt that survival rates in their series were similar to those following radical surgery, but reported no control group of patients to justify this opinion. Certainly there appears to be little to suggest any improvement in survival with this technique. Radiation therapy has also been used as an adjuvant to nodal dissection. Creagan reported the only randomized study in 1978 comparting patients given postoperative radiation therapy to those managed by node dissection alone [150]. In this small trial of 55 patients, no improvement in the disease – survival with adjuvant irradiation was detected. This lack of significant benefit may be explained by (1) conventional fractionation, and (2) the low rate of failure with lymphadenectomy alone. Further investigation of this matter in high-risk patients (large or multiple nodes) may be warranted.

3. Palliative treatment

Hilaris in 1963 pointed out the benefits of palliative irradiation in the patient with malignant melanoma, noting an overall rate of improvement in his series of 57% using conventional fractionation [151]. This initial report has been amplified by Katz and others [152]. In light of the systematic failure of approximately 29% of stage I patients and 81% of stage II patients, this valuable palliative resource should not be ignored [153].

Future prospects in the management of this disease with irradiation center upon further basic radiobiologic and clinical studies of fractionation, radiosensitizers [154], radioprotectors, hyperthermia [155–158], particle radiotherapy [159],

Table 2.

Author	Type of lesion	5-year survival	local control
Harwood [135]	SSM	1/6	6/6
Hellriegel [146]	all types	65/95	
Jorgsholm [147]	all types		9/15

and cytotoxic drugs. Already there is evidence that suggests benefit in animals and in man from combined hyperthermia and radiation treatment in melanoma. Perhaps in the future the prospects of treating melanoma with irradiation will be improved.

References

1. Carswell, R., cited by Urega, O.B., Pack, E.T. 1966. On the antiquity of melanoma. Cancer 19: 607–610.
2. Pemberton, O. 1867. Clinical Illustrations of Various Forms of Cancer. Longmans, Green, Reader, and Dyer, London.
3. Elwood, J.M., Lee, J.A.H. 1975. Recent data on the epidemiology of malignant melanoma. *Sem. Oncol.* 2: 149–154.
4. Cosman, B., Heddle, S.B., Crikelair, G.F. 1976. The increasing incidence of melanoma. Plast. Recontr. Surg. 57: 50–56.
5. Schreiber, M.M., Bozzo, P.D., Moon, T.E. 1981. Malignant melanoma in Southern Arizona: Increasing incidence and sunlight as an etiologic factor. Arch. Dermatol. 117: 6–11.
6. Lee, J.A.H., Carter, A.P. 1970. Secular trends in mortality from malignant melanoma. J.N.C.I. 45: 91–97.
7. Luce, J.K., McBride, C.M., Frei, E., III. 1973. Melanoma. In Cancer Medicine. (J.F. Holland, E. Frei, III, eds.). Les & Frebiger, Philadelphia, pp. 1823-1844.
8. Gussack, G.S., Reintgen, D., Cox, E., Fusher, S.R., Cole, T.B., Seigler, H.F. 1983. Cutaneous melanoma of the head and neck: A review of 399 cases. Arch. Otolaryngol. 109: 803–808.
9. Hinds, M.W., Kolonel, L.N. 1980. Malignant melanoma of the skin in Hawaii, 1960–1977. Cancer 45: 811–817.
10. Krementz, E.T., Sutherland, C.M., Carter, R.D. *et al.* 1976. Malignant melanoma in the American Black. Ann. Surg. 183: 533–542.
11. Lancaster, H.O. 1956. Some geographical aspects on the mortality from melanoma. Med. J. Aust. 2: 1082–1087.
12. Anaise, D., Steinitz, R., BenHur, N. 1978. Solar radiation: a possible etiologic factor in malignant melanoma in Israel. Cancer 42: 299–304.
13. Urbach, F. 1983. Sunlight and melanoma. J. Dermatol. Surg. Oncol. 9: 679–689.
14. Williams, R.R., Stegens, N.L., Goldsmith, J.R. 1977. Association of cancer site and type with occupation and industry from the Third National Cancer Survey Interview. J.N.C.I. 59: 1147–1185.
15. Lee J.A.H., Strickland, D. 1980. Malignant melanoma: Social status and outdoor work. Br. J. Cancer 42: 757–763.
16. Sober, A.J., Lew, R.A., Fitzpatrick, T.B. *et al.* 1979. Solar exposure patterns in patients with cutaneous melanoma. Clin, Res. 27: 573A.
17. Shaw, H.M., Milton, G.W., Farago, G. *et al.* 1978. Endocrine influences on survival from malignant melanoma. Cancer 42: 669–677.
18. Bhawan, J. 1979. Melanocytic nevi. A review. J. Cutan. Pathol. 6: 153–169.
19. Mihm, M.C., Jr., Clark, W.H., Jr. Reed, R.J. 1975. The clinical diagnosis of malignant melanoma. Sem. Oncol. 2: 105–118.
20. Fitzpatrick, T.B., Blichrest, B.A. 1977. Simple sign to differentiate benign from malignant pigmented cutaneous lesions. N. Engl. J. Med. 296: 1518.
21. Spitz S. 1948. Melanomas in childhood. Am. J. Pathol. 24: 591–609.
22. Paniago-Pereira, C., Maize, J.C., Ackerman, A.B. 1978. Nevus of large spindle cells and/or epitheloid cells (Spitz's nevus). Arch. Dermatol. 114: 1811–1823.

262

23. Clark, W.H., Jr., Mihm, M.C. 1969. Lentigo maligna and lentigo maligna melanoma. Am. J. Pathol. 55: 39–67.

‹ 24. Bodenham, D.C. 1975. Malignant melanoma of the head and neck. In: Cancer of the Head and Neck (R.G. Chambers, ed.). Excerpta Medica, Amsterdam, pp. 85–91.

‹ 25. Conley, J., Hamaker, R.C. 1977. Melanoma of the head and neck. Laryngoscope 87: 760–764.

‹ 26. Byers, R.M., Smith, J.L., Russell, N., Rosenberg, V. 1980. Malignant melanoma of the external ear. Am. J. Surg. 140: 518–521.

27. Day, C.L., Sober, A.J., Kopf, A.W. *et al.* 1981. A prognostic model for clinical stage I melanoma of the upper extremitiy: The importance of anatomic subsites in predicting recurrent disease. Ann. Surg. 193: 436–440.

28. Brownstein, M.H., Helwig, E.B. 1972. Patterns of subcutaneous metastasis. Arch. Dermatrol. 105: 862–868.

29. Guiliana, A.E., Moseley, H.S., Morton, D.L. 1980. Clinical aspects of unknown primary melanoma. Ann. Surg. 191:98–104.

30. Garg, R., McPherson, T.A., Lentle, B. *et al.* 1979. Usefulness of an elevated serum lactate dehydrogenase value as a marker of hepatic metastases in malignant melanoma. Can. Med. Assoc. J. 120: 1114.

31. Murray, J.L., Lerner, M.P., Nordquist, R.E. 1982. Elevated gluatmyl transpeptidase levels in malignant melanoma. Cancer 49: 1439–1443.

32. Thomas, J.H., Panoussopoulous, D., Liesmann, G.E. *et al.* 1979. Scintiscans in the evaluation of patients with malignant melanoma. Surg. Gynecol. Obstet. 149: 574–576.

33. Evans, R.A., Bland, K.I., McMurtrey, M.J. *et al.* 1980. Radionuclide scans not indicated for clinical stage I melanoma. Surg. Gynecol. Obstet. 150: 532–534.

34. Kirkwood, J.M., Myers, J.E., Vlock, D.R. *et al.* 1982. Tomographic gallium-67 citrate scanning: Useful new surveillance for metastatic melanoma. Ann. Intern. Med. 97: 694–699.

35. Bydder, G.M., Kreel, L. 1981. Body computer tomography in the diagnosis of malignant melanoma metastases. C.T. 5: 21–24.

36. Musumeci, R., Acerbil, L., Balzarina, G.P. *et al.* 1972. Lymphographic evaluation of 116 cases of malignant melanoma. Tumor 58: 1–12.

37. Cox, K., Hare, W.S.C., Bruce, P.T. 1966. Lymphography in melanoma. Cancer 19: 637–647.

38. Reintgen, D.S., Sullivan, D., Coleman, E., Briner, W., Croker, B.P., Seigler, H.F. 1983. Lymphoscintography for malignant melanoma: surgical considerations. Am. Surg. 49, 12: 672–678.

39. Roses, D.F., Ackerman, A.B., Harris, M.N. *et al.* 1979. Assessment of biopsy techniques and histopathologic interpretations of primary cutaneous malignant melanoma. Ann. Surg. 189: 294–297.

40. Little, J.H., Davis, N.C. 1974. Frozen section diagnosis of suspected malignant melanoma of the skin. Cancer 34: 1163–1172.

41. Epstein, E., Bragg, K., Linden, G. 1969. Biopsy and prognosis of malignant melanoma. J.A.M.A. 208: 1369–1371

42. Clark, Jr., W.H., From, L., Bernadina, E.A., Mihm, Jr., M.C. 1969. The histogenesis and biologic behavior of primary human malignant melanomas of the skin. Cancer Res. 29: 705–726.

43. Balch, C.M., Murad, T.M., Soong, S.J. *et al.* 1978. A multifactorial analysis of melanoma: Prognostic histopathologic features comparing Clark's and Breslow's staging methods. Ann. Surg. 118: 732–742.

44. Breslow, A. 1975. Tumor thickness, level of invasion, and node dissection in stage I cutaneous melanoma. Ann. Surg. 182: 572–575.

45. Breslow, A. 1979. Prognostic factors in the treatment of cutaneous melanoma. J. Cutan. Pathol. 6: 208–212.

46. Wanebo, H.J., Fortner, J.G., Woodruff, J. *et al.* 1975. Selection of the optimum surgical

treatment of stage I melanoma by depth of microinvasion: Use of the combined microstage technique (Clark-Breslow). Ann. Surg. 188: 302–315.

47. Day, Jr., C.L., Lew, R.A., Mihm, Jr., M.c. *et al.* 1981. A multivariate analysis of prognostic factors for melanoma patients with lesions 3.65 mm in thickness. The importance of revealing alternate Cox models. Ann. Surg. 195: 44–49.

48. Day, Jr., C.L., Mihm, Jr., M.C., Lew, R.A. *et al.* 1982. Prognostic factors for patients with clinical stage I melanoma of intermediate thickness (1.51–3.99 mm). A conceptual model for tumor growth and metastasis. Ann. Surg. 195: 35–43.

49. Van der Esch, E.P., Cascinelli, N., Preda, F. *et al.* 1981. Stage I melanoma of the skin: Evaluation of prognosis according to histologic characteristics. Cancer 48: 1668–1673.

50. Beahrs, O.II., Myers, M.H. 1983. Manual for staging of cancer, American Joint Committee on Cancer . J.B. Lippincott, Philadelphia, pp. 117–123.

51. Ames, F.C., Sugarbaker, E.V., Ballantyne, A.S. 1976. Analysis of survival and disease control in stage I melanoma of the head and neck. Am. J. Surg. 132: 484–491.

52. Das Gupta, T.K. 1977. Results of treatment of 269 patients with primary cutaneous melanoma: A five-year prospective study. Ann. Surg. 186: 201–209.

53. Knutson, C.D., Hori, J.M., Watson, F.R. 1981. Melanoma of the head and neck. Am. J. Surg. 124: 470–473.

54. Handley, W.S. 1907. The pathology of melanotic growths in relation to their operative treatment. Lancet 1: 927–10003.

55. Wilson, R. 1958. Malignant melanoma – a follow-up study. West. J. Surg. Obstet. Gynecol. 66: 19–31.

56. McNeer, G., Cantin, J. 1967. Local failure in the treatment of melanoma. Am. J. Roentgen, Rad. Ther. Nucl. Med. 99: 790–808.

57. Jones, W.M., Williams, W.J., Roberts, M.M. *et al.* 1968. Malignant melanoma of the skin: Prognostic value of clinical features and the role of treatment in 111 cases. Br. J. Cancer 22: 437–451.

58. Shingleton, W.W., Seigler, H.F., Stocks, L.H. *et al.* 1975. Management of recurrent melanoma of the extremity. Cancer 35: 574–579.

59. Elias, E.G., Didolkar, M.S., Goel, T.P. *et al.* 1977. A clinicopathologic study of prognostic factors in cutaneous malignant melanoma. Surg. Gynecol. Obstet. 144: 327–334.

60. Karakousis, C.P., Holyoke, E.D. 1980. Biologic behavior and treatment of intransit metastasis of melanoma. Surg. Gynecol. Obstet. 150: 29–32.

61. Milton, G.W., Shaw, H.N., Farago, G.A. *et al.* 1980. Tumor thickness and the site and time of first recurrence in cutaneous malignant melanoma (stage I). Br. J. Surg. 67: 543–546.

62. Cascinelli, N., Van der Essche, E.P., Breslow, A. *et al.* 1980. Stage I melanoma of the skin: the problem of resection margins. Eur. J. Cancer 16: 1079–1085.

63. Golomb, F.M. 1983. Discussion of two papers entitled 'Optimal resection margin for cutaneous melanoma' and 'Patients perception of the cosmetic impact of melanoma resection'. Plast. Reconstr. Surg. 71: 76–78.

64. Cosimi, A.B., Sober, A.J., Mihm, M.C., Fitzpatrick, T.B. 1984. Conservative surgical management of superficially invasive cutaneous melanoma. Cancer 56: 1256–9.

65. Bagley, F.H., Cady, B., Lee, A., Legg, MA. 1981. Changes in clinical presentation and management of malignant melanoma. Cancer 47: 2126–34.

66. Patel, J.K., Didolkan, M.S., Pickren, J.W., Moore, R.H. 1978. Metastatic pattern of malignant melanoma. A study of 216 autopsy cases. Am. J. Surg. 135: 807–10.

67. Olson, R.M., Woods, J.E., Soule, E.H. 1981. Regional lymph node management and outcome in 100 patients with head and neck melanoma. Am. J. Surg. 142: 470.

68. Day, C.L., Mihm, M.C., Lew, R.A., Kopf, A.W., Sober, A.J., Fritzpatrick, T.B. 1982. Cutaneous malignant melanoma: Prognostic guidelines for physicians and patients. C.A. 32(2): 113–122.

69. Balch, C.M. 1980. Surgical management of regional lymph nodes in cutaneous melanoma. J. Am. Acad. Dermatol. 3(5): 511–24.

70. Simons, J.N. 1972. Malignant melanoma of the head and neck. Am. J. Surg. 125: 485–488.

71. Harris, T.J., Hinckley, D.M. 1983. Melanoma of the head and neck in Queensland. Head Neck Surg. 5(3): 197–203.

72. Storm, F.K., Eilber, F.R. 1981. The value of lymphadenectomy in melanoma of the head and neck. In: Head and Neck Oncology: Controversies in Cancer Treatment (A.R. Kagan, J.W. Miles, zds.). G.K. Hall, Boston, pp. 127–138.

73. Balch, C.M., Milton, G.W., Shaw, H.M., Soong, S.J. 1985. Elective lymph node dissection: Pros and cons. In: Cutaneous Melanoma (C.M. Balch, G.W. Milton, H.M. Shaw, S.J. Soong, eds.). Lippincott, Philadelphia, pp. 131–157.

74. Kapelanski, D.P., Block, G.E., Kaufman, M. 1979. Characteristics of the primary lesion of malignant melanoma as a guide to prognosis and therapy. Ann. Surg. 189: 225–235.

75. Balch, C.M. 1982. Pathology, prognostic factors and surgical treatments of cutaneous melanoma. Curr. Concepts Oncol. 4: 8.

76. Sim, F.H., Taylor, W.F., Ivins, J.C. et al. 1978. A prospective randomized study of the efficacy of routine elective lymphadenectomy in management of malignant melanoma: preliminary results. Cancer 41: 948–956.

77. Day, C.L., Sober, A.J., Lew, R.A. et al. 1981. Malignant melanoma patients with positive nodes and relatively good prognosis: Microstaging retains prognostic-significance in clinical stage I melanoma patients with metastasis to regional nodes. Cancer 47: 955–962.

78. Fortner, J.G., Woodruff, J., Schottenfeld, D. 1977. Biostatistical basis of elective node dissection for malignant melanoma. Ann. Surg. 186: 101–103.

79. Conley, J.J., Pack, G.T. 1963. Melanoma of the head and neck. Surg. Gynecol. Obstet. 116: 15–28.

80. Lingemen, R.E. et al. 1977. Neck dissection: Radical or conservative, Ann. Otol. 86: 737.

81. Bocca, E., Pignataro, O., Oldini, C., Cappa, C. 1984. Functional neck dissection: An evaluation and review of 843 cases, Laryngoscope 94: 942.

82. Molinari, R., Cantu, E., Chicsa, F., Grandi, C. 1980. Restrospective comparison of conservative and radical neck dissection in laryngeal cancer. Ann. Otol. 89: 578–581.

83. Seigler, H.F., Cox, E., Mutzner, F. et al. 1979. Specific active immunotherapy for melanoma. Ann. Surg. 190: 366–372.

84. Everall, J.D., O'Doherty, C.J., Ward, J. et al. 1975. Treatment of primary melanoma with intralesional vaccinia before excision. Lancet 2: 583–586.

85. Casterman-Elias, S., Simar, L., Vanijck, R. et al. 1977. Immunosurgical treatment of stage I malignant melanoma. Cancer Immunol. Immunother. 2: 179–187.

86. Rosenberg, S.A., Rapp, H., Terry, W. et al. 1982. Intralesional BCG therapy of patients with primary stage I melanoma. In: Immunotherapy of Human Cancer (W.D. Terry, S.A. Rosenberg, eds.). Elsevier North Holland, New York, pp. 289–291.

87. Comis, R.I. 1976. DTIC (NSC-45388) in malignant melanoma: A perspective. Cancer Treat. Rep. 60: 165–176.

88. Luce, J.K. 1972. Chemotherapy of malignant melanoma. Cancer 30: 1604–1616.

89. Bellet, R.E., Mastrangelo, M.J., Laucius, J.F. et al. 1976. Randomized perspective trial of DTIC (NSC-45388) alone versus BCNU (NSC-409962) plus vincristine (NSC-67574) in the treatment of metastatic malignant melanoma. Cancer Treat. Rep. 60: 595–600.

90. Luce, J.K., Thurman, W.G., Isaacs, B.L. et al. 1970. Clinical trials with the antitumor agent 5-(3,3,-dimethy-1-triazeno) imidazole-4-carboxamide (NSC 45388). Cancer Chemother. Rep. 54: 119–124.

91. Rochlin, D.B., Wagner, D.E., Wilson, W.L., Weber, A.P. 1970. Results of phase I and II studies with imidazole-carboxamide-dimethyl-triazene (Abstr. 768). Tenth Int. Cancer Congress, Houston.

92. Burke, P.J., McCarthy, W.H., Milton, G.W. 1971. Imidazole carboxamide therapy in advanced malignant melanoma. Cancer 27: 744–750.

93. Wagner, D.E., Ramirez, G., Weiss, A.J., Hill, G.J. 1972. Combination phase I-II study of imidazole carboxamide. Oncology 26: 310–316.

94. Czarnetzki, B.M., Macher, E. 1981. DTIC (dacarbazine)-induced hepatic damage. Arch. Dermatol. Res. 270: 375–376.

95. Frosch, P.J., Czarnetzki, B.M., Macher, E. et al. 1979. Hepatic failure in a patient treated with DTIC for malignant melanoma. J. Cancer Res. Clin. Oncol. 95: 281–286.

96. Greenstone, M.A., Dowd, Pm., Mikhailidis, D.p., et al. 1981. Hepatic vascular lesions associated with dacarbazine treatment. Br. Med. J. 182: 1744–1745.

97. Feaux de Lacroix, W., Runne, U., Hauk, H. et al. 1983. Acute liver dystrophy with thrombosis of hepatic veins: A fatal complication of Dacarbazine treatment, Cancer Treat, Rep. 67: 779–784.

98. Rzmirez, G., Wilson, W., Grage, T. et al. 1972. Phase II evaluation of 1,3-bis(2-chloroethyl-nitrosourea) (BCNU; NSC-409962) in patients with solid tumors. Cancer Chemother. Rep. 56: 787–790.

99. Ahmann, D.L., Hahn, R.G., Bisel, H.F. 1972. A comparative study of 1-(2-chloroethyl)-3-cyclo-hexyl-1-nitrosourea (NSC-79037) and imidazole carboxamide (NSC-45388) with vincristine (NSC-67574) in the palliation of disseminated malignant melanoma. Cancer Res. 32: 2432–2434.

100. Ahmann, D.L., Hahn, R.G., Bisel, H.F. 1974. Evaluation of 1-(2-chloroethyl-3-4-methyl-cyclo-hexyl)-1-nitrosourea (methyl-CCNU, NSC-95441) versus combined imidazole carboxamide (NSC-45388) and vincristine (NSC-67574) in palliation of disseminated melanoma. Cancer 33: 615–618.

101. Van Amburg, A.L., Presant, C.A., Burns, D. 1982. Phase II study of chlorozotocin in malignant melanoma: A Southeastern Cancer Study Group report. Cancer Treat. Rep. 66: 1431–1433.

102. Ahmann, D.L., Hahn, R.G., Bisel, H.F. et al. 1975. Comparative study of methyl-CCNU (NSC-95441) with cyclophosphamide (NSC-26271) and 5-(3,3-dimethyl-1-triazeno) imidazole-4-carboxamide (NSC-45388) with vincristine (NSC-67574) in patients with disseminated melanoma. Cancer Chemother. Rep. 59: 451–453.

103. Cauverqne, J., Clavel, B., Klein, T. et al. 1978. Chemotherapy of malignant melanoma. Bull. Cancer 65: 107–109.

104. Wittes, R.E., Wittes, J.T., Golbey, R.B. 1978. Combination chemotherapy in metastatic melanoma. Cancer 41: 415–421.

105. Rersas, S., Athanasiou, A., Flynn, M.D. et al. 1982. Combined chemotherapy with vindesine and DTIC in advanced malignant melanoma. Proc. Am. Soc. Clin. Oncol. 1: 169.

106. Gerner, R.E., Moore, G.E., Dickey, C. 1975. Combination chemotherapy in disseminated melanoma and other solid tumors in adults. Oncology 31: 22–30.

107. Goodnight, J.E., Jr., Moseley, H.S., Eilber, F.R. et al. 1979. Cis-dichloro-diammineplatinum (II) alone and combined with DTIC for treatment of disseminated malignant melanoma. Cancer Treat. Rep. 63: 2005–2007.

108. Friedman, M.a., Kaufman, D.A., William, J.E. et al. 1979. Combined DTIC and cis-dichloro-diammineplatinum (II) therapy for patients with disseminated melanoma: A Northern California Oncology Group study. Cancer Treat. Rep. 63: 493–495.

109. Byrne, J.M., Reynolds, P.M. 1982. Phase II study of cyclophosphamide, vincristine and DTIC + BCG in the treatment of malignant melanoma. Aust. N.Z. J. Med. 12: 263–266.

110. Samson, M.K., Baker, L.H., Cummings, G. et al. 1982. Clinical trial of chlorozotocin, DTIC, and dactinomycin in metastatic malignant melanoma. Cancer Treat. Rep. 663: 371–373.

111. Carey, R.W., Green, M.R., Anderson, J. 1983. Vinblastine-dimethyltriazenoimidazole carboxamide (DTIC)-cis-platinum (VDP): Active regimen in metastatic melanoma. Proc. Am. Soc. Clin. Oncol. 2: 237.

266

112. Ahn, S.S., Giuliano, A., Kaiser, L. *et al.* 1983. The limited role of BOLD chemotherapy for disseminated malignant melanoma. Proc. Am. Soc. Clin. Oncol. 2: 228.

113. Cohen, S.M., Ohnuma, T., Cheung, T. *et al.* 1983. Bleomycin, carmustine, vincristine, and dacarbazine in patients with metastastic melanoma. Clin Treat. Rep. 67: 947–948.

114. York, R.M., Lawson, D.H., McKay, J. 1983. Treatment of metastatic malignant melanoma with vinblastine, bleomycin by infusion and cisplatin. Cancer 52: 2220–2222.

115. Mechl, Z., Nekulova, M., Sopkova, B. *et al.* 1983. The VBD regimen (vinblastine-bleomycin-cis-platinum) with high doses of cisplatinum in the therapy of advanced malignant melanoma. Proc. 13th Int. Cong. Chemother., part 246, pp. 22–25.

116. Pugh, R., Jacobs, E., Bateman, J.*et al.* 1974. In: Proceedings of the 11th International Cancer Congress, Florence.

117. Cruz, A.B., Jr., Armstong, D.M., Aust, J.B. 1974. Treatment of advanced malignancy with CCNU (1-(2-chlomethyl)-3-cyclohexyl-1-nitrosourea (NSC 74037). A phase II cooperative study. Proc. Am. Assoc. Cancer Res. and Am. Soc. Cun. Oncol. 15: 184.

118. DeWasch, G., Bernheim, J., Michel, J. *et al.* 1976. Combination chemotherapy with three marginally effective agents, CCNU, vincristine and bleomycin in the treatment of Stage III melanoma. Cancer Treat. Rep. 60: 1273–1276.

119. Seigler, H.F., Lucas, S., Pickett, N.J., Huang, A.T. 1980. DTIC, CCNU, Bleomycin, and Vincristine (BOLD) in Metastatic Melanoma. Cancer 46(1): 2346–2348.

120. Wick, M.M., Byers, L., Frei, E., I.I.I. 1977. L-Dopa: Selective toxicity for melanoma cells in vitro. Science 197: 468–469.

121. Nathason, L., Hall, F.C., Fiarber, S. 1967. Biological aspects of human malignant melanoma. Cancer 20: 650–655.

122. Myhre, E. 1963. Malignant melanoma in children, Acta Pathol. Microbiol. Scand, 59: 184–188.

123. Sadoff, L., Winkley, J., Tyson, S. 1973. Is malignant melanoma an endocrine dependent tumor? Oncology 27: 244–257.

124. Shiu, M.H., Schottenfield, D., Maclean, B., Fortner, J.G. 1976. Adverse effect of pregnancy on melanoma. Cancer 37: 181–187.

125. George, P.A., Fortner, J.G., Pack, G.T. 1960. Melanoma with pregnancy. Cancer 13(4): 854–859.

126. McCarty, K.S., Jr., Wortman, J., Stowers, S. *et al.* 1980. Sex steroid receptor analysis in melanoma. Cancer 46: 157–164.

127. Zava, D.T., Goldhirsch, A. 1983. Estrogen receptor in malignant melanoma: fact or artefact? Eur. J. Cancer Clin. Onol. 19(8): 1151–9.

128. Johnson, R.O., Bisel, H.F., Andrews, N. *et al.* 1966. Phase I clinical study of 6-methylpregn-4-ene-e, 11, 20-trione (NSC-17256). Cancer Chemother. Rep. 50: 671–673.

129. Lopex, R., Karakousis, C.P., Didolkar, M.s. *et al.* 1978. Estramustine phosphate (estracyt) in advanced malignant melanoma. Cancer Treat. Rep. 62: 1329–1332.

130. Didolkar, M.S., Catane, R., Lopez, R., Holyoke, E.D. 1978. Estramustine phosphate (estracyt) in advanced malignant melanoma resistant to DTIC treatment, Proc. Am. Assoc. Cancer Res. 19: 381.

131. Fisher, R.I., Young, R.C., Lippman, M.C. 1978. Diethylstilbestrol therapy of surgically non-resectable malignant melanoma. Proc. Am. Assoc. Cancer Res. 19: 339.

132. Beretta, G., Tabiadon, D., Fossati, P. 1979. Clinical evaluation of medroxiprogesterone acetate (MAP) in malignant melanoma. Cancer Treat. Rep. 63: 1200.

133. Creagan, E.T., Schutt, A.J., Ahmann, D.L. *et al.* 1982. Phase II study of high-dose megestrol acetate in patients with advanced malignant melanoma. Cancer Treat. Rep. 66: 1239–1240.

134. Meyskens, F.L., Jr., Voakes, J.B. 1980. Tamoxifen in metastatic malignant melanoma. Cancer Treat. Rep. 64: 171–173.

135. Harwood, A.R., Cummings, B.J. 1981. Radiotherapy for malignant melanoma: a reappraisal. Cancer Treat. Rev. 8: 271–282.

136. Dewey, D.L. 1971. The radiosensitivity of melanoma cells in culture. Br. J. Radiol. 44: 816–816.
137. Hornsey, S. 1972. The radiation response of human malignant melanoma cells in vitro and in vivo. Cancer Res. 32: 650–651.
138. Habermalz, H.J., Fisher, J.J. 1976. Radiation therapy of malignant melanoma. Experience with high individual treatment doses. Cancer 38: 2258–2262.
139. Overgaard, J. 1980. Radiation treatment of malignant melanoma. Int. J. Radiat. Oncol. Biol. Phys. 6: 41–44.
140. Hornsey, S. 1970. The relationship between total dose, number of fractions and fraction size in the response of malignant melanoma in patients. Br. Radiol. 51: 905–909.
141. Lobo, P.A., Liebner, E.J., Chao, J.J.-H., Kanji, A.M. 1981. Radiotherapy in the management of malignant melanoma. Int, J. Radiat. Oncol. Biol. Phys. 7: 21–16.
142. Trott, K.R., von Lieven, H., Kummermehr, J., Skopal, D., Lukacs, S., Braun-Falco, O., Kellerer, A.M. 1981. The radiosensitivity of malignant melanomas. Part II: Clinical studies. Int. J. Radiat. Oncol. Biol. Phys. 7: 15–20.
143. Harwood, A.R. 1982. Conventional radiotherapy in the treatment of lentigo maligna and lentigo maligna melanoma. J. Am. Acad. Dermatol. 6(3): 310–316.
144. Harwood, A.R. 1983. Lentigo maligna melanoma yields to radiotherapy. Report of the American Society of Therapeutic Radiologists. J.A.M.A. 249(3): 323–327.
145. Braun-Falco, O., Lucas, S., Schoefinius, H. 1975. Zurbehandlung der melanosis cercusmscripta praecancerosa. Dubreuilh. Hantartz 26: 207–210.
146. Hellriegel, W. 1963. Radiation therapy of primary and metastatic melanoma. Ann. N.Y. Acad. Sci. 100: 131–141.
147. Jorgsholm, B., Engdahl, I. 1955. Malignant melanoma. Acta Radiol. 44: 417–433.
148. Dickson, R.J. 1958. Malignant melanoma: a combined surgical and radiotherapeutic approach. 79: 1063–1070.
149. Nitter, L. 1962. The treatment of malignant melanonce with special reference to the possible effect of radiotherapy. Acta Radiol. 46: 547–562.
150. Creagan, E.T., Cupps, R.E., Ivins, I.C. et al. 1978. Adjuvant radiation therapy for regional nodal metastasis from malignant melanoma. A randomized study. Cancer 42: 2206–2210.
151. Hilaris, B.S., Raben, M., Calabrese, A.S. et al. 1963. Value of radiation therapy for distant metastases from malignant melanoma. Cancer 16: 765–773.
152. Katz, H.R. 1981. The results of different fractionation schemes in the palliative irradiation of metastatic melanoma. Int. J. Radiat. Oncol. Biol. Phys. 7: 907–911.
153. McNeer, G., Das Gupta, T. 1964. Prognosis in malignant melanoma. Surgery 56: 512–518.
154. Guichard, M., Tenforde, T., Curtis, S., Malaise, E.P. 1982. Effect of combined misonidazole and accelerated neon ions on a human melanoma transplanted into nude mice. Radiology 142: 219–23.
155. Perez, C.A., Kopeckey, W., Rao, D.V., Baglan, R., Mann, J. 1981. Local microwave hyperthermia and irradiation in cancer therapy: preliminary observations and directions for future clinical trials. Int. J. Radiat. Oncol. Biol. Phys. 7: 765–72.
156. Kim, J.H., Hahn, E.W., Ahmed, S.A. 1982. Combination hyperthermia and radiation therapy for malignant melanoma. Cancer 50: 478–482.
157. Corry, P.M., Spanos, W.J., Tilchen, E.J. et al. 1982. Combined ultrasound and radiation therapy treatment of human superficial tumors. Radiology 145: 165–169.
158. Noell, U.R.T., Woodward, K.T., et al. 1980. Microwave-induced local hyperthermia in combination with radiotherapy of human malignant tumors. Cancer 45: 638–646.
159. Verhey, L.J., Munzenrider, J.E. 1982. Proton beam therapy. Ann. Rev. Biophys. Bioeng. 2: 331–57.

16. Lymphomas of extranodal head and neck sites

CHARLOTTE JACOBS

Introduction

Although the otolaryngologist treats mainly cancers of squamous histology, non-Hodgkin's lymphomas represent a substantial number of newly diagnosed head and neck cancers [1, 2]. Cervical adenopathy is one of the most common presenting signs of non-Hodgkin's lymphomas, but up to 10% of patients present with lymphomas in extranodal head and neck sites – Waldeyer's ring or other extralymphatic sites, including oral cavity, larynx, salivary gland, paranasal sinus, thyroid, and orbit. The signs and symptoms of a non-Hodgkin's lymphoma in an extranodal head and neck site may be similar to those of a head and neck squamous cancer, and only by biopsy can the distinction be made. However, occasionally a pathologist will have difficulty distinguishing between a poorly differentiated carcinoma and a non-Hodgkin's lymphoma. Newer immunohistologic techniques have been helpful in making this distinction. The histologic classification of the non-Hodgkin's lymphomas has undergone recent change, and familiarity with the currently used classification systems is important in understanding the natural history and expected outcome of patients with lymphomas. Based on retrospective analysis of series of patients with extranodal and neck lymphomas at various institutions, appropriate staging procedures can be recommended. Finally, the therapy of the non-Hodgkin's lymphomas is rapidly changing, and survival data continue to improve. The recommended optimal therapy varies with histology, stage of disease, and head and neck site. This review will cover the presentation, histology, staging and treatment of extranodal head and neck lymphomas.

Presentation

Non-Hodgkin's lymphomas of head and neck sites occur at a mean age of 58 years [3–8], and there is no difference in age at presentation for various sites.

C. Jacobs (ed) Cancers of the head and neck.
© *1987, Martinus Nijhoff Publishers, Boston. ISBN 0–89838–825–2. Printed in the Netherlands.*

Males are affected more frequently than females with a ratio of 1.6:1 [3–11]. The exceptions to this include the salivary glands in which there is a male to female ratio of 1:1 [3], lymphomas of the orbit, with a female to male ratio of 2.4:1 [12], and primary thyroid lymphomas, which favor women with a female to male ratio of 3.5:1 [13, 14].

From a review of 779 patients with head and neck lymphomas (excluding thyroid and orbit) [3, 6, 7, 9, 11, 15–17], Waldeyer's ring was the most common region involved (Table 1). Of Waldeyer's ring, the tonsil represented 36%, naso-pharynx – 16%, base of tongue – 10%, and other Waldeyer's sites – 4%. Of the extralymphatic sites at presentation, the nasal cavity and paranasal sinuses were most common at 16%, followed by salivary glands – 8%, oral cavity – 6%, larynx – 1%, and other extralymphatic sites – 4%. Twenty-one percent of patients had multiple areas of involvement within the head and neck region [3].

The presenting symptoms of head and neck lymphomas are similar to those of squamous cell carcinoma. Approximately 80% of patients with a tonsillar lym-phoma complained of a sore throat or 'a lump in the throat' [3]. Patients with lymphomas of the nasopharynx complained of nasal obstruction or decreased hearing 75% of the time [3]. Sixty-seven percent of patients with lymphoma in the base of tongue presented with symptoms of dysphagia or sore throat [3]. For patients with involvement of the nasal cavity or paranasal sinus, 85% complained of nasal obstruction or sinusitis. The majority of patients with salivary gland lymphomas complained of a mass. Of the entire group, only 15% presented with complaints of neck adenopathy, and only 5% had systemic symptoms (fever, night sweats, weight loss) [3].

For primary thyroid lymphomas, the most common presenting symptoms include a neck mass – 73%, dysphagia – 36%, and hoarseness – 27% [13, 18]. Patients with lymphomas of the orbit present predominately with complaints of

Table 1. Head and neck lymphomas – sites of presentation[a]

Primary site	No. of patients	(%)
Tonsil	326	(36%)
Nasopharynx	145	(16%)
Nasal cavity, paranasal sinus	142	(16%)
Base tongue	87	(10%)
Salivary glands	74	(8%)
Oral cavity	59	(6%)
Other extralymphatic sites	37	(4%)
Other Waldeyer's sites	34	(4%)
Larynx	6	(1%)
Total	779	

[a] References 3, 6, 7, 9, 11, 15–17.

swelling; other signs and symptoms include visual change, epiphora, proptosis, ptosis, and discomfort [12]. In one series, the most common sign of orbital lymphoma was exophthalmos, and the most common physical finding with conjunctival lymphoma was a palpable mass [19].

Histologic classification

There are multiple histologic subtypes of the non-Hodgkin's lymphomas, and they influence the choice of staging procedures, the expected sites of involvement, therapy, and outcome. Multiple different histologic classification systems have been utilized, but the most widely reported is the Rappaport System [20] (Table 2).

Rappaport Classification System

The Rappaport System is based on two distinct histologic features of the lymphoid tissue – the cell type (well-differentiated lymphocytic, poorly-differentiated lymphocytic, histiocytic, mixed lymphocytic histiocytic or undifferentiated) and the architectural pattern (nodular, diffuse). Using the Rappaport System, two distinct prognostic groups can be defined [21]. Patients in the 'unfavorable' group include nodular histiocytic (NH), diffuse histiocytic (DH), diffuse lymphocytic poorly-differentiated (DLPD), diffuse mixed lymphocytic histiocytic (DM), diffuse undifferentiated (DU), lymphoblastic [22], and Burkitt's lymphoma [23]. Thus

Table 2. Histologic classification of the non-hodgkin's lymphomas

Modified Rappaport classification [20]	Working formulation [29]
Favorable	Low grade
Diffuse lymphocytic, well-differentiated	Small lymphocytic
Nodular lymphocytic, poorly-differentiated	Follicular predominateley small cleaved cell
Nodular mixed lymphocytic histiocytic	Follicular mixed small cleaved and large cell
Unfavorable	Intermediate grade
Nodular histiocytic	Follicular predominately large cell
Diffuse poorly differentiated lymphocytic	Diffuse small cleaved cell
Diffuse mixed lymphocytic histiocytic	Diffuse mixed small and large cell
Diffuse histiocytic	Diffuse large cell
	High grade
(Diffuse histiocytic)	Large cell immunoblastic
Lymphoblastic	Lymphoblastic
Diffuse undifferentiated	Diffuse small noncleaved cell
Burkitts	
Non-Burkitts	

the unfavorable group includes most patients with diffuse lymphomas with the exception of diffuse lymphocytic well-differentiated. The 'favorable' group includes patients with nodular lymphocytic poorly-differentiated (NLPD), nodular mixed lymphocytic histiocytic (NM), and diffuse lymphocytic well-differentiated (DLWD) lymphomas.

A review of 1232 patients [3–9, 11, 15–11, 14] (Table 3) showed that the majority of head and neck lymphomas were of unfavorable histologies. Half of the patients had nodular or diffuse histiocytic lymphomas, and 25% had diffuse lymphocytic poorly-differentiated lymphomas. The most common favorable lymphoma was nodular lymphocytic poorly-differentiated, but it only represented 8% of the group. In our series [3] histology varied with site of presentation. All patients with lymphomas of the nasal cavity or paranasal sinus had unfavorable histologies, whereas over half of the patients with salivary gland lymphomas had favorable histologies.

A review of 87 patients with lymphomas of the thyroid [13, 14, 25] demonstrated that unfavorable histologies, predominantly diffuse histiocytic lymphoma, account for the majority of cases (Table 4). A high percentage of glands also contained histologic evidence of Hashimoto's thyroiditis [14]. In contrast, lymphomas of the orbit have mainly lymphocytic histologies, and of 84 patients [12, 26–28], 40% had DLWD, 35% had DLPD, and only 10% had diffuse histiocytic lymphoma. Kim reported that of lymphomas originating in the conjunctiva, all were of lymphocytic histology [19].

Table 3. Head and neck lymphomas – histologic classification[a]

Histology[b]	No. of patients	(%)
Unfavorable		
Nodular or diffuse histiotcytic	618	(50%)
Diffuse lymphocytic poorly-differentiated	302	(25%)
Diffuse mixed lymphocytic histiocytic	84	(7%)
Diffuse undlfferentiated	19	(2%)
Lymphoblastic	20	(2%)
Burkitt's	5	(1%)
Unclassified	17	(1%)
Favorable		
Nodular lymphocytic, poorly-differentiated	99	(8%)
Diffuse lymphocytic, well-differentiated	48	(4%)
Nodular mixed lymphocytic histiocytic	20	(2%)
Total	1232	

[a] References 3–9, 11, 15–1, 24.
[b] Rappaport System [20].

Working Formulation

With new knowledge about the characteristics of lymphoma cells and their immunologic make-up, many new classification systems have been described, and the old Rappaport System has been challenged. In order to standardize the classification of lymphomas, the National Cancer Institute funded a study by prominent pathologists which resulted in a new classification system – the Working Formulation (Table 2). This classification system is similar to the Rappaport System, but it divides the lymphomas into three major subgroups which have similar clinical course. This system is highly reproducible and is rapidly becoming the most commonly used classification system.

Immunohistochemistry

The pathologist and otolaryngologist may have difficulty distinguishing a benign lymphoid infiltrate from a lymphoma even with a good biopsy specimen. The distinction can often be made on fresh frozen tissue and is based on the fact that the majority of non-Hodgkin's lymphomas are either B or T cell malignancies [30]. The B cell lymphomas usually express a single class of light chains which helps distinguish them from reactive hyperplasia in which the cell population has a mixture of kappa and lambda immunoglobulin light chains [31]. To distinguish a T cell lymphoma from reactive hyperplasia, one can use a panel of T cell antigens to find aberrant phenotypes [32].

Another problem for the otolaryngologist and pathologist may be the dis-

Table 4. Histologic classification of thyroid and orbital lymphomas

Histology[c]	Thyroid[a]	Orbit[b]
Unfavorable		
Nodular and diffuse histiocytic	69 (79%)	8 (10%)
Diffuse lymphocytic, poorly-differentiated	4	29 (35%)
Diffuse mixed, lymphocytic histiocytic	5	4
Diffuse undifferentiated		3
Lymphoblastic		
Favorable		
Nodular lymphocytic, poorly-differentiated	2	5
Diffuse lymphocytic, well-differentiated	4	34 (40%)
Nodular mixed, lymphocytic histiocytic	3	1
Total	87	84

[a] References 13, 14, 25.
[b] References 12, 26–28.
[c] Rappaport classification [20].

tinction between an undifferentiated or anaplastic cancer and a high grade lymphoma. This difference in histology can often be determined by the use of pan leukocyte antibodies which are sensitive for cells of bone marrow origin [33, 34]. The combination of this procedure with anti-keratin antibodies for carcinomas and anti-S100 protein antibodies for amelanotic melanomas, can be very useful in making the distinction.

Staging

Pretreatment evaluation

Pretreatment evaluation should begin with a review of all pathologic material. Following this, a complete physical examination with indirect laryngoscopy should be performed with special attention to all lymph node bearing areas, the liver and spleen (Table 5). The size of the lesion and its extent should be accurately measured with the help of plain films, tomograms, and computerized tomography (CT). For patients with orbital lymphomas, it is essential to have an ophthamologic evaluation and CT scanning. For patients with lymphoma, a thyroid scan is useful and usually shows cold nodules [13]. Thyroid function tests should be obtained since many patients with thyroid lymphomas are hypothyroid [14]. A complete blood count with a differential and platelets may reflect involvement of the spleen or bone marrow, and occasionally abnormal circulating cells can be seen. Liver function tests with special attention to the serum alkaline phosphatase and serum lactic dehydrogenase (LDH), should be performed. The LDH is a prognostic indicator for the lymphomas of unfavorable histology [35]. A standard chest X-ray is usually adequate to determine mediastinal or parenchymal disease, but if there is any question of involvement, a chest CT scan should be performed. In one series of patients with thyroid lymphoma [13], 66% of patients had an abnormal chest X-ray with the majority showing tracheal deviation. A CT scan of the abdomen is useful in evaluating potential involvement of the liver and occasionally of the spleen. It is useful in evaluating the upper abdominal and mesenteric nodes, but the subdiaphragmatic lymphogram is much more accurate in detecting disease in the retroperitoneal lymph nodes. In addition, the lymphogram dye remains in the lymph nodes for up to 2 years, and by obtaining a plain film on followup visits, the physician can assess the status of retroperitoneal lymph nodes.

Because of the propensity for lymphomas to involve the bone marrow, a percutaneous needle bone marrow biospy should be performed in the posterior iliac crest. An aspirate is not sufficient to diagnose lymphoma in the bone marrow, since lymphoma tends to involve the paratrabecular regions. In our series [3], 25% of patients with favorable histologies had bone marrow involvement. We found that only 18% of patients with unfavorable histologies of extranodal and neck presentations had positive bone marrows. An association between involvement of Waldeyer's ring and the gastrointestinal tract has been described by Banfi [36], who found an 11% incidence of involvement of the GI tract in patients with head and neck lymphomas, and Brugere [6] who found a 3% incidence of GI tract involvement at presentation and a 20% involvement at time of relapse. Thus an upper gastrointestinal series and small bowel follow-through is recommended for patients with lymphomas of Waldeyer's ring.

In our series [3] 30% of patients with disease in the paranasal sinuses relapsed in the central nervous system, and thus a lumbar puncture is recommended as part of the staging of these patients. A lumbar puncture is also recommended for certain subgroups of lymphoma patients who have a high risk for central nervous system involvement at presentation or relapse: patients with unfavorable histologies and bone marrow or testicular involvement [37], patients with undifferentiated lymphomas [38], and patients with lymphoblastic lymphomas [22].

A routine staging laparotomy is not recommended for this group of non-Hodgkin's lymphomas because of the increased accuracy of currently available diagnostic tests and recent changes in therapeutic programs.

Staging System

When the initial evaluation is complete, the patient is assigned a stage, using the Ann Arbor Staging System, the same system used for Hodgkin's disease [39], (Table 6). This system is based on sites of lymph node involvement or dissemination to other organs and the presence or absence of systemic symptoms. The 'E' lesion was designated to indicate extralymphatic involvement of tissue adjacent to a lymph node, not considered metastatic disease. Thus, lymphomas involving the oral cavity, salivary glands, larynx, nasal cavity, and paranasal sinuses would be designated 'E' lesions as opposed to Waldeyer's ring, which represents lymphatic tissue.

Table 5. Initial staging evaluation for patients with head and neck lymphomas

Review pathology slides
Complete physical examination, indirect laryngoscopy
CT scan of head and neck site
Complete blood count with differential
Liver function tests
Chest X-ray
Lymphogram
CT scan of abdomen
Bone marrow biopsy
Upper gastrointestinal series (Waldeyer's ring)
Lumbar puncture (paranasal sinus)

From a series of over 1,000 patients with head and neck lymphomas [3–9, 11, 15–17, 24], excluding thyroid and orbit, the stages were as follows: stage I – 34%, II – 35%, III – 16%, IV – 18% (Table 7). The majority of patients did not have B symptoms. Patients with lymphoma of the thyroid have predominately early stage disease, with 86% of patients staged as stage I or IIE disease following their initial evaluation [13, 18, 25]. In a series of 49 patients with orbital lymphomas [26, 27, 40, 41], 65% were found to have stage I disease, and 33% were found to have stage IV disease. The majority of patients with stage IV disease were so on the basis of a positive bone marrow [41]. Approximately 10% of patients had bilateral orbital involvement at presentation.

The Ann Arbor Staging System has been criticized as inadequate for staging the head and neck lymphomas since it does not incorporate size or local extent in its definition of stage. The TNM system is felt by some investigators to be more useful for head and neck lymphomas, and a relationship between distal relapse rate and tumor size utilizing the TNM system has been described [9]. However, in our own series [3] the T status did not influence disease-free survival or survival, whereas, the Ann Arbor System was useful in predicting disease-free survival for the unfavorable histologies.

At completion of treatment and during the follow-up period, it is critical that all prior sites of involvement be re-evaluated on a regular basis. In addition, other potential sites of extension should be routinely evaluated utilizing the chest X-ray, plain film of the abdomen (if a lymphogram was performed), complete blood counts, and liver function tests. In addition, the physician should be attuned to complaints which may indicate spread to the gastrointestinal tract or central nervous system.

Table 6. Ann Arbor staging system [39]

Stage I:	Involvement of a single lymph node region (I) or of a single extralymphatic organ or site (IE)
Stage II:	Involvement of two or more lymph node regions on the same side of the diaphragm (II) or localized involvement of an extralymphatic organ or site and of one or more lymph node regions on the same side of the diaphragm (IIE)
Stage III:	Involvement of lymph node regions on both sides of the diaphragm (III); this may be accompanied by localized involvement of an extralymphatic organ or site (IIIE) or by involvement of the spleen (IIIS) or both (IIISE)
Stage IV:	Diffuse or disseminated involvement of one or more extralymphatic organs or tissues with or without lymph node enlargement
Symptoms:	A – Absence of systemic symptoms
	B – Unexplained fever, night sweats, or weight loss of more than 10% body weight

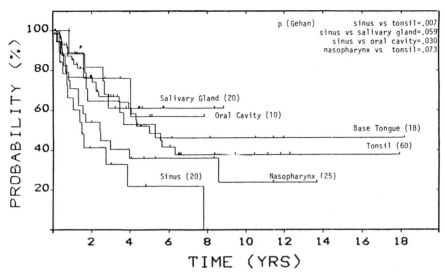

Figure 1. Survival of non-Hodgkin's lymphomas of the head and neck by site.

Therapy

Multiple factors are taken into consideration in determining the optimal treatment program: primary site of involvement, histology, stage of disease, and individual patient considerations.

The primary site of involvement of head and neck lymphomas does influence the freedom from relapse time and survival (Figure 1). In our series of 156 patients, the 5-year survival was influenced by site: salivary gland – 61%, oral cavity – 57%, tonsil – 49%, base of tongue – 47%, nasopharynx – 36% and paranasal sinuses – 12%.

Table 7. Head and neck lymphomas – initial stage

Stage[a]	No. of patients (%)		
	All sites[b]	Thyroid[c]	Orbit[d]
I, IE	346 (34%)	27 (47%)	32 (65%)
II, IIE	365 (35%)	22 (39%)	1
III, IIIE	136 (16%)	6 (11%)	–
IV	182 (18%)	2 (4%)	16 (33%)
Total	1029	57	49

[a] Ann Arbor Staging System [39].
[b] References 3–9, 11, 15–17, 24.
[c] References 13, 18, 25.
[d] References 26, 27, 40, 41.

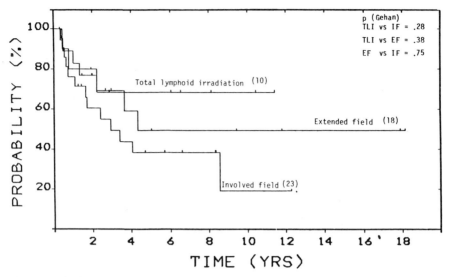

Figure 2. Survival of unfavorable lymphomas, stage I and II, based on radiation field.

Histology as well influenced survival (Figure 2). For favorable histologies, the 5-year survival was 69%, as compared to 39% for patients with unfavorable histologies. In the following sections general guidelines will be given for the management of head and neck lymphomas, although each case must be individualized.

Unfavorable lymphomas – stages I/II

For patients with unfavorable lymphomas of early stage, radiation therapy has been the primary mode of therapy. The appropriate dose delivered with a linear accelerator is 4000 to 5000 rad for involved sites and 4000 rad for uninvolved sites – a lower dose than is necessary for the treatment of squamous cell cancers. Patients are treated four or five times weekly at a dose rate of 1000 rad per week. The radiation port most commonly used is the Waldeyer's field, consisting of opposed lateral fields which encompass the nasopharynx and oropharynx, adjacent base of skull, preauricular, submandibular, and upper cervical nodes with a posterior margin encompassing the posterior cervical nodes [4]. The 'mini-mantle' field encompasses the cervical, supraclavicular, infraclavicular, and axillary lymph nodes. The mediastinum, which is not frequently a site of extension in these diseases, is shielded [4]. Treatment programs are defined as follows: involved field – radiation limited to known sites of disease, extended field – radiation to involved sites and the next contiguous lymph node group, total lymphoid irradiation – sequential treatment of Waldeyer's, mini-mantle, abdominal, and pelvic fields.

In most series, patients with head and neck lymphomas have been treated with involved or extended field radiation therapy only. In our series, patients with stages I and II unfavorable lymphomas had no difference in 5-year survival based on radiation field: total lymphoid irradiation – 60%, extended field irradiation – 50%, involved field irradiation – 39% (Figure 2).

In trying to design the optimal treatment program, the initial sites of relapse should be determined. From a series of 360 patients with stages I and II head and neck lymphomas who relapsed following radiation [3, 5–11, 24], 73% relapsed at distal sites, 14% locally and 13% in regional sites (Table 8). This would suggest that chemotherapy may be the most appropriate addition to current treatment programs. The excellent outcome reported for patients with early stage non-Hodgkin's lymphomas treated with chemotherapy alone [42], suggests that chemotherapy should be used in the management of these patients, either alone or with involved field radiation. Because of the high incidence of central nervous system involvement with the paranasal sinus, we recommend prophylactic treatment of the central nervous system with chemotherapy ± irradiation. There is as yet no long-term data to indicate whether this approach will be efficacious. It is important to stress that the lymphomas of unfavorable histology can be rapidly fatal if not treated aggressively, and it is difficult to salvage a patient who has failed their first treatment program.

Unfavorable histologies – stages III/IV

For patients with stages III and IV unfavorable lymphomas, chemotherapy is the treatment choice. There are a variety of combinations from which to choose, and among those, two of the most frequently used regimens are CHOP (cyclophosphamide, adriamycin, vincristine, prednisone) [43] and M-BACOD (methotrexate, bleomycin, adriamycin, cyclophosphamide, vincristine, dexomethasone) [44]. With these, cure rates may range from 25 to 50%. The role of radiation in these patients is usually as an adjunct for sites of bulky disease.

Table 8. Initial sites of relapse for stages I and II head and neck lymphomas[a]

Site of relapse	No. of relapsing patients	
Distal	264	(73%)
Local	49	(14%)
Regional	47	(13%)
Total	360	

[a] References 3, 6–11, 24.

Lymphoblastic lymphomas

Lymphoblastic lymphoma, a high-grade lymphoma, may present in head and neck extranodal sites, although it usually presents in young people with a mediastinal mass. The disease rapidly spreads to bone marrow and meninges, and thus, regardless of stage, patients need to be treated with aggressive chemotherapy programs including central nervous system prophylaxis. With aggressive treatment, 60% of patients can be cured [45].

Favorable histologies – stages I/II

Only a small percentage of patients will present with stage I or II disease of favorable histology. For those patients radiation therapy alone is appropriate. Most radiation therapists use involved or extended field, although the optimal radiation field has not yet been determined. With this approach, survival is approximately 90% at 9 years [46]. Chemotherapy has not been shown to be advantageous when added to radiation for the management of these patients [47].

Favorable histologies – stages III/IV

Patients with stages III and IV lymphomas of favorable histology have a long survival regardless of treatment. Chemotherapy options includes single agent chemotherapy with chlorambucil or combination chemotherapy with CVP (cyclophosphamide, vincristine, prednisone), and with either of these, 60 to 80% of patients will achieve a complete remission with a survival of approximately 80% at 5 years [48]. However the majority of patients will have relapsed one or multiple times during this period of time. Because the favorable histologies have such an indolent nature, selected patients may have therapy delayed until they become symptomatic [49].

Orbital lymphomas

For patients with localized lymphomas of the orbit, radiation therapy is the treatment of choice. Doses of 3500 to 4000 rad are necessary for local control. Damage to the retina and optic nerve is infrequent below 5000 rad. The lens is the structure that is most susceptible to radiation damage and as little as 400 rad can cause cataract formation. The lacrimal glands can be damaged, and a rare patient will complain of dry eyes. Specialized techniques have been devised to minimize long-term toxicity to the orbit [12, 40]. Most investigators report excellent response of orbital lymphomas to radiation with no local recurrences [12, 40], and in one series of 19 patients in which seven patients recurred, two did so in the opposite orbit, three in cervical lymph nodes and two systemically [12]. Factors which are associated with adverse prognosis include orbital bone erosion, stage IV disease, and unfavorable histologies [26]. Patients with stages III and IV disease should be treated with appropriate chemotherapy depending on their histologic subtype.

Thyroid lymphomas

For patients with stages I and II thyroid lymphoma, 5-year survival rates as high as 75 to 85% have been reported [14]. In a series from Stanford [18], eight patients with early stage disease were treated with 4300–5200 rad in 4 to 5 ½ weeks with 6 MV photons. Five patients were treated with a mantle field and three with a mini-mantle. All patients with stage I disease were alive without evidence of recurrence, and two patients with stage II disease relapsed in distal sites. The authors concluded that high-dose regional radiation is highly effective for thyroid lymphomas.

In a series from the Mayo Clinic [13], 34 patients had stage I/II disease. Of those, approximately one-third were treated to the neck only with 2400 to 6000 rad, and 28 patients were treated additionally to the mediastinum. At 5 years the survival was 57% with the disease-free survival of 59%. The disease-free survival tended to be higher for patients who received extended field radiation than for those who received radiation to the neck only; for stage I patients disease-free survival tended to be superior for those whose disease did not extend beyond the capsule; disease-free survival tended to be better for those patients with no residual disease following surgical excision than for those with residual disease. None of these differences reached statistical significance. Fourteen patients recurred, and most failed in multiple sites both locally and distally. There were several prognostic factors that indicated a high risk of recurrence, including hoarseness, stridor, an enlarged mediastinal mass on chest X-ray, and tracheal deviation. Based on their results, the authors recommended treatment to the thyroid and mantle of no greater than 4000 rad without laryngeal or cervical spinal cord blocks. They questioned the potentially beneficial role of surgical excision prior to radiation and suggested a role for subdiaphragmatic radiotherapy or adjuvant chemotherapy in the treatment of early stage thyroid cancer. These recommendations differ slightly from the Stanford group who found a high cure rate with higher doses of radiotherapy to extended fields alone, regardless of surgical excision.

For patients with thyroid cancer of stages III and IV, chemotherapy should be recommended with the type dependent on the histology.

282

Conclusions

The otolaryngologist is often the first physician to evaluate a patient with a head and neck lymphoma. It is often difficult to distinguish lymphomas from squamous cell carcinoma on clinical grounds. An adequate excisional or incisional biopsy is necessary to determine the diagnosis and the histologic subtype. If the diagnosis is still in question, further immunohistochemical studies will be of value. Prior to planning therapy, an extensive pretreatment evaluation is necesary to determine the stage of disease. Based on stage, histology, and primary site, appropriate programs involving radiation and/or chemotherapy can be recommended. When lymphomas are recognized early and treated properly, a high cure rate and/or survival can be expected.

References

1. Bonadonna, G., Molinari, R., Banfi, A. 1981. Hodgkin and non-Hodgkin lymphoma presenting in the head and neck. In: Cancer of the Head and Neck (J.Y. Suen, E.N. Myers, eds.). Churchill Livingstone, New York.
2. Schnitzer, B., Weaver, D.K. 1979. Lymphoreticular disorders. In: Tumors of the Head and Neck (J.G. Batsakis, ed.). Williams and Wilkins Co, Baltimore.
3. Jacobs, C., Hoppe, R.T. 1985. Non-Hodgkin's lymphomas of head and neck extranodal sites. Int. J. Radiat. Oncol. Biol. Phys. 11: 357–364.
4. Hoppe, R.T., Burke, J.S., Glatstein, E., Kaplan, H.S. 1978. Non-Hodgkin's lymphoma. Involvement of Waldeyer's ring. Cancer 42: 1096–1104.
5. Bajetta, E., Buzzoni, R., Rilke, F., Valagussa, P. et al. 1983. Non-Hodgkin's lymphomas of Waldeyer's ring. Tumori 69: 129–136.
6. Brugere, J., Schlienger, M., Gerard-Marchant, R. et al. 1975. Non-Hodgkin's malignant lymphomata of upper digestive and respiratory tract: Natural history and result of radiotherapy. Br. J. Cancer 31: 435–440.
7. Plantenga, K.F., Hart, G., van Heerde, P., Tierie, A.H. 1981. Non-Hodgkin's malignant lymphomas of upper digestive and respiratory tracts. Int. J. Radiat. Oncol. Biol. Phys. 7: 1419–1427.
8. Shimm, D.S., Dosorets, D.E., Harris, N.L. et al. 1984. Radiation therapy of Waldeyer's ring lymphoma. Cancer 54: 426–431.
9. Mill, W.B., Lee, F.A., Franssila, K.O. 1980. Radiation therapy treatment of stage I and II extranodal non-Hodgkin's lymphoma of the head and neck. Cancer 45: 653–661.
10. Wang, C.C. 1969. Malignant lymphoma of Waldeyer's ring. Radiology 92: 1335–1339.
11. Wong, D.S., Fuller, L.M., Butler, J.J., Schullenberger, C.C. 1975. Extranodal non-Hodgkin's lymphomas of the head and neck. A.J.R. 123: 471–481.
12. Fitzpatrick, P.J., Macko, S. 1984. Lymphoreticular tumors of the orbit. Int. J. Radiat. Oncol. Biol. Phys. 10: 333–340.
13. Blair, T.J., Evans, R.G., Buskirk, S.J. et al. 1985. Radiotherapeutic management of primary thyroid lymphomas. Int. J. Radiat. Oncol. Biol. Phys. 11: 365–370.
14. Hamburger, J.I., Miller, J.M., Kini, S.R. 1983. Lymphoma of the thyroid. Ann. Intern. Med. 99: 685–693.
15. Fierstein, J.T., Thawley, S.E. 1970. Lymphoma of the head and neck. Laryngoscope 88: 582–593.

16. Clark, R.M., Fitzpatrick, P.J., Gospodarowicz, M.K. 1983. Extranodal malignant lymphomas of the head and Neck. J. Otolaryngol. 4: 239–245.

17. Shidnia, H., Hornback, N.B., Lingeman, R., Barlow, P. 1985. Extranodal lymphoma of the head and neck area. Am. J. Clin. Oncol. 8: 235–243.

18. Clark, L.Y., Hoppe, R.T., Burke, J.S., Kaplan, H.S. 1981. Non-Hodgkin's lymphoma presenting as thyroid enlargement. Cancer 48: 2712–2716.

19. Kim, Y.H., Fayos, H.V. 1976. Primary orbital lymphoma: A radiotherapeutic experience. Int. J. Radiat. Oncol. Biol. Phys. 1: 1099–1105.

20. Rappaport, H. 1966. Tumors of the hematopoetic system. In: Atlas of Tumor Pathology, Section III, Fascicle 9. Armed Institute of Pathology, Washington, DC.

21. Jones, S.E., Fuks, Z., Bull, M. et al. 1973. Non-Hodgkin's lymphomas IV. Clinicopathologic correlation in 405 cases. Cancer 31: 806–823.

22. Nathwani, B.N., Kim, H., Rappaport, H. 1976. Malignant lymphoma, lymphoblastic. Cancer 38: 964–983.

23. Ziegler, J.L., 1979. Management of Burkitt's lymphoma: an update. Cancer Treat. Rev. 6: 95–105.

24. Horiuchi, J., Okuyama, T., Matsubara, S. et al. 1982. Extranodal non-Hodgkin's lymphoma in the head and neck: Irradiation and clinical course. Acta Radiol. Oncol. 21: 383–399.

25. Burke, J.S., Butler, J.J., Fuller, L.M. 1977. Malignant lymphomas of the thyroid. Cancer 39: 1587–1602.

26. Bennett, C.L., Patterman, A., Bitran, J.D. et al. 1986. Staging and therapy of orbital lymphomas. Cancer 57: 1204–1208.

27. Jereb, B., Lee, H., Jakobiec, F.A., Kutcher, J. 1984. Radiation therapy of conjunctival and orbital lymphoid tumors. Int. J. Radiat. Oncol. Biol. Phys. 19: 1013–1019.

28. Knowles, D.M., Jakobiec, F.A. 1980. Orbital lymphoid neoplasms: A clinicopathologic study of 60 patients. Cancer 46: 576–589.

29. The Non-Hodgkin's Lymphoma Pathologic Classification Project. 1982. National Cancer Institute sponsored study of non-Hodgkin's lymphomas: Summary and description of a working formulation for clinical usage. Cancer 49: 2112–2135.

30. Lukes, R.J., Taylor, C.R., Parker, J.W., Lincoln, I.L. 1978. A morphologic and immunologic surface marker study of 299 cases of non-Hodgkin's lymphomas and related leukemias. Am. J. Pathol. 90: 461–485.

31. Levy, R., Warnke, R., Dorfman, R.F., Haimovich, J. 1977. The monoclonality of human B-cell lymphomas. J. Exp. Med. 145: 1014–1028.

32. Weiss, L.M., Crabtree, G.S., Rouse, R.V., Warnke, R.A. 1985. Morphologic and immunologic characterization of 50 peripheral T cell lymphomas. Am. J. Pathol. 118: 316–324.

33. Warnke, R.A., Weiss, L.M. 1985. A practical approach to the immunodiagnosis of lymphomas emphasizing differential diagnosis. Cancer Surveys 4: 348–358.

34. Warnke, R.A., Gatter, K.C., Falini, B. et al. 1983. Diagnosis of human lymphoma with monoclonal anti-leukocyte antibodies. N. Engl. J. Med. 309: 1275–1281.

35. Fisher, R.I., Hubbard, S.M., DeVita, V.T. et al. 1981. Factors predicting long-term survival in diffuse mixed, histiocytic, or undifferentiated lymphoma. Blood 58: 45–51.

36. Banfi, A., Bonadonna, G., Ricci, S.B. et al. 1972. Malignant lymphomas of Waldeyer's ring: Natural history and survival after radiotherapy. Br. Med. J. 3: 140–143.

37. MacKintosh, F.R., Colby, T.V., Podolsky, W.J., Burke, J.S., Hoppe, R.T., Rosenfelt, F.P., Rosenberg, S.A., Kaplan, H.S. 1982. Central nervous system involvement in non-Hodgkin's lymphoma: an analysis of 105 cases. Cancer 49: 586–595.

38. Bunn, P.A., Schein, P.S., Banks, P.M., DeVita, V.T. 1976. Central nervous system complications in patients with diffuse histiocytic and undifferentiated lymphoma: leukemia revisted. Blood 47: 3–10.

39. Carbone, P.P., Kaplan, H.S., Musshoff, K., Smithers, D.W., Tubiana, M. 1971. Report of the committee on Hodgkin's disease staging classification. Cancer Res. 31: 1860–1861.

40. Austin-Seymour, M.M., Donaldson, S.S., Egbert, P.R. *et al.* 1985. Radiotherapy of lymphoid diseases of the orbit. Int. J. Radiat. Oncol. Biol. Phys. 11: 371–379.

41. Lazzarino, M., Morra, E., Rosso, R. *et al.* 1985. Clinicopathologic and immunologic characteristics of non-Hodgkin's lymphomas presenting in the orbit. Cancer 55: 1907–1912.

42. Miller, T.P., Jones, S.E. 1983. Initial chemotherapy for clinically localized lymphomas of unfavorable histology. Blood 62: 413–418.

43. McKelvey, E.M., Gottlieb, J.A., Wilson, H.E. *et al.* 1976. Hydroxyldaunomycin (adriamycin) combination chemotherapy in malignant lymphoma. Cancer 38: 1484–1493.

44. Skarin, A.T., Canellos, G.P., Rosenthal, D.S. *et al.* 1983. Improved prognosis of diffuse histiocytic and undifferentiated lymphoma by use of high dose methotrexate alternating with standard agents (M-BACOD). J. Clin. Oncol. 1: 91–98.

45. Coleman, C.N., Cohen, J.R., Burke, J.S., Rosenberg, S.A. 1981. Lymphoblastic lymphoma in adults: Result of a pilot protocol. Blood 4: 679–684.

46. Paryani, S.B., Hoppe, R.T., Cox, R.S., Colby, T.V., Rosenberg, S.A., Kaplan, H.S. 1983. Analysis of non-Hodgkin's lymphomas with nodular and favorable histologies, stages I and II. Cancer 52: 2300–2307.

47. Monfardini, S., Banfi, A., Bonadonna, G. *et al.* 1980. Improved five-year survival after combined radiotherapy-chemotherapy for stage I-II non-Hodgkin's lymphoma. Int. J. Radiat. Oncol. Biol. Phys. 6: 125–134.

48. Rosenberg, S.A., 1979. Non-Hodgkin's lymphoma - selection of treatment on the basis of histologic type. N. Engl. J. Med. 301: 924–928.

49. Portlock, C.S., Rosenberg, S.A. 1977. Chemotherapy of the non-Hodgkin's lymphomas: the Stanford experience. Cancer Treat. Rep. 61: 1049–1055.

Index

288

THE LIBRARY
UNIVERSITY OF CALIFORNIA